Pescar, Susan C.
     Where does it hurt? : a guide to
symptoms and illnesses / Susan C. Pescar
and Christine A. Nelson. -- New York :
Facts on File, 1983.
     313 p.

     Bibliography : p. 303-304
     Includes index.
     ISBN 0-87196-741-3

WHERE DOES IT HURT?

A Guide to Symptoms and Illnesses

WHERE DOES IT HURT?

A Guide to Symptoms and Illnesses

Susan C. Pescar and Christine A. Nelson, M.D.

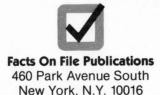

Facts On File Publications
460 Park Avenue South
New York, N.Y. 10016

Where Does It Hurt?

Library of Congress Cataloging in Publication Data

Pescar, Susan C.
  Where Does It Hurt?

  Previously published as: Symptoms & illnesses /
Susan C. Pescar. © 1983
    Bibliography: p.
    Includes index.
    1. Symptomatology. 2. Medicine, Popular. I. Nelson,
Christine A. II. Title.
  RC69.P47 1984   616.07′2   83-5663
  ISBN 0-87196-741-3

PRINTED IN THE UNITED STATES OF AMERICA

10   9   8   7   6   5   4   3   2   1

DEDICATION

To MAL and MARGIE BOUGHEN

My dear and special friends,
thank you for sharing yourselves,
your family and your love
with me and my family.
And, Mal, thank you for
showing *all of us* what the words
courageous, valiant and brave
really mean.
I will always remember.
With love,

SUSAN C. PESCAR

To JOHN J. PROCKNOW, M.D.

Your accomplishments
have been inspirational
and your dedication as a physician
to be admired.
I thank you for your
support, encouragement and love.
With love,

CHRISTINE A. NELSON, M.D.

ACKNOWLEDGEMENTS

Very special thanks and a great deal of credit must be given to the following people who devoted an enormous amount of time and hard work to the development and completion of this book: **ELEANORA SCHOENEBAUM**, Editorial Director, Facts on File, Inc., New York; **SUSAN COHAN**, freelance copy editor, New York; and **SALLY HERTZ**, Special Sales Manager, Facts on File, Inc., New York. They and **OTHERS AT FACTS ON FILE, INC.**, New York, made tremendous personal sacrifices on behalf of this book. The efforts of each and every person were greatly appreciated.

The following people must also be thanked for the many hours they gave and countless personal sacrifices they made to help research, type and/or compile information for this book: **Arlene West Pescar; Valerie Pescar Swigart; Robert Swigart; Paula Nelson Chirumbolo; Craig Pescar; Barbara Nesthus; Henry and Charlotte Ludwig;** and **Kathy Channell.** Without their help this book could not have been completed.

CONTENTS

SECTION ONE

IMPORTANT: THE KEY TO USING THIS BOOK

Where Does It Hurt? is carefully designed to be an easy-to-use, helpful and useful resource for you. Emphasis in medical care today is on two vital factors—(1) the prevention of illness or injury and (2) the early detection of an illness or other health condition when it occurs. In this way, it is hoped that many illnesses or health problems can be avoided and others successfully treated because of prompt diagnosis.

We have all said, or heard others say, "I wonder if I have the flu?" "Could this be appendicitis?" "Do you think my ankle is broken?" "Oh, it's just a common cold, isn't it?" Or, "I heard on the radio that we have an epidemic of Bornholm disease—known as 'devil's grippe.' What in the world is that?"

We have also said, or heard others say, "I have this persistent pain in my knee, and my knee swells off and on. I wonder if I should have it checked?" "I keep getting these headaches, and they make me really sick to my stomach. Do you suppose there's something seriously wrong?" The list goes on and on.

Such reasoning is typical. In fact, when we don't feel well, we usually approach the situation in one of two ways:

• We wonder if (or worry that) we may have a certain illness or health problem and want more information about that specific condition. In this situation we want to know if the symptoms being experienced match

3

those of the illness or problem. Sometimes, too, we may simply want more information about the symptoms and effects of a particular illness or problem.

• We have identified some of our symptoms but have little or no idea what they might mean. We don't know whether these symptoms are actually insignificant or whether they are associated with a potentially serious illness or health problem. In this case we want to know to which illness, disease, condition or problem the symptoms point. Most importantly, we need to know if the symptoms require medical evaluation.

Because we tend to approach our health concerns in these two ways— either by starting from the technical name of the illness or health problem or by wondering about the symptoms we are experiencing—*Where Does It Hurt?* provides you with both approaches.

Section Two is a list of illnesses, diseases, conditions and health problems presented in alphabetical order for easy reference. If you think you may have a certain illness or problem or simply want to know more about its symptoms and effects, then all you have to do is go to Section Two. Each illness or problem is briefly described there, with a discussion of its causes (if known), details of the symptoms associated with it and notes about its potential seriousness. The following is a sample of how diseases/disorders are handled in Section Two.

HERPES SIMPLEX TYPE 2 (GENITAL HERPES)

Painful, recurrent virus infection, with blisters or ulcers on or near the genital area...

Symptoms: Water-filled blisters that may crust over or become ulcers, located on or near the genitals (penis in males and vulva or vagina in females). First infection is usually...

Cause: Infection with Herpes simplex type 2 virus. A sexually transmitted (venereal) disease except in...

Severity of Problem: Intensely painful, but usually not otherwise a problem in the adult. However, can be insidious and life...

Contagious? Yes. Extremely contagious when disease is active...

Treatment: No known cure or effective treatment. Pain relief is sometimes necessary (physician prescription), and sitz baths may be helpful. Encouraging research developments...

Prevention: Avoid sexual contact with a person who has active herpes (lesions present). Use of condom protection even when the virus is inactive is highly recommended to prevent...

Discussion: Genital herpes is the most common sexually transmitted disease today. It is at an epidemic level. The virus usually resides in the tissues of the genital tract and . . .

Section Three is a "Quick-Reference Symptoms Guide." Major symptoms are listed in alphabetical order in large, bold type (for example, **FEVER**). Under each major symptom heading is a general discussion of that major symptom, so you can better understand its possible significance. After the discussion of the major symptom is a list that includes more specific symptoms or sets of symptoms. These are followed by the illnesses or health problems that each symptom or group of symptoms most often matches. (All illnesses and problems are listed in alphabetical order, not in their order of seriousness.)

For example, if your major symptom is fever, then you would go to the major heading **FEVER** in the "Quick-Reference Symptoms Guide" (Section Three). Under **FEVER** you would first find the symptom or set of symptoms that best matches the ones you are experiencing (such as "Fever with Abdominal Pain"). You would then review each of the possible causes listed (such as "See: Appendicitis, Colitis, etc." by turning to Section Two. After reading the entry for each possibility, you will have a better idea about which problem or problems you most likely have. This is essentially a process of elimination.

Following is a sample of part of a major symptom category, so you can see how they are handled in Section Three.

FEVER

Fever is an abnormal elevation of body temperature and is usually a sign of illness. But remember—fever, no matter how high or low, *is not* a disease of itself. It is, in fact, just one of many indicators of the potential cause and seriousness of a problem.

While most often fever signals an infection, the body temperature can rise to as high as 103 F with something as normal as vigorous exercise on a hot day. Other noninfectious causes of fever include several forms of arthritis, some cancers, hyperthyroidism and . . .

Fever Without Other Symptoms
See: ROSEOLA; SEIZURE—FEBRILE

Fever with Abdominal Pain
See: APPENDICITIS; CHOLECYSTITIS—ACUTE; COLITIS—ULCERATIVE; DIVERTICULAR DISEASE—DIVERTICULITIS; GALLSTONES; SALMONEL-LOSIS—TYPHOID FEVER; etc

The purpose of *Where Does It Hurt?* is not to encourage self-diagnosis or self-treatment. Self-diagnosis can be risky and often dangerous. This

book cannot replace the judgment of a trained physician. However, each of us makes an evaluation of our physical well-being throughout our lives. It is this evaluation that directs our actions. Do we wait to see if the symptoms go away? Do we call for a doctor's appointment? Do we seek immediate medical intervention?

A case in point. Think about the last time you experienced abdominal discomfort or pain. At first you may have ignored it, thinking it was possibly indigestion or a sensitive stomach. If the discomfort persisted or worsened, then you might have wondered if you had a case of the flu or a touch of food poisoning. If these symptoms still persisted and others followed—such as vomiting, diarrhea, fever—you probably started to become more concerned, wondering if the symptoms were more significant than you originally thought. At this point, you had to make a decision: See whether the original symptoms worsened or additional ones occurred; seek medical advice; or seek immediate medical care.

No one wants to overreact or underreact when it comes to evaluating a situation and making a decision. We want our decisions to be educated and well-informed. Therefore, we very much need to know if a set of symptoms has great significance and deserves our attention, or if the symptoms represent little cause for concern. The intent of *Where Does It Hurt?* is to provide you with a helpful, easy-to-use tool to assist you in better evaluating the significance of symptoms. It also hopes to answer some of the questions each of us has about certain illnesses or health problems.

The more we know about and understand the symptoms of illnesses or health problems, the better equipped we are to play a more active role in the evaluation and decision-making process. Hopefully, with more knowledge, we will be able to help ourselves by preventing potentially serious or definitely serious problems or by detecting them early. With prompt diagnosis and proper treatment or management, many serious conditions can be avoided entirely, while the impact of others can be lessened.

The human body is extremely complex, and to really understand it would require infinitely more specialized education and training than a lay person possesses. Often there are very subtle, fine-line differences between various illnesses and health problems. Only a physician is capable of ruling out certain problems and pinpointing the illness or condition a particular set of symptoms typifies. The physician also has the tool of a physical examination and medical tests at his or her disposal to verify a diagnosis.

It is highly recommended that before turning to Sections Two and Three you first read "Multi-Systems Problems (The Chain-Reaction Phenomenon)" and "How to Better Describe Symptoms to Your Doctor" (both in Section

One). In this way, you will have a better understanding of the body's systems and their interaction. You will also prepare yourself to better and more specifically explain the symptoms and feelings you are experiencing.

Remember, this book can in no way replace your personal physician. He or she knows you, your family and your personal medical history and is trained to diagnose medical problems and recommend specific treatment when indicated.

Where Does It Hurt? **does not in any sense reflect the total range of illnesses, diseases, conditions and health problems known today, nor does it include every symptom of every illness or problem. Its intent is to present the major symptoms that together are associated with particular illnesses or problems. In this way, you can better distinguish between conditions that are more serious and potentially serious, and those that are more minor and less worrisome.**

The point is, the early detection of potentially serious health problems is of prime importance and most often has a significant impact on the success of treatment and the avoidance of unnecessary complications. *Where Does It Hurt?* answer many of the questions you have about the symptoms and effects of certain illnesses and health problems, and it can assist you in making more informed decisions when you must evaluate such a problem.

Multi-Systems Problems
(The Chain-Reaction Phenomenon)

We have all heard the terms *primary* and *secondary,* but they take on a slightly different significance when applied to disease entities, illnesses and health conditions. There are health problems that essentially affect multiple organ systems. In other words, a certain problem, condition or illness may have its major effect on one organ system but will also have some minor to major effect on one or more other organ systems.

For example, there are both "primary hypertension" and "secondary hypertension." Eighty-five percent of people with diagnosed hypertension have "primary" hypertension. Although the cause of their elevated blood pressure is unknown, it is still the central, basic problem (increased pressure in the arteries, often associated with the collection of fatty substances on the insides of the blood vessels). Primary hypertension can most often be managed through diet, exercise and medication. In 15 percent of those diagnosed as having hypertension, however, the hypertension is "secondary" to another problem—

the primary problem. Secondary hypertension may result in those people with a primary renal (kidney) disorder, heart disease, endocrine disorders and other conditions.

The distinction between primary and secondary hypertension is important to the treatment of the disorder. If the hypertension is secondary to a renal disease, then treatment of the kidney problem (the primary condition) is vital to lessening or alleviating the elevated blood pressure. Treating only the secondary hypertension would prove to be helpful, but it would not directly attack the main problem. In the same sense, uncontrolled primary hypertension may lead to a secondary renal disorder. In this case, management and treatment of the primary hypertension should reduce or alleviate the risk of the secondary kidney problem if permanent damage has not already occurred.

The point is, many health problems have a significant effect on multiple organ systems. Sometimes this phenomenon shows up in the symptoms we experience and is confusing to non-medical persons, because symptoms that are seemingly unassociated occur—when in fact they are related.

It is easier to understand the human body if we compare it to a finely tuned and maintained machine having many parts, with major as well as minor components. The human body also has many parts, among them major components that are vital to efficient operation—organ systems such as the heart and vascular system, the hepatic system (liver), endocrine system (glands) and renal system (kidneys), to name a few.

Sometimes something goes wrong with a small part of the machine, but this does not have a lasting effect on the machine as a whole. Let's say its oil needs changing. Without fresh oil, the machine does not function quite as well, but as soon as the oil has been changed, it runs perfectly again. The same is true of the impact of most minor illnesses or health problems on the body.

However, if a major component of the finely tuned machine experiences a significant problem, this may affect the functioning of the other major components and the machine as a whole. Again, this is true of the human body, where the peformance and functioning of major organ systems depend on one another and are inherently interrelated.

Too often we tend to view the human body's various organ systems as totally independent and distinct entities, functioning separately and not having any remarkable effect on each other. Unfortunately, this is far from the truth.

If someone has a disorder involving the thyroid (part of the endocrine system), it seems perfectly logical to assume that the performance of all organs and body functions will be normal except for the thyroid. It is then most perplexing to talk to someone with a thyroid problem that is presently out of control. What he or she may describe (heart palpitations; heat intolerance; excessive sweating; weakness; warm, moist skin; excessive thirst; increase in appetite with weight loss; blurred vision; shaky hands; dizziness; intermittent labored breathing; and urinary frequency) sounds as if *many* organ systems and body functions are out of control. How could one little organ cause all of these seemingly unrelated symptoms?

Let's look at another example. If a major artery to the heart becomes blocked (coronary artery disease), this may result in less oxygen being fed to the heart muscle. The heart will then have trouble functioning properly, and permanent damage may occur. (Remember, the heart, like all muscles, needs oxygen and nutrients.)

Now the heart is unable to efficiently pump oxygen-enriched blood to the other organs and areas of the body. Because of this, the liver and kidneys may have to work harder to cleanse the blood and expel toxic substances. The lungs may have to work harder to deliver more oxygen, so the person must breathe harder in an attempt to meet the body's pressing need. One organ system after another may become involved, each being stressed. Then, of course, all of these secondary problems put more stress on the cardiovascular system—and a vicious cycle of demands and needs occurs. This takes place because all organ systems interrelate and rely on one another to some minor or major extent.

This chain-reaction phenomenon also accounts for a variety of complex symptoms and often makes for a difficult medical diagnosis. Considering this chain-reaction phenomenon (or domino effect), a great deal of emphasis in medicine today is on the early management and treatment of illnesses or conditions—so that complications can be prevented or managed before they worsen. Essentially, then, "complications" often refer to the secondary problems that may occur because of the effects of the primary problem.

Thus, it is important to remember that the human body is a complex, interrelated mechanism. It may have unique components that perform special and specific jobs, but its overall functioning and health are very much dependent on all systems working efficiently and in unison.

There are countless illnesses or health problems that may, at some point, affect the functioning of other organ systems besides the primary organ system involved. These include diabetes, thyroid disease, adrenal gland malfunction and other endocrine problems; cardiovascular disease, including heart disease and stroke; most of the cancers; hypertension; renal (kidney) disorders; blood diseases or disorders; lung disease; connective tissue diseases like rheumatoid arthritis; inflammatory bowel disease; and alcoholism and drug abuse.

Our life-styles also play a significant role both in the prevention of illness and injury, as well as in our body's ability to combat problems when they occur and bounce back rapidly. Lack of adequate exercise, poor nutritional habits, being overweight or underweight, smoking, abusing alcohol or other drugs (including prescribed, over-the-counter and illegal), being overly stressed, lacking adequate rest or generally abusing our bodies in any way all jeopardize our overall health and well-being.

All of these factors make us more susceptible to illness, accident or injury, and each of us can avoid or manage most (if not all) of them. Each of the health hazards mentioned above can, by itself, cause serious problems. When you start combining two or more of them, then the risk for serious health problems increases strikingly. And the statistical risk rises as each additional hazard joins the group.

What is even more striking is the fact that each of these health hazards caused by poor life-style can affect multiple organ systems and destroy overall health. Cancer, heart disease, stroke, and liver and kidney disorders are only a few of the problems that can occur as a result of these health hazards alone.

Therefore, we should keep in mind the potential overall impact that our life-style and personal habits can have on our organ systems and general well-being. And we should consider the chain-reaction phenomenon that can occur in our bodies in response to our actions (or lack thereof) and our personal choices. It really isn't a simple matter of "slightly" injuring one organ system. When a great enough insult takes place and serious damage or problems occur, many organ systems may get involved. These kinds of complications can have serious to grave results.

Again, the important thing is to do everything possible to prevent serious threats to our health and life. Secondly, it is imperative that we learn all we can about recognizing potentially troublesome or significant problems as early as possible, so prompt management and treatment can begin. In this way, we may be able to stop a problem before it becomes serious or lessen its severity, and we better our odds for successful management and treatment.

Infections:
Special Considerations

Infections are problems that everyone "knows" about but few people actually understand. The fact is, while many infections are minor and limited to a small area or a single organ and/or organ system, others involve many or all of the body systems to a greater or lesser extent.

Infections limited to one area of the body are called *localized* infections, while those that involve several or all areas and organ systems are called *generalized* or *systemic* infections. It is vital to remember that a localized infection can easily become a systemic infection if not treated promptly. When this occurs, the infection spreads to other areas of the body and can then become quite serious or life-threatening.

One of the most devastating forms of infection is known as sepsis or septicemia (commonly called "blood poisoning"). In this severe type of infection, the microorganism (the tiny "germ" that causes the infection) invades the bloodstream from one area of the body and is then carried to all parts of the body. The microorganism multiplies rapidly and can cause a localized infection in any organ, as well as a generalized blood infection. This spread of infection to organ after organ can occur rapidly as the blood carries the infection throughout the body.

This rapid spread of infection often leads to sudden, overwhelming shock. Organ systems can deteriorate rather quickly at this point. If not treated swiftly, septic shock will most often result in death. Treatment involves very intensive medical intervention in a hospital. Because of the underlying potential for serious, massive systemic infection, even minor infections require proper medical attention.

Infections are described in two ways—by their location and by the microorganisms that cause them. Interestingly, the relative risk of experiencing a serious problem from an infection depends on both of these factors. One other important factor is the effectiveness of each individual's defense system in controlling the spread of infection.

Besides sepsis (generalized infection), there are other infections that, although limited to a specific organ system, are potentially life-threatening. Because of their seriousness, these illnesses cause secondary damage to other areas of the body as well. Some of these infections include meningitis (infection of the coverings of the brain and spinal cord), serious forms of pneumonia (lung infection), certain types of kidney infections, some infections of the skin and underlying tissues, and infections of the bones and joints. These and certain other more rare conditions must be recognized promptly and treated correctly in order to prevent lasting complications or even death.

There are many—almost countless—micoorganisms that can potentially cause infection in humans. However, the ones we hear about most are infections caused by bacteria and viruses, with those caused by fungi and parasites a bit less common. The problems each of these groups of "germs" causes have certain characteristics (symptoms and signs) that often make it possible to recognize the invading microorganism(s) without laboratory tests—although tests are frequently done to verify the initial diagnosis so appropriate treatment is not delayed.

Bacteria and Viruses

People sometimes wonder why no attempt is made to eliminate all the bacteria and viruses in the world. Doing so, however, would also eliminate all other forms of life—sooner or later. We often forget that microorganisms are not *all* bad. The fact is, some cause harm, some do not, and some are actually good. *Bacteria,* for example, are always found in the mouth, as well as in the mucous membranes of the eyes, respiratory tract, urinary tract and digestive system. Some of these bacteria are considered "normal flora" and aid in the digestion or breakdown of foods. Other "normal flora" protect the body from the invasion of certain dangerous germs.

Occasionally, a "bad" microorganism—called a pathogen—is found on the surface of the mucous membranes and at just the right moment invades the blood and adjacent tissues. At other times, the infection is caused by the introduction of pathogenic (infection-producing) bacteria into the body through the skin (a cut, for example), the nose and respiratory tract, or the mouth and digestive tract. The infective agents then establish themselves in the tissue(s) of the body, sometimes causing mild, localized symptoms and other times causing severe, overwhelming infection.

Bacterial infections include such specific diseases as streptococcal sore throat ("strep throat"), impetigo, erysipelas, diphtheria, pertussis (whooping cough), typhoid fever, tuberculosis, cholera, dysentery, gas gangrene, tetanus, some sexually transmitted diseases, botulism, plague and even leprosy. In addition, certain types of meningitis, pneumonia, urinary tract infection, bone and joint infections, and less serious infections like skin, wound and ear infections can be caused by a variety of bacterial organisms.

A closer look at this group of organisms and the infections they cause clearly shows that great progress has been made in the prevention and treatment of many, if not all, of these diseases. Until 30 years ago serious bacterial infections were a major cause of death and/or disability around the world. The discovery (and further development) of antibiotics, better nutrition, improvements in personal hygiene, aseptic (sterile) conditions in hospitals and surgery, and immunizations have extended life expectancy by 20 to 25 years (past age 45) in many prosperous countries. Suddenly there was a way to prevent and/or effectively treat bacterial infections that had previously killed or permanently damaged. (These diseases can still be deadly in countries where antibiotics, immunizations, sanitation techniques, personal hygiene and advanced medical care are not readily available to the vast majority of the population.)

In addition to the countless bacteria that can cause disease, there are approximately 200 human *viruses* that can potentially cause infection. Viruses are tiny organisms too minuscule to be seen without a powerful electron microscope. Unlike bacteria, viruses cannot be destroyed by the usually available antibiotics. Some viruses also have the capability to lie dormant (inactive) in the tissues of the body, causing recurrent disease. Herpes simplex type 2 (genital herpes) is an excellent example of this kind of viral infection. The person with herpes may experience an episode that will subside—only to flare up periodically throughout his or her lifetime. Many viruses, however, do not have the capacity to lie dormant but simply "run their course."

Viruses cause specific diseases such as measles, rubella, mumps, polio, influenza, chickenpox and shingles, and certain sexually transmitted diseases. They are also responsible for the vast majority of infections of the respiratory tract (common cold, sore throat, conjunctivitis, ear infections, laryngitis, pneumonia) and digestive tract (gastroenteritis and hepatitis). Viruses cause many cases of meningitis and encephalitis, as well as certain other overwhelming infections.

The most widely known and experienced of these viral diseases is the common cold (upper respiratory infection). To be more exact, the common cold can be the result of one of a vast number of viruses! It is estimated that, in any given week during the winter months, approximately 15 percent of the population will suffer from the common cold. There are so many viruses that can cause the common cold that we can and do continue to get colds over and over again. Unfortunately, there is no way to combat the common cold: It is one of the viral diseases that must "run its course." The only thing we can do is make ourselves more comfortable and seek medical care when it appears that we may have something more than a cold. Those people with chronic health problems, however, must be more cautious and often require medical management of the common cold, so it does not develop into something more serious for them.

This is not to say that no progress has been made against viral diseases. Immunizations against many devastating viral diseases have saved countless lives and spared others from what would have been lifelong chronic problems. Yet a large number of viral diseases still cannot be prevented through immunization and are the subjects of ongoing medical research. Antiviral drugs are also being studied, still with little success, but with signs of progress being made.

Vaccines (immunizations) against viruses have been developed, first by using dead viruses to try to stimulate body immunity, then by developing modified, weaker doses of live viruses. Now, the most commonly used viral vaccines are live weakened viruses, which actually give a person a slight case of the disease. This allows the body to produce antibodies against the virus. Once we have these antibodies, we are protected from an infection in the future, even from the full-strength disease virus itself. If that same virus subsequently tries to invade the body, the antibodies that were made before promptly recognize the virus and rapidly destroy it. Immunizations against measles, rubella (German measles), mumps and polio can prevent these formerly common viral diseases; and vaccination against smallpox has effectively eradicated it throughout the world. Vaccines are also available to prevent certain viral diseases that are limited to tropical countries and less-developed areas of the world.

Fungi and Parasites

Fungus infections are somewhat less common than those caused by viruses and bacteria, and they generally tend to be more bothersome than life-threatening. Certain skin problems such as athlete's foot are caused by fungi, which can also cause deep infections, especially in people who have abnormal immune systems. However, a few fungus infections cause generalized disease in people with normal immune systems as well. These diseases are usually caught by contact with the organisms, which live in the soil in certain areas of the world. Diseases like histoplasmosis and coccidiodomycosis cause lung infection, which can initially look like tuberculosis. Yeast infections of the skin (diaper rash in infants and vaginitis in women) are also common fungus conditions.

Some fungus infections are easily recognized and treated. Others can be difficult to diagnose and may require long treatment with special drugs. In people with inadequate immune systems, fungus infections can cause death.

Parasites are small organisms that usually live part of their life cycles in human beings and the remainder in other animals. They most commonly cause problems in the digestive tract (especially diarrhea) but can also cause generalized or systemic disease. Many different kinds of "worms" are parasites and can be treated with special medications. Giardia is a fairly common parasite of the digestive system, and toxoplasmosis is a systemic parasitic disease. Many of these problems can be difficult to recognize, and treatment can be uncomfortable but successful.

The Immune System—Working from Within

Our bodies play a significant role in combating all types of infections. In a real sense, we have an army working from within—our immune system and its sophisticated search-and-destroy capabilities. We are able to resist many microorganisms because we have some built-in protection (called innate immunity), and we also can develop immunity against organisms with which we have come into contact (called acquired immunity). This special immune system protects us against many types of microorganisms, whether bacterial, viral, fungal or parasitic.

Let's take a bacterial infection as a simple example of how the immune system might work. Suppose you cut your hand while gardening one day. Bacteria invade the cut and start multiplying rapidly. The body's defense system responds by sending more blood to the area infected with the bacteria. This results in what we see as swelling and redness and what we often feel as pain. What we *don't* see or feel is that white blood cells are mobilizing and multiplying their forces to attack the bacteria. (For the body to be able to send more white cells to the area of infection, it must first release large numbers of white cells into the blood. This action, which makes the white-cell count elevated, is the reason a blood test may be helpful in determining if there is a hidden infection.) The white cells surround and devour the bacteria. Pus is really a combination of bacteria, white blood cells and blood protein that has leaked out of the cut—the by-product of this local defense system's fight against infection.

If some of the bacteria escaped into the bloodstream or nearby tissue, another part of the immune system is activated. The lymph nodes, which contain special cells that develop antibodies against the invading bacteria, also play a role in trying to control infection. Often these nodes swell as they participate in the battle to destroy the bacteria. So both the local forces (the white blood cells and the body's production of inflammation) and systemic forces (the development of antibodies) act together to destroy and control infection. These processes take time, however, and with serious infections, antibiotics are given to assist in the destruction of the bacteria.

This same basic response occurs when any microorganism invades. Our body's protective system responds and attacks, sometimes so efficiently and effectively that we are not even aware that an invasion took place. At other times, however, we become quite sick as the microorganism spreads into the tissues and throughout the body, attacking various organ systems along the way. The defense system has been overwhelmed and needs prompt and intensive medical support.

Recognizing and Treating Infection

We are all familiar with the signs of localized infection. There is usually pain or discomfort that heralds the onset of the infection. Swelling, tenderness, redness and warmth of the area are also part of the inflammation process— the body's defense against infection. If the infection becomes more severe and begins to spread, we may notice fever, generalized aches and pains, a feeling of being sick, and tenderness and swelling of the lymph nodes near the place where the infection started.

If the infection spreads further, we may feel progressively worse all over and have increasingly serious symptoms that point to the sites where the infection is the most severe. For example, pneumonia usually starts with a cough and mild discomfort. As it worsens, the coughing becomes more severe, fever and chest pain develop, and breathing difficulty may occur.

Many people wonder why a doctor wants to perform laboratory tests even when he or she is fairly sure of the location and type of microorganism causing an infection. Although certain symptoms point toward "groups" of germs or germ types, the doctor cannot be absolutely sure if the problem is viral, bacterial, fungal or parasitic in certain situations. When an infection is serious, knowing exactly which microorganism is causing it is vital in order for the physician to prescribe proper treatment. If it is a virus, antibiotics would not be effective. If the cause is bacterial, then the physician would want to know which antibiotic would be most effective. This can be determined when the exact type of bacteria is identified in the laboratory. Treatment to eradicate fungi or parasites also depends upon the type of organism responsible for the illness. Once this is known, the doctor can prescribe the best drug.

The Bottom Line on Infection

It is vitally important to identify an infection as early as possible so treatment (where indicated) can be started *before* the infection gets out of control. The fact is, no organ or body tissue is totally immune to all infections. Because of this we must be sure that we (and our children) receive the recommended immunizations available today, practice proper personal hygiene, follow sound nutritional plans, identify potentially problematic infections early and seek appropriate medical care when necessary. In this way, we play an important role in assisting our body's protective system in fighting invaders and ensuring better health and a longer life.

How to Better Describe
Symptoms to Your Doctor

Diagnosing an illness or a health problem is very much like putting together the pieces of an intricate, complex and sometimes perplexing puzzle. It is often the kind of puzzle where many pieces are quite similar and exhibit only very subtle differences. To assemble the puzzle requires skill, experience and the ability to distinguish between subtleties.

The pieces of the diagnostic puzzle come together as more and more information is gathered. What most people don't realize is how very important they themselves are in assisting the physician and facilitating a more specific and accurate diagnosis. The more detailed and descriptive we can be about what we are experiencing, the more clues we give the doctor. Essentially, then, it is our description of symptoms that gives direction to the doctor's initial efforts.

Let's go back for a moment. Imagine how very difficult it is to identify a problem involving someone who cannot tell you what is bothering him or her. If you are a parent or have ever been around an infant or a not-yet-talking small child, then you know how helpless you feel and how frustrating it can be when you hear the child cry and cry—unable to explain what hurts. Think about how many times you said, or heard others say, "Oh, I only wish he could tell me *what is wrong!*"

When a parent calls the doctor, the doctor first asks what *overt symptoms* the child is exhibiting (for example, fever, vomiting, diarrhea). The doctor also asks how the child is *acting*. Because the child cannot verbally describe the origin of the problem, his or her actions must essentially convey the message. Is the child pulling his legs up to his stomach? Is she rubbing her ears? Is he blinking constantly or rubbing his eyes? Is her breathing irregular or strained?

As the child grows older and becomes more verbal, he or she can give you more information. Interestingly, though, the child still cannot distinguish between the major symptom(s) and secondary ones. For example, a 3 year old may complain about his stomach hurting. Indeed, he may have an ear infection, but what he describes is what he regards as more bothersome to him. In effect, the pain in his ear (the primary symptom) is not as bothersome to him as his stomachache (a secondary symptom). In some cases, the child may have heard people talk about stomachaches and so assumes this must be what is wrong with him. That is, he associates (and confuses) what he has heard with the meaning of "sickness" and decides that, since he is sick, it must be his stomach!

Or a child may complain about her eyes hurting "real bad." You start to wonder if she needs corrective glasses. Once she is evaluated by the doctor, you are told she has the flu. The fact is, she was experiencing aching everywhere—but for her, it was her eyes hurting that proved most bothersome.

As we become more aware of our bodies and learn more about ourselves, we become better able to distinguish our major symptoms from more minor ones. This ability to discriminate and accurately describe what we are experiencing is extremely helpful to the physician.

Some experts estimate that if the doctor is a skilled questioner and the patient's responses are honest, precise and descriptive, an accurate diagnosis can be reached as often as 75 percent of the time by means of this "question-and-answer" process alone. This is called the "history" or, more often, the "history of the present illness," of the well-known history and physical examination (referred to as an "H and P").

Taking the History, Especially the History of the Present Illness

What you tell the doctor, then, gives him or her the clues needed to pursue a diagnosis. Your description of your chief sysmptom(s) and secondary symptoms, as well as your responses to the physician's questions, are vital. The fact is, the history is probably the single most important aspect of the diagnostic process.

Like the intricate and complex puzzle with so many pieces looking alike, countless diseases and health problems have certain symptoms in common. Often there is a very fine line or a very subtle difference between the type or pattern of symptoms associated with one problem as compared with another. Your ability to specifically describe the symptoms you are having can make a major difference in how the doctor will proceed in terms of ordering diagnostic tests and/or pursuing a course of action.

Reaching a specific diagnosis is often a process of elimination. The doctor begins to rule out certain possibilities as you describe your symptoms in detail and directs his or her efforts at those problems that are more likely the culprits. It is therefore vital that you be candid and straightforward about what you are experiencing.

At times, people tend to downplay their symptoms. They simply don't want to sound like complainers. Others lessen the severity or extent of their symptoms out of fear that something really serious might be wrong. The problem is, this misleads the doctor, who must believe what patients are saying. Still others exaggerate their symptoms out of fear that no one will take them seriously. Again, this points the doctor down the wrong path.

The symptoms we experience are really our body's way of communicating with us. Like the actions of the nonverbal child, which the doctor must interpret, our symptoms are our body's way of telling us something that we must then interpret and describe. It is therefore very important that we not downplay or exaggerate, but instead detail our symptoms as specifically as humanly possible.

Let's take pain as an example and review the kind of detailed descriptions that would be of greatest assistance to your doctor.

Your Major Symptom or Chief Complaint
Although we are using pain as an example, by just saying "pain," we would not be telling the doctor enough. What kind of pain? Is it dull, deep,

only on the surface, sharp, shooting, severe, throbbing, burning, boring, squeezing, a feeling of pressure?

Timing

Is the pain constant, off and on, every hour, every day or once a month? Does it come and go sporadically? Is the pain always the same, or is it different each time you feel it?

Location

Where is the pain exactly? Be as specific as possible. The leg is a rather large area—and so is the abdomen, chest, back or head. If the pain is in the chest, where in the chest is it located—the upper right side, the middle under the breastbone, on the lower left side under the rib cage? For knee pain, is it exactly in the knee, or just above it? And is the pain on the surface or deep inside?

When the pain occurs, does it start at one location and radiate (or move) to another? Or does it only hurt in one specific area? You can also show the doctor where the pain occurs, but try to be as specific as possible about exactly where it hurts most. If the pain radiates to another area, then show the doctor the path it takes.

Causative Factors

The doctor is interested in things that may "bring on" the problem or those that give more clues to what is going on. For example, does the pain occur before, during or after meals? Only while exercising? Only after exercising? Before, during or after any certain activity? Was there anything that changed in your schedule or normal routine prior to the start of the pain?

Associated Symptoms

The doctor knows that certain secondary symptoms are associated with a chief complaint and point more clearly to its origin. These questions about associated symptoms are usually asked systematically—first, overall questions, then those that review all the body systems and functions, often starting at the head and ending at the toes. It is usually helpful for you to go through these steps in your own mind so you can more specifically answer the doctor's questions. In addition to your major symptom(s) or chief complaint(s), the physician might ask the following:

Overall body questions: Do you have a feeling of being more tired than usual? Do you sleep more than usual, or are you having trouble sleeping? Overall weakness? General achiness? Changes in energy level—more or less energy than usual? Depressed or down-in-the-dumps? Aches, pains or stiffness in the joints? Loss of or increase in appetite? Any changes in the skin—rash, dryness, oiliness, flakiness? Fever? Chills? Hot flashes?

Head: Headaches? Dizziness? Blurry vision? Earache? Ringing in the ears? Eye discomfort—itching, burning, pain upon movement of the eyes? Postnasal drip? Nasal congestion? Sore mouth or tongue? Sneezing? Bad breath?

Throat and neck: Sore throat? Stiff neck? Lumps in the neck? Swollen neck or throat? Neckache or pain? Hoarseness or constant throat clearing? Any trouble swallowing? Choking episodes?

Chest: Coughing? Dry, irritating cough or loose cough with mucus? Tightness or pain in chest with cough? Chest pain? Where? Does it hurt when you breathe, and where? Is there anything that makes the chest pain better or worse? Any palpitations or irregular heartbeat? Does the heart seem to skip a beat, beat too fast, too slow or erratically?

Stomach, lower abdomen and urinary tract: Any pain or discomfort in the stomach? Any pain before, during or after meals? Any change in dietary habits? Heartburn or nausea? Feeling of fullness too soon after starting to eat? Gas or grumbling intestines? Constipation? Diarrhea? Any rectal bleeding? Blood or mucus in bowel movements? Any problems with urination? Burning, pain, loss of control of urine? Inability to urinate, even if you feel the need? Do you get up in the night to urinate? How often? Is that different from your normal routine, or has it increased over time? If male, is there any pain in the testicles? Any premature ejaculation, impotence or other sexual problems? If female, any discharge or bleeding between periods? Vaginal burning or itching? Loss of urine with laughing or coughing? Sexual problems? Menstrual cramps or premenstrual symptoms? Irregular periods?

Back, legs and arms: Any discomfort or pain in the back? Any stiffness? Any joint pain or stiffness? Weakness in legs or arms? Numbness or tingling in arms, legs, hands or feet?

What Have You Done About the Problem?

The doctor will want to know what steps you have taken to try to alleviate or lessen the symptoms or problem. Have you rested? Stayed off your feet? Taken any over-the-counter medications (these include vitamins, too)? If so, exactly what, how much and for how long? Have you changed your diet or eating habits? Increased or decreased your activity? Changed your environment? Have you applied heat or cold to a painful or uncomfortable area? Have you seen another professional, such as a chiropractor, nutritionist, health food expert, healer? If so, what has been done for you?

Have You Experienced These Symptoms Before?

The doctor will ask whether this is a recurring problem. Have you experienced these or similar symptoms before? How long did the symptoms last?

How long ago? What happened? Did the symptoms just suddenly stop, or slowly lessen? Was there anything different about this latest episode, as compared to the previous episodes?

Has Anyone Else Around You Had Similar Symptoms?

Do you have any reason to believe what you have is contagious? Have others around you (for example, in your family) experienced the same symptoms? If nausea and vomiting are involved, have you eaten out or been to a large gathering where food was served? If so, have any others who were there had any similar symptoms? Has anyone with similar symptoms recently been diagnosed as having a disease that frightens you?

Performing the Physical Examination

Some physicians take the "history" first, then do the "physical examination," while others ask questions while completing the examination. This is most often a matter of personal preference. As previously noted, it is estimated that an accurate diagnosis can be reached as much as 75 percent of the time by the history aspect of the evaluation alone if the physician is an excellent questioner and the patient is precise, descriptive and honest about his or her symptoms. Once a careful physical examination has been performed, it is estimated that an accurate diagnosis can now be reached 85 percent to 95 percent of the time. Therefore, the physical examination can increase the accuracy of diagnosis by 10 percent to 20 percent.

The extent of any physical exam will very much depend on the reason(s) for performing it. The annual physical examination (or the routine physical, as it is sometimes called) is usually quite extensive. Its purpose is to determine overall health and well-being and to identify any health problems as early as possible, so potentially serious conditions can be treated or managed long before they become serious threats.

However, when you call a doctor with specific symptoms, the extent of the examination will often be determined in part by the symptoms described. Nonetheless, almost all physicals include the taking of "vital signs"—the temperature, pulse, respiratory rate, blood pressure, and measurements of height and weight (as well as head circumference or size in infants). During almost all visits, the physician will also check major body systems, such as the head and neck, heart, lungs and abdomen, regardless of the complaint. He or she may omit certain parts of the usual examination, depending on the main problem and how long it has been since your last complete examination.

During a *complete* physical examination, the doctor will usually do the following:

Head and Neck
- Feel the surfaces for lumps, swelling or any abnormality.
- Feel the lymph nodes in the front, sides and back of neck.
- Check the thyroid gland for size, lumps or enlargement.
- Look for any abnormalities of the mouth, gums, throat, teeth and nose.
- Check ears for abnormal buildup of wax, or infection in the ear canals or behind the eardrums.
- Check eyes to see if they move in unison and function correctly.
- See if the eyes appear watery, inflamed or crusty.
- Check the functioning of the pupils.
- Look directly at blood vessels in the back of the eye using a special instrument.
- Some physicians perform hearing and vision screening tests, while others may order or recommend that they be done elsewhere. Still others do not include these in the routine examination unless a problem is suspected.

Chest
- Perform a breast examination for both sexes (although this should be done more routinely in women).

Lungs
- Check whether the chest moves normally.
- Note if any breathing trouble is present (either with breathing in or breathing out).
- Listen to lungs in front, sides and back. Are there any unusual noises?

Heart
- Listen to the heart, both as it fills with blood and as it empties (pumps) blood.
- Listen for heart rhythm, checking for extra beats, a rate that is too fast or slow, or a heartbeat that is very irregular.
- Check the circulation by feeling the pulses in the arms, legs and feet, and check to see that blood flow to the skin is normal.
- Check the skin (especially the lips or nails) for any signs of blueness.

Abdomen

- Listen to the bowel sounds and check for sounds that suggest aneurysm.
- Check the abdomen for unusual swelling or bloating.
- Feel the abdomen for any tenderness, soreness, muscle tension or deep masses.
- Check the size of the liver, spleen and other organs. Feel for deep masses or tenderness.

Back

- Check for straightness and any abnormalities.
- Feel for any tenderness over the kidneys or other areas of the back.
- Note any skin changes, rashes or redness.

Genitalia

- *In males*: Check external genitalia—penis, scrotum, testicles. Check for lumps, hernia and other abnormalities.
- *In females*: Check external genitalia—vulva, labia, clitoris, vaginal opening. Perform pelvic examination and Pap smear.

Rectum

- Check the external rectal area for hemorrhoids and fissures (cracks).
- Perform a rectal examination, feeling for masses (and, in males, the size of the prostate gland).
- Check for masses, abnormal tightness or laxity, tenderness.

Arms, Legs, Hands and Feet

- Look for swelling, varicose veins, redness or skin changes.
- Determine if there are any structural abnormalities.

Neurological Examination

This examination can be very extensive or quite limited. It usually includes at least the following:

- Check the cranial nerves and how they function, including vision, smell, eye movements, facial expressions, hearing, balance, swallowing, gag reflex, movement of the tongue, some movements of the shoulders.
- Check for sensations such as touch, pain, temperature, vibration sense and position sense.
- Test muscle strength and coordination.

• Check reflexes in both arms and legs.
• Check posture, balance and gait.

Diagnostic Tests

Routine physical evaluations most often include a complete blood count (called a CBC) and an analysis of the urine (called a UA). The CBC involves testing the blood for anemia (too few red blood cells or too little hemoglobin, the substance in the blood that carries oxygen) and for whether or not the white blood cells are normal in number and type. It also includes an evaluation of the platelets (particles in the blood that are important for normal blood clotting). The urinalysis involves testing urine for blood, protein, sugar, ketones and acidity, and looking under the microscope for signs of infection (pus cells and bacteria), red blood cells, crystals and clumps of cells called casts. These studies help determine if there are problems with the kidneys and may detect certain other conditions as well.

Diagnostic testing is also performed to verify an initial diagnosis of a suspected illness or health problem, to help determine the proper course of treatment or to further identify an illness or condition when the history and physical examination do not provide enough information to make a definite diagnosis. After the results of initial testing, the doctor sometimes needs to do even more testing to reach a particularly difficult diagnosis.

Because so many illnesses and health problems have so many symptoms in common, the doctor often requests a series of diagnostic tests that screen for other possible problems in order to confirm his or her suspicions, even though the doctor is fairly certain about the basis for the illness. This assures that appropriate treatment can be given without delay, since the tests verify the initial diagnosis and rule out other possibilities.

At times, too, doctors order laboratory tests and X rays because patients demand them—because they are not satisfied with a diagnosis based on the history and physical examination alone. Other times, diagnostic tests are ordered as a protection against legal liability. Because of the numbers of lawsuits for malpractice and the public demand that doctors not be "wrong," some doctors feel it is a necessity to verify a diagnosis with a laboratory test rather than take a risk that they might have missed something, misdiagnosed a problem or overlooked an additional hidden or disguised problem (where a laboratory test or X ray would provide the only clue to its detection).

The Bottom Line on Symptoms

Again, overt symptoms are essentially our body's way of communicating with us—its means of telling us that something is amiss or needs attention. Therefore, we should pay attention to our body's messages, whether the need is for more rest, more exercise, reducing stress, following a more nutritionally balanced diet, treating a minor illness or seeking medical attention for a more major problem.

When you need to call your doctor (to see if you need to be seen), or when you are seeing your doctor about a problem, determine ahead of time your chief complaint(s) or major symptom(s), so you can describe them in detail.

Ask yourself the questions presented in this section, so you are better prepared to respond to your physician's questions. It is vital that you be specific, precise, honest and straightforward. This includes saying, "I don't know," or "I haven't been aware of (or noticed) that," when this is the case. In other words, don't make up answers to "please" the doctor—simply reply as best and as specifically as you can. This is all you can ask of yourself and all anyone can ask of you.

This book will be of greatest benefit to you in helping you learn the skill of distinguishing between major and minor symptoms and develop the ability to describe them in detail. Most important, you will be better able to play a more active and positive role in assisting your personal physician, who needs your help and cooperation to make a correct diagnosis. This is one of the areas of medical care where you can and do make a significant contribution.

SECTION TWO

DISEASES

ABORTION—INDUCED, COMPLICATIONS OF

Termination of pregnancy.

Symptoms: Infection: fever, abdominal pain, chills, excessive bleeding, foul odor to vaginal discharge. Perforation of the uterus: severe abdominal pain, shock.

Cause: Sometimes complications occur because of poor surgical techinique (sloppy, not sterile), especially when abortions are performed in non-medical settings. Other times, complications occur even under the best of circumstances.

Severity of Problem: Some complications are minor, others life-threatening. Infection, bleeding and perforation of the uterus are among the most serious immediate complications. Some women who have had repeated induced abortions have difficulty with spontaneous abortions in later pregnancies, and some have difficulty in conceiving. A few deaths still occur each year following induced abortions.

Contagious? No.

Treatment: For all known or suspected complications of induced abortion, seek medical attention immediately. Perforation of the uterus requires intensive medical support and either surgical repair or removal of the uterus. Infection must be treated immediately, usually with intravenous antibiotics.

Prevention: Be sure the doctor (in a clinic or hospital) who is to perform the abortion is well qualified and reputable. Be alert to signs of complications and get medical help immediately if you experience them.

Discussion: Most abortions induced before 16 weeks of gestation are performed by dilating the cervix and emptying the uterus by either suctioning or scraping away the contents. Termination of pregnancies after 16 weeks usually requires injection of a salt solution into the uterus or admistration of a drug to cause contractions of the uterus and a period of active labor in order to expel the fetus. Complications occur in few women who have abortions performed by skilled physicians.

ABORTION—SPONTANEOUS (ALSO KNOWN AS "MISCARRIAGE")

Unintentional loss of the fetus before the 20th week of pregnancy.

Symptoms: First sign is vaginal bleeding. Second sign is usually pain in the lower abdomen (due to opening of the cervix).

Cause: The vast majority of the time, spontaneous abortion is caused by serious structual malformations in the fetus that make it impossible for the fetus to survive. This appears to be nature's way of terminating pregnancy. Other causes include severe chronic hypertension, hypertensive vascular disease, hyperthyroidism, abnormal uterus, serious infection, maternal trauma, incompetent cervix, uncontrolled diabetes, hormonal deficiencies and the effects of teratogens.

Severity of Problem: Approximately 15 percent to 20 percent of pregnancies end in spontaneous abortion. It is important to seek the advice of a physican if any symptoms occur. Spontaneous abortion can also threaten the woman's well-being if severe, uncontrolled bleeding occurs.

Contagious? No.

Treatment: If bleeding occurs, lie down immediately. Call your personal physician for advice. Little can be done if the problem is due to structural malformation in the fetus. If due to another cause, treatment would depend on the condition or problem identified.

Prevention: The possibility of preventive measures depends on the cause.

Discussion: Approximately 15 percent to 30 percent of women will experience some vaginal bleeding during pregnancy, which may or may not signal a threatened abortion. Severe bleeding and/or pain indicate the need for immediate medical intervention.

ABSCESS

Local infection with a collection of pus and much inflammation.

Symptoms: Depends on the location of the abscess (see entries for particular locations for specifics).

Cause: Infection by bacteria, often a staphylococcus.

Severity of Problem: Mild if abscess is small and on the surface (see ABSCESS—BOIL for more information); can be life-threatening if it is deep in the body tissues and not treated appropriately. The bacteria can invade the blood and cause a general infection (see SEPTICEMIA).

Contagious? Depends on the type of abscess and its location.

Treatment: Administration of antibiotics and sometimes drainage of the pus.

Prevention: Not very effective. However, spread of skin abscesses (boils) can be successfully controlled.

Discussion: An abscess is a collection of pus formed when the body's defense system begins to fight an infection. When bacteria infect an area, blood rushes to that area, which becomes red, hot and sore. White blood cells gather to fight the infection, forming pus and swelling. If the pus is under pressure, the abscess may rupture and drain. People with poor immunity, those who have diabetes mellitus and those who are chronically ill are more prone to infections and abscess formation.

ABSCESS—BOIL

Collection of pus under the skin, starting in a hair follicle.

Symptoms: Hard, dark-red, painful swelling under the skin. Over several days pus forms in the center, leaving a yellowish soft spot.

Cause: Infection by bacteria, generally a staphylococcus.

Severity of Problem: Usually mild but painful. Can spread to other body parts and invade the bloodstream, causing generalized infection (see SEPTI-CEMIA). Boils on the face, especially around the nose, are particularly risky.

Contagious? Yes. The bacteria can be spread to others and/or to new areas of your own body, causing boils and other kinds of infections.

Treatment: Apply heat to the tender area and do not squeeze or manipulate, especially if boil is on the face. Wash hands and the area around the boil well and often with soap and water to avoid spread. Call your doctor to discuss whether an antibiotic is needed and whether the boil requires draining. Multiple boils require medical attention and antibiotics.

Prevention: Wash carefully, especially if in contact with someone with boils or impetigo. Do not pick pimples.

Discussion: Most often found on hairy parts of the body where there is irritation and rubbing (for example, the neck, the belt line). Can spread to new areas of the body if not treated appropriately.

ABSCESS—PERITONSILLAR (QUINSY)

Severe tonsil infection with formation of pus collection inside the tonsil.

Symptoms: Fever and symptoms of tonsillitis (severe sore throat, difficulty swallowing, nausea, headache, generalized aches and pains), followed by worsening of pain in throat. Increasing difficulty swallowing, with feeling of lump in one side of the throat. Thickening of voice, pain with neck movement. Enlargement of one tonsil, with tenderness and pushing of the structures of the throat to one side by swelling. Lymph node on the infected side under the jaw tender and swollen.

Cause: Severe bacterial infection of the tonsils, with invasion of the tonsil by the bacteria. Pus forms inside, leading to swelling. Usually caused by a combination of bacteria, including streptococcus and staphylococcus.

Severity of Problem: Very serious infection. Requires immediate medical care.

Contagious? Not as such, but underlying infection is, if caused by streptococcus.

Treatment: Hospitalization and intravenous antibiotics. Warm salt water gargles, pain relief. Drainage of the abscess in the tonsil by surgery when pus formation is present and abscess is soft. Tonsillectomy is usually recommended after the acute infection has cleared.

Prevention: Prompt treatment of tonsillitis.

ABSCESS—TOOTH

Inflammation and infection of the pulp of a tooth may progress to a collection of pus at the base of the tooth.

Symptoms: Pain in a tooth or the jaw; swelling and tenderness of the jaw; sensitive tooth. Mild to moderate fever; sometimes general aching.

Cause: Usually mouth bacteria that invade unhealthy tissue.

Severity of Problem: Painful; can lead to loss of a tooth or to infection of the bone near the tooth.

Contagious? No.

Treatment: Rinse the mouth often with warm salt water. Use aspirin or acetaminophen for pain. Call or see a dentist as soon as possible. Antibiotic treatment is necessary. Dental treatment is needed if the tooth is to be saved. Extraction of an abscessed tooth is often required.

Prevention: Get regular dental care and treatment. Use good dental care practices. See your dentist at the earliest sign of tooth pain or sensitivity.

Discussion: Infection may extend to the bone, or the pus may drain into the mouth. If not treated, the tooth will be lost. Most often occurs in people with poor dental hygeine and many decayed teeth, or when inflammation of the tooth pulp has not been treated.

ACHALASIA

Difficulty swallowing due to malfunction of the circular muscle at the opening into the stomach from the esophagus.

Symptoms: Initially, difficulty swallowing (called dysphagia), along with a sensation of food sticking behind the breastbone or above the stomach. At the start, this is occasional, but it increases in frequency. There may or may not be pain in the chest, back or shoulder along with the difficulty swallowing. Regurgitation of food, bad taste in mouth, bad breath may be associated. Weight loss may occur if swallowing problem is severe.

Cause: Lack of coordination of the muscles and nerves involved in swallowing. The circular muscle between the esophagus and stomach does not open to allow food into the stomach, so the lower end of the esophagus enlarges. Food gathers there and can only be pushed on by swallowing large volumes of liquids or by straining at the end of swallowing. In an unusual form of this problem, the muscles at the end of the esophagus enlarge and go into spasm as well, producing actual pain with swallowing. The reason this happens is not known.

Severity of Problem: Initially bothersome, but eventually can lead to enough blockage to swallowing to be extremely uncomfortable and can lead to weight loss.

Contagious? No.

Treatment: At the early stages people learn to swallow by drinking large amounts of liquids and straining at the end of swallowing. This ultimately does not work and also leads to weight loss because the liquids interfere with eating enough food. With increasing problems, treatment consists of enlarging the end of the esophagus using a swallowed balloon to stretch the muscle. This may need to be done repeatedly. About 20 percent to 25 percent of victims are not helped by this and may require surgery to correct the condition.

Prevention: None known.

Discussion: This problem can occur at any age but is most common in men, starting between the ages of 30 and 50.

ACNE

A common skin disease usually seen in adolescents, acne is basically an inflammation of the skin related to overactive sebaceous (oil) glands.

Symptoms: Small, red pimples located on face, neck, back and chest in adolescents. Blackheads and whiteheads; occasional inflamed and infected pimples. Oily skin. Skin outbreaks that come and go.

Cause: Exact cause is unknown, although hormonal changes, especially overproduction of male hormones (called androgens) seems to play a role. Inflammation of acne pimples seems related to leakage of sebum (oil) into the surrounding skin and smoldering infection due to skin bacteria. While certain foods in the diet of some individuals seem to play a role, their role is less significant than most people think.

Severity of Problem: Can be very mild, with only a few pimples and blackheads now and then, or very severe, with deep pustules, cysts and scars that persist for life. There is a slight family tendency to the deeper form of acne, which is much more common in boys than in girls.

Contagious? No.

Treatment: For mild acne wash the skin well once or twice a day, using a somewhat drying but not too harsh soap. The goal is to reduce but not eliminate the oiliness of the skin. (Blackheads are *not* dirt and should not be scrubbed too much.) As acne gets more severe, treatment includes use of a mild peeling agent, which irritates the skin enough to cause it to peel slightly. Benzoyl peroxide is commonly used for this. With severe acne with pustules and much skin inflammation, expert help from a dermatologist is important to control the skin inflammation and limit the amount of scarring if possible. Treatment may include special peeling agents, retinoic acid, ultraviolet light therapy, careful skin surgery to open the pustules and cysts, and antibiotic therapy. Pimples, blackheads and pustules should not be squeezed except by a doctor.

Mild, controlled sun exposure, enough to produce slight peeling, can help some victims. Diet changes (with avoidance of fatty foods, sweets, chocolate, etc.) are commonly tried and vastly overrated.

Prevention: None known.

Discussion: In its simplest form, acne is characterized by small pimples found over the oily parts of the body (face, neck, shoulders, chest and back). These pimples may have small blisters on the top that contain white material or may look black (blackheads) because of exposure of the oil to air. If the oil glands with the oily secretions are squeezed, the oil leaks into the skin and causes inflammation. Normal skin bacteria play a role in this inflammation process. Larger pustules form, with much redness, pain and swelling. As these pustules grow, they may develop into thickened cysts. This deep form of acne leaves permanent scars.

Acne usually starts at puberty and is more common in boys than in girls. It can occur at other times in life, related to hormonal changes and use of certain medications. It can be controlled and improved with good, professional skin care. In most cases, the chances of scarring and severe skin disease can be greatly reduced with good dermatologic skin treatment. If scars do form, skin surgery called dermabrasion can be useful.

ACOUSTIC NEURINOMA

Tumor located inside the brain on or near the cranial nerve that controls hearing and balance (the auditory or acoustic nerve).

Symptoms: Hearing loss in one ear, tinnitus (ringing or noises heard in one ear), and sometimes dizziness and loss of balance. The hearing loss is gradual and may go unnoticed until the tinnitus starts.

Cause: There are no known factors that seem to increase the risk for this tumor. The tumor is benign (noncancerous) and grows very slowly.

Severity of Problem: Without treatment the tumor grows gradually and leads to complete hearing loss in the affected side and sometimes severe dizziness. It usually does not grow quickly enough to cause severe increase in brain pressure and other nervous system abnormalities.

Contagious? No.

Treatment: Removal of the tumor by surgery is the treatment of choice. This will usually cure the dizziness, but hearing may be completely destroyed in that ear.

Prevention: None known.

Discussion: Acoustic neurinomas are usually small tumors that can be successfully removed without leaving further damage than deafness in the affected side. One of the least damaging brain tumors.

ALCOHOLISM

Disease in which a person is compelled to drink alcoholic beverages. Physical addiction to alcohol is also a part of the disease.

Symptoms: Psychological and physical dependence on alcohol; steady or "binge" drinking; elaborate schemes to obtain alcohol or hide that it was consumed. As complications develop, symptoms may include some or all of the following: defective memory; frequent accidents and injuries; unusual (sometimes obviously intoxicated) behavior; poor nutrition; liver disease; failure to function in job or family life; blackout spells.

Cause: Probably many causes, including psychological problems that allow a person to become dependent on a chemical to alter mood. There may be a physical and family tendency to become addicted to this and other drugs.

Severity of Problem: Can lead to chronic, life-threatening physical complications. Can destroy family and other relationships as disease becomes severe.

Contagious? No.

Treatment: Intensive treatment to first detoxify, then reeducate and offer psychological support. Severe problems can best be handled in the hospital, while less severe problems can be handled with outpatient care alone. Ongoing self-help groups are particularly helpful to people who have an alcohol problem.

Discussion: Alcoholism is the third leading cause of death in the United States. It affects people of all socioeconomic backgrounds and all ages, including children and teen-agers. There is a tendency for alcoholics to use other drugs besides alcohol. The difference between "social drinking" and alcohol dependence can be subtle.

ALLERGIC REACTIONS AND DISORDERS (ATOPY)

An allergic reaction is basically an overreaction of the body's defense system. Normally, the body fights "foreign" invaders by developing antibodies against them. In allergic disorders this development of antibodies is excessive—out of proportion to the danger of the substance. There are many types of allergic reactions and disorders, which will be discussed in the following entries.

Symptoms: Depends on the type of reaction and its severity. In contact dermatitis and eczema, for example, a skin rash that itches is found. In allergic rhinitis the person is bothered by mild to severe nasal congestion and sneezing. In asthma there is difficulty breathing, and in anaphylactic shock the person collapses and may die. Review each of those entries for more information.

Cause: Exaggerated body defense reaction to an "allergen"—a substance the body recognizes as "foreign" and dangerous. The body develops antibodies against the invader, so when it is exposed again in the future, it reacts in a specific way (for example, with a rash, nasal congestion, wheezing, intestinal upset).

Severity of Problem: Varies with the type of disorder and the individual. Some allergic reactions are bothersome and mild, while others can and do kill people.

Contagious? No.

Treatment: Again, depends on cause and severity. Refer to entries for individual types of reactions listed for more information.

Prevention: Avoid contact with any known allergen.

Discussion: A person can come into contact with an allergen by inhaling it, eating it or absorbing it through the skin or mucous membranes. The allergen causes a cell called a mast cell to release a chemical, histamine. Histamine then causes various symptoms, depending on the person and the type of allergen. Many people develop one or more allergies in their lifetimes. Estimates vary from 10 percent to 30 percent of the population, with allergic disorders ranging from mild to life-threatening. The tendency to have allergic reactions, which is called atopy, runs in families.

ALLERGIC REACTIONS AND DISORDERS (ATOPY)— ALLERGIC DERMATITIS (ECZEMA, ATOPIC DERMATITIS)

Chronic rash caused by allergic (also called atopic) reaction to substances the body perceives as "foreign."

Symptoms: Dry, red, irritated skin, with cracking and bleeding at times. Thickening of skin occurs over time. Pain and itching can be severe. Most often located on hands, elbow creases, behind knees and on ankles and feet, although it can occur elsewhere.

Cause: Contact with substance(s) to which a person is sensitive (most commonly through skin contact or food allergy). The body recognizes the substance as "foreign" and develops a reaction against it. The reaction may persist over an extended time, even after the contact has been eliminated.

Severity of Problem: Can vary from minor and bothersome to very serious. Severe, extensive forms of eczema increase the risk of serious infection.

Contagious? No.

Treatment: Reduce contact with soap and water; use moisturizing creams for mild problems. If a specific offending agent is know, avoid contact with it. Problems that persist in spite of this should be evaluated by a physician. Steroid creams and lotions may be prescribed.

Prevention: Avoid contact with materials known to cause reactions.

Discussion: Eczema may begin in infancy and either go away completely or persist through childhood and into adulthood. In adults, women are most often afflicted and usually have eczema on the hands.

ALLERGIC REACTIONS AND DISORDERS (ATOPY)— ALLERGIC RHINITIS (HAY FEVER)

Constant or recurring inflammation and irritation of the lining of the nose and upper respiratory tract as a result of allergy, usually to something inhaled or present in the air.

Symptoms: Watery discharge from the nose that can be very pronounced. Itching of the nose and often of the eyes may be very bothersome. There are bursts of sneezing. Night and morning dry cough can result from postnasal drip and drainage of the clear secretions into the back of the throat. A crease-like indentation may be seen over the top of the nose in children and adults with this problem because of the repeated scratching of the nose.

Cause: Allergic reaction to one or more substances with which the person has come into contact. Most often the contact is with a pollen or irritating substance "in the air," although foods and other materials may also cause trouble.

Severity of Problem: Variable, from only occasionally bothersome to a constant, severe problem.

Contagious? No.

Treatment: The most successful treatment is identifying the substance that causes the reaction, then avoiding it. If this is not possible, antihistamine drugs taken by mouth may be helpful. These can be purchased without a prescription. For severe cases that are "perennial"—present year round— more potent medication may be necessary.

Prevention: Avoid exposure to substances known to cause or worsen the problem.

Discussion: Allergic rhinitis is one of the most common allergic reactions and may start in infancy or childhood. It may come and go, with peaks during certain seasons, or be present much or all of the time. It can be distinguished from a common cold by the lack of fever and the fact that, with this problem, the nasal secretions tend to stay very watery. Can lead to complications of sinusitis and otitis media, both acute and serious. May be seen in persons with asthma and other allergic symptoms.

ALLERGIC REACTIONS AND DISORDERS (ATOPY)— ASTHMA

Chronic disease marked by reversible narrowing of the medium and small-sized airways, leading to breathing difficulty and wheezing.

Symptoms: Tight cough, feeling of tightness in the chest, shortness of breath and wheezing noise on breathing out are the most common symptoms. These symptoms come and go. In severe attacks, coughing may lead to vomiting.

Cause: Most of the time, asthma is caused by allergy or sensitivity to something with which the person has come into contact. This can be in the form of dust or pollen or pollutants that have been inhaled, or it can be in the form of foods or medications that have been swallowed. Infection may trigger an attack, and stress or emotional tension may make an attack worse. Certain medications can also cause the airway spasm that leads to wheezing.

Severity of Problem: Can vary from mild, with only rare attacks, to severe, with constant wheezing and progressive lung disease. Deaths from asthma are rare but still occur.

Contagious? No.

Treatment: Must be treated by a physician. Cough and wheeze, which is caused by spasm of the airways, are treated with several different types of medications, which may need to be taken around the clock or only occasionally. Sometimes medications that are inhaled are also needed for good control. For acute attacks, injections of epinephrine and other emergency measures may be needed. Severe attacks must be treated in a hospital and may require oxygen and other vigorous support. Infection must be treated if present. Part of treatment is identifying the cause of attacks, then avoiding or controlling exposure to the offending substance.

Prevention: The tendency to have asthma cannot be avoided, but attacks can be prevented or lessened by controlling exposure to things known to bring on wheezing. Complications of chronic lung disease can be controlled or prevented by careful control of asthma in its early stages.

Discussion: Asthma may start in infancy or as late as adulthood. There is a tendency for allergic asthma to occur in certain families, and many asthmatics have other allergic symptoms as well (such as allergic rhinitis, eczema, hives). Sometimes asthma is called "chronic bronchitis." Some asthmatics must take medications every day to control their problem, while others only need it with attacks of wheezing. People with asthma are prone to developing pneumonia and atelectasis (collapse of the lung).

ALLERGIC REACTIONS AND DISORDERS (ATOPY)— CONTACT DERMATITIS

Rash or skin irritation that results from contact with an object or material to which the person is sensitive. May be an acute, one-time thing or a chronic condition.

Symptoms: In an acute reaction, pain and itching, redness and a rash over a certain area of the body. Sometimes blistering occurs. With long-term contact the rash often becomes scaly and "weeps" a yellowish liquid. There may be a pattern of the rash that helps identify its cause.

Cause: Skin contact with a substance that is irritating and to which the person is sensitive.

Severity of Problem: Bothersome and uncomfortable; usually localized to one area and not severe.

Contagious? No.

Treatment: Eliminate contact with the offending substance. Apply a soothing solution such as Burow's solution (see your physician or pharmacist). With chronic, bothersome problems, see a doctor. Treatment often includes the use of steroid cream or lotion and an oral antihistamine to aid sleep and reduce itching.

Prevention: Avoid contact with known irritants or allergens.

Discussion: Contact dermatitis can occur as an acute, one-time outbreak of rash or be chronic due to repeated contact with an offending substance. Common offenders include poison plants (poison ivy, poison oak, poison sumac), perfumes, cosmetics, dyes (for example, in shoes), jewelry (usually with nickel used as the base metal), soaps and cleaners, wool, etc. Sometimes the pattern of the rash on the skin is most helpful in figuring out the cause.

ALLERGIC REACTIONS AND DISORDERS (ATOPY)— URTICARIA (HIVES)

Skin rash with varying sized and shaped welts and blotches, usually caused by contact with something to which the person is allergic.

Symptoms: Red blotches on the skin that may swell and develop unusual shapes. Some of the blotches may have a whitish welt in the center and itch intensely. The rash may be limited to a small area of the skin or spread over the body. The rash tends to come and go, with new blotches developing often. There may be swelling of the lips and face and generalized itching as well.

Cause: Usually an allergic reaction to a substance with which the person has had contact. This can be something touched or inhaled or eaten. Often related to medication or food. Sometimes infection causes hives, and in certain situations the cause of the hives may never be determined.

Severity of Problem: Uncomfortable, with intense itching. Can be serious and life-threatening if swelling of the lips and throat occurs.

Contagious? No.

Treatment: Keep the skin cool to prevent excessive itching. Contact a doctor about medication to relieve the itching and reduce the rash (antihistamines are sometimes effective for this). If breathing difficulty or swelling of the lips or throat occurs along with hives, go to an emergency facility for immediate treatment.

Prevention: If the cause of the hives is known, avoid contact with that substance. If bee sting or insect allergy is involved, desensitization injections might be recommended by your doctor. Avoid taking any medication that produced hives in the past.

Discussion: Some people who get hives have only one episode and never have another. Others have many attacks; the cause may be uncertain. After two to three attacks, most doctors recommend a search for the cause. The rash of hives can come and go for as long as two weeks, even if contact with the offending substance is eliminated and antihistamine medications are taken.

ALOPECIA—MALE PATTERN BALDNESS

A very common form of permanent baldness (alopecia), most often seen in men.

Symptoms: Painless loss of hair, beginning at the sides in the front and extending further backward. May progress quickly or slowly, may be mild or severe. No underlying problems found. There may be seborrhea, with dandruff and greasiness of the scalp associated.

Cause: Tendency to have this is hereditary, usually inherited from the mother's side of the family. Heredity determines both the time it starts and its severity.

Severity of Problem: Can be a mild problem with little loss of hair, or can be extensive. Usual problems are emotional.

Contagious? No.

Treatment: No cure and no treatment will stimulate regrowth of hair. (Many quack claims are available.) For severe problems, surgical hair implant may be recommended.

Prevention: None.

Discussion: While male pattern baldness is most often a problem of males, it occasionally occurs in women. Women can also suffer another similar type of baldness with generalized severe thinning of all the head hair. This is also a permanent hair loss without effective cure.

AMENORRHEA

Absence of menstrual periods during the time when a woman usually has menstrual cycles.

Symptoms: With *primary amenorrhea* menstrual cycles have never started. In *secondary amenorrhea* menstrual cycles cease unexpectedly. There may be other symptoms, depending on cause.

Cause: *Primary amenorrhea* usually results from a hormonal lack. This is seen with tumors or disorders of the pituitary gland; ovarian problems that make the ovaries not respond to pituitary homones; and disorders of the hypothalamus (an area of the brain with a definite but poorly understood relationship to the pituitary gland). Amenorrhea can also result from abnormalities of the uterus, imperforate hymen and chromosomal abnormalities.

Secondary amenorrhea (temporary) is common and may result from pregnancy (the most common cause!); stopping birth control pills; emotional stress; excessive gain or loss of weight; vigorous exercise (this is common in young athletes); certain endocrine disorders (hypothyroidism, Cushing's disease, Addison's disease); tumors; certain ovarian problems; and "psychogenic" (emotional) causes.

Severity of Problem: Amenorrhea is a symptom of an underlying problem but of itself is not serious, except for the psychological stress caused by failure to menstruate. Severity (and permanence) of the underlying problem is variable.

Contagious? No.

Treatment: Depends on cause but usually involves attempting to restart menstrual cycles after pregnancy has been ruled out as a cause. May involve treatment with hormones for short or long periods of time.

Prevention: Only as is possible for the underlying causes: good diet, stress control, sensible weight-loss programs.

Discussion: Primary amenorrhea is, by definition, lack of menstrual cycles after age 16. Temporary episodes without periods are *extremely* common in young women under stress.

ANAPHYLACTIC SHOCK

Immediate, life-threatening allergic reaction, with shock and severe difficulty breathing. Requires *immediate* medical care.

Symptoms: Sudden trouble breathing, severe itching and swelling of the lips, tongue and throat, as well as skin; cough, wheezing and feeling of suffocation; may be followed by sudden collapse and loss of consciousness; death may occur within minutes.

Cause: An immediate allergic reaction to a foreign substance (for example, a bee sting, an injected medication, a food).

Severity of Problem: A life-threatening emergency.

Contagious? No.

Treatment: Call paramedics immediately. Keep person calm. Begin cardiopulmonary resuscitation (CPR) if respiratory and/or cardiac arrest occur.

Prevention: If you have known allergies to medications or other substances, avoid these things at all cost and be alert to early symptoms of anaphylaxis (itching, breathing trouble, hives). Ask your doctor about a kit that contains epinephrine if you have serious, life-threatening allergies.

ANEMIA

A condition in which there are too few red blood cells in the body. The term *anemia* is also used to refer to conditions in which there is too little or abnormal hemoglobin, the pigment in the red blood cells that carries oxygen.

Symptoms: Often there are no symptoms if the problem is mild. As the anemia gets more severe, there is easy fatigability, weakness and paleness. In some forms there is also jaundice and enlargement of the liver and spleen. When anemia becomes very severe, or occurs suddenly, symptoms of heart failure might be experienced.

Cause: There are very many possible causes, with some of them common and others very rare. General catagories of causes are: nutritional (iron deficiency, pernicious anemia, folic acid deficiency); blood loss; hereditary anemias with abnormal hemoglobins; hemolytic anemias (the red blood cells are fragile or abnormally shaped, so they break easily); aplastic (failure of the bone marrow to produce red blood cells); and anemia of chronic disease (seen in many generalized diseases, such as infection, arthritis, kidney disease, liver disease, etc.).

Severity of Problem: Variable, from mild and without symptoms, to severe and life-threatening.

Contagious? No.

Treatment: Depends on cause. If nutritional, replacing the deficiency will cure the problem. Looking for and treating causes of blood loss are important. The hereditary forms cannot be cured, but transfusions and other care are often needed.

Prevention: Avoiding dietary deficiencies for the nutritional forms. Genetic counseling may be a good idea for those with hereditary forms of anemia, so they understand how the disease is inherited and what the risks are for their future children.

Discussion: Anemia is one of the most common diseases or conditions. We will discuss certain of the most common forms in detail below. It is always important that the cause for the anemia be detected—treating anemia with iron or vitamins is not appropriate unless your physician has determined that the cause is iron or vitamin deficiency.

ANEMIA—APLASTIC ANEMIA

A severe form of anemia in which the bone marrow fails to produce red blood cells, as well as white blood cells and platelets (tiny particles which are important in blood clotting).

Symptoms: Severe paleness, weakness and fatigue. Frequent, severe infections. Bleeding episodes with both deep internal bleeding and bruising and bleeding into the skin.

Cause: Certain drugs are known to cause bone marrow failure and aplastic anemia. Radiation is also a factor. In more than half of cases, however, no cause is found.

Severity of Problem: Usually a fatal disease, from severe bleeding or infection.

Contagious? No.

Treatment: Blood transfusions, treatment of infection are very important. Sometimes transplantation of bone marrow from a matching donor is effective. There are certain drugs that have been tried, but which have been disappointing.

Prevention: Avoiding drugs known to cause apastic anemia unless essential for treatment of a serious condition, avoiding unnecessary radiation exposure (diagnostic x-rays are not usually thought to be involved) are always wise. However, since most causes are not known, prevention is not really possible.

Discussion: Aplastic anemia is quite rare. Other causes of severe anemia and low white blood cells and platelets are more common and include leukemias and other cancers.

ANEMIA—IRON DEFICIENCY

Lack of hemoglobin and red blood cells because of lack of enough iron in the body to make hemoglobin.

Symptoms: Weakness, pale color to the skin and chronic fatigue. Compulsion to eat things other than food (for example, laundry starch, clay, ice, dirt) is very common. When the disease is severe, there is irritability, loss of concentration and, in children, behavior disturbances. Difficulty breathing and palpitations (because of early heart failure) can occur with very severe forms.

Cause: In *adults*, chronic blood loss is the most common cause. This can be through excessive menstrual flow in women, or with hidden bleeding, usually in the intestine (from an ulcer, cancer, gastritis, polyp, for example). In pregnancy additional iron is needed, because extra blood must be made, for both mother and fetus.

In *young children,* especially those under 2 years old, the most common cause of iron deficiency anemia is lack of enough iron in the diet. This is usually caused by drinking too much milk without eating foods that supply iron. Milk anemia produces another problem, which is irritation of the intestine and chronic, small amounts of bleeding, which adds further to the problem.

Severity of Problem: Can be mild and unnoticed until a blood test is done, or severe and resulting in heart failure.

Contagious? No.

Treatment: One of the most important aspects of treating iron deficiency is to identify the cause and treat it. Treating the anemia but not finding that the cause is an ulcer or cancer is not very helpful for a person.

The treatment for this type of anemia is iron taken by mouth. Iron treatment should be supervised by a doctor and is usually continued for at least three months after the anemia has disappeared, so the body's iron stores can be replenished. Iron available in over-the-counter vitamins is not enough to treat true anemia. Diet changes to include foods that are high in iron are part of long-term treatment, as is reduction of milk drinking to less than a quart of milk a day in children.

Prevention: Dietary iron deficiency can be prevented by eating a balanced diet that includes foods that are high in iron. In infants and children, avoiding cow's milk in the first year of life and limiting the amount of milk after that to less than one quart a day later are important.

ANEMIA—SICKLE-CELL

Hereditary disorder in which the hemoglobin (the pigment in the blood that carries oxygen) is abnormal.

Symptoms: Repeated episodes of pain in the abdomen, arms or legs in a black person, usually starting in infancy or childhood. Weakness, paleness and fatigue. Jaundice is usually present (seen in the whites of the eyes) but gets worse when the pain episodes, called crises, happen.

Cause: The body makes an abnormal hemoglobin called hemoglobin S. This hemoglobin makes the red blood cells fragile and easily distorted, especially when there is lack of oxygen. The red blood cells change shape, to look like "sickles," and are destroyed by the body, causing the anemia.

This disease is inherited as a recessive trait—one abnormal gene from the father and one from the mother. People who "carry" the abnormal gene have mild anemia but don't usually have other symptoms. They are said to have "sickle-cell trait."

Severity of Problem: Sickle-cell anemia is a serious, non-curable disease. After many episodes of crisis (sickling episodes), there is a tendency to have kidney failure. There is a serious risk for overwhelming infection (septicemia) with a certain bacteria, pneumococcus, especially in childhood. People with this disease can die from hemorrhage into the brain, often in childhood. However, most live into adulthood, but with many problems. Gallstones are common.

Contagious? No.

Treatment: Episodes of crisis—destruction of red blood cells—are treated with plenty of liquids, oxygen, pain medications and transfusions of blood if needed. Since the risk for septicemia is high, fevers usually are treated in the hospital with intravenous antibiotics, after infection is searched for.

Prevention: The only prevention is the avoidance of two people with sickle-cell trait having children. (Their risk of having a child with the disease is one in four with each pregnancy, and half of their children will also carry the abnormal gene.)

Discussion: Screening tests exist to detect people who carry the abnormal sickle-cell gene and have been made widely available. This problem can exist along with other types of hereditary abnormal hemoglobins. Sickle-cell problems are seen almost exclusively in the black population.

ANEMIA—THALASSEMIA

Hereditary anemia in which the body is unable to make a certain portion of the hemoglobin pigment (the substance in the red blood cells that carries oxygen).

Symptoms: In *thalassemia minor* there are no symptoms, and the problem is detected during a routine check of the blood count or because a person looks slightly pale.

In *thalassemia major* severe paleness from infancy, with jaundice in some children. The liver and spleen become enlarged early in life, and gallstones are common. The anemia is often severe enough to cause heart failure, with shortness of breath, weakness and edema.

Cause: Thalassemia is a hereditary defect in which the body cannot make the correct amounts of a portion of the hemoglobin. *Thalassemia minor* is the form of the disease in which the person has only one of the abnormal genes in a pair, while in *thalassemia major* there is complete inability to make the normal hemoglobin, because both genes of the gene pair are abnormal. This trait occurs most often in people of Mediterranean background, certain Chinese and some blacks.

Severity of Problem: *Thalassemia minor* is a mild condition with no serious consequences other than mild anemia and the ability to pass on the abnormal thalassemia gene to children. *Thalassemia major* is a serious chronic disease that is often fatal in childhood.

Contagious? No.

Treatment: No treatment is needed for thalassemia minor, and iron treatment should usually be avoided. Thalassemia major must be treated with repeated blood transfusions throughout life.

Prevention: Only possible by preventing pregnancy when both partners are so-called carriers of the thalassemia gene (both have thalassemia minor). This is not always satisfactory, and their carrier state may not be known. The risk for two carriers having a child with thalassemia major is one out of four for each pregnancy, and the risk is one in two for thalassemia minor.

Discussion: The anemia of thalassemia minor is similar to iron deficiency and is often confused with it. It is important that the distinction be made and that people with thalassemia minor not be treated with excessive doses of iron.

ANEURYSM

Outpouching of the wall of a blood vessel, usually an artery, due to a weakness in the wall of the artery. Can happen in large or small arteries, with varying effects.

Symptoms: Symptoms usually are caused by rupture of the aneurysm rather than by the outpouching itself. Severe, sudden pain (most commonly located in the abdomen, chest or brain). Loss of consciousness, collapse, shock; death may follow if a large aneurysm ruptures.

Cause: Most often, diseases of the blood vessels, such as arteriosclerosis or infection. Weakness of the muscle of the artery wall or damage to the blood vessel from physical trauma can lead to aneurysm.

Severity of Problem: Can lead to death if aneurysm ruptures.

Contagious? No.

Treatment: If ruptured, immediate medical care and vigorous support are indicated. Call paramedics if rupture is suspected. Surgery is the only effective treatment. It may involve replacement of the weakened blood vessel section with a graft, or occasionally repair is possible.

Prevention: None.

Discussion: Aneurysm is a serious problem because of the constant risk of the weakened blood vessel wall's rupturing. It can occur in children and young adults due to an inherited weakness of the blood vessel but is more common in middle-aged and elderly people.

ANGINA PECTORIS

Pain in the chest. Refers to pain that originates in the heart.

Symptoms: Sudden pain in the chest, often with or after exercise, stress or eating. Frequently described as crushing, located under the breastbone; may radiate down the arm or into the shoulder, most often the left. Sometimes felt as "indigestion" or heartburn. There may be faintness, shortness of breath, paleness. Usually lasts less than five minutes.

Cause: Sudden lack of adequate blood supply to the heart muscle. Often brought on by exercise, eating or stress. A common cause is underlying arteriosclerosis or other form of cardiovascular disease, which results in narrowing of the arteries that supply the heart with its nourishment.

Severity of Problem: Potentially life-threatening. Increasing pain or frequency of pain can signal worsening of the disease. Can lead to progressive loss of ability to function without pain or shortness of breath.

Contagious? No.

Treatment: Should be evaluated by a physician if angina is suspected. Avoid unusual or preventable stress if possible. Medication (either long-lasting or short-acting) is often used to help relieve the symptoms.

Prevention: Appropriate diet in early life, as well as ongoing attention to nutrition. Avoid stress where possible.

Discussion: Chest pain should never be taken lightly but rather regarded as a signal that there may be a problem. People with known heart disease may have symptoms. Prompt medical evaluation and treatment can spell the difference between life and death.

ANOREXIA NERVOSA

Very complex eating disorder usually starting in the adolescent years.

Symptoms: Dramatic weight loss with or without apparent reduction in the amount of food eaten. Sometimes self-induced vomiting occurs, and some people actually eat voraciously before they vomit. As malnutrition becomes severe, hair loss, menstrual irregularity, low blood pressure and slow heartbeat occur.

Cause: A very complicated psychological and physical problem that usually starts in the teen-age years but can continue into adulthood. Markedly more common in girls than in boys.

Severity of Problem: Life-threatening as malnutrition increases. People with this problem can die from the effects of malnutrition, from infection or from suicide.

Contagious? No. However, it is becoming more common because of the emphasis on thinness in Western society.

Treatment: Requires intense medical and psychiatric care, usually in a hospital. Treatment is very complex.

Prevention: None known, although early recognition of the problem can prevent the life-threatening complications.

APPENDICITIS

Inflammation of the appendix, a small structure attached to the end of the large bowel.

Symptoms: Abdominal pain that usually starts near the umbilicus, then may move ("localize") to the lower right side. Loss of appetite, nausea and low fever are common. Usually no diarrhea, although mild constipation may occur. (Do not take a laxative if these symptoms are present.)

Cause: Not completely certain, but thought to be related to blockage of the opening of the appendix by a small piece of stool, followed by infection of the obstructed appendix, with formation of pus.

Severity of Problem: If not recognized and treated early, the appendix can rupture and lead to serious infection of the lining of the abdomen. Generalized infection can follow.

Contagious? No.

Treatment: Surgical removal of the appendix as soon after the problem is recognized as possible. If rupture has occurred, antibiotic treatment is also needed.

Prevention: None known.

Discussion: Most commonly seen in children, although the problem can happen in adults. Appendicitis is very difficult to recognize in very young children and often goes unnoticed until the appendix has burst and serious infection has started. Some people believe that chronic appendicitis with intermittent abdominal pain occurs, but this is quite controversial. At the time of abdominal surgery performed for other reasons, the appendix is often removed as a precaution, because it does not have any known function, and there is always a risk of appendicitis.

ARTERIOSCLEROSIS

So-called "hardening of the arteries," this condition is a result of atherosclerosis (accumulation of fatty deposits inside the arteries). The blood vessels become narrowed and hardened and may go into spasm.

Symptoms: Can be without symptoms at first, then with gradual development of problems, depending on which blood vessels are narrowed. May be associated with high blood pressure, angina pectoris, cramps and pains in the legs after exercise, dizziness and headaches, and abnormal kidney function.

Cause: The deposits of fatty material, with hardening of the deposits with calcium and then spasm of the arteries with partial or complete obstruction. Hypertension, diabetes mellitus and obesity increase the risk for arteriosclerosis. Some people with a high content of fatty substances (triglycerides and cholesterol) in their blood are also prone to this condition.

Severity of Problem: Variable, but usually worsens over time. Can lead to serious, life-threatening complications.

Contagious? No.

Treatment: In the early stages certain people can be helped tremendously by drugs that relax the spasms in the arteries. Stress relief and exercise also help with relieving the spasm. Some people require surgery to clean out the obstructed arteries or to replace the narrowed section with a graft.

Prevention: Although there is no absolute way to prevent this problem, there are measures that may keep the disease from progressing. If you are overweight, try to reduce. Start a doctor-prescribed exercise program. If you smoke, stop; if you don't, don't start. Eat a well-balanced diet and reduce the content of fats in your diet if your doctor so recommends.

Discussion: Complications of this problem, which is one of the features of the aging process, are among the most common causes of death and disability in the United States. While it is not truly hereditary, certain families have a much greater tendency for development of arteriosclerosis in early and middle adulthood.

ARTHRITIS—DEGENERATIVE JOINT DISEASE (OSTEOARTHRITIS)

Chronic, progressive stiffness and deformity of joints without any generalized symptoms.

Symptoms: Stiffness of one or more joints of the body, usually in the morning or after a time of being inactive. Then enlargement of the joint, with little deformity. Joint pain becomes worse after prolonged exercise or overuse, followed by limited motion of the joint and grating sensation upon movement. No redness or excessive warmth of joint, no fever or generalized body symptoms. There may be small nodules on hands and deformity of hands, especially of the tips of the fingers.

Cause: Thought to be due to degeneration of the cartilage and joint surfaces. May be due to aging or may be a result of past injury to a joint.

Severity of Problem: Can vary from mild and bothersome discomfort to severe stiffness and limited function.

Contagious? No.

Treatment: Rest and local heat; exercises to keep joints less stiff, but without overstressing; medications to control pain and reduce inflammation (aspirin and other anti-inflammatory drugs may be used). Injection of cortisonelike drugs into the joints in severe cases. Weight reduction if the victim is obese.

Prevention: Avoid abuse of joints and becoming overweight. Get prompt, proper treatment for joint injuries.

Discussions: A particularly common problem. Very bothersome, but control of pain and maintenance of good function are quite possible.

ARTHRITIS—GOUT

Acute inflammation of a joint because of deposits of uric acid crystals.

Symptoms: Sudden onset of severe pain, redness, swelling and tenderness of a joint, often at night. Most common joint affected is big toe, although other joints can be affected. After inflammation has subsided, the skin over the joint peels and itches.

Cause: Deposit of uric acid crystals in a joint. Thought to be related to sudden rises or falls in the blood uric acid level. Uric acid levels can be high because of a hereditary problem with handling uric acid or because of other problems or diseases (such as reduced urine production because of dehydration; fasting; destruction of body tissue or tumor, as seen in cancers under treatment; kidney disease; certain drugs).

Severity of Problem: Acute attacks are very painful. Can lead to deposits of uric acid in other areas of the body and to chronic arthritis. Uric acid can form kidney stones.

Contagious? No.

Treatment: Prompt medical care is needed. A medication, colchicine, is used to rapidly reduce the arthritis and the blood level of uric acid. Gout requires heat to the joint, pain relievers, determination of cause. High liquid intake will help the kidneys to eliminate excessive uric acid.

Prevention: Treatment of underlying causes of increased uric acid production; use of medications that cause rapid excretion of uric acid when tumors are treated. Plenty of liquids when on a diet; awareness of complications of drug treatment for certain problems.

Discussion: Over 90 percent of gout sufferers are men over the age of 30. Some hereditary tendency. Alcohol excess may precipitate an attack in people who are at risk.

ARTHRITIS—JUVENILE RHEUMATOID

Inflammatory disease of the joints as well as other body organs, starting childhood.

Symptoms: Several types of pictures: Systemic form starts with high fevers, generalized weakness, swelling of lymph nodes and spleen, loss of appetite and a rash. May take weeks to months for any joint swelling to occur and is hard to recognize. In pauciarticular (few joints) form, swelling, pain and limited motion of one or several joints are noticed. Fever, general weakness and loss of appetite also occur. Joints are usually knee, elbow, ankle or wrists. Back and neck may be stiff. In polyarticular form early morning stiffness, swelling and redness of many joints—especially the joints of the hands and feet, as well as the larger joints of both arms and legs—are found. Usually fever, appetite loss and weight loss also occur. Pain can be very severe, and the child can become almost immobile.

Cause: Unknown

Severity of Problem: Usually a progressive disease that leads to some chronic stiffness and deformity of joints. Growth may not be as rapid as normal. Some childran have only a few long-term problems with joint deformity and stiffness.

Contagious? No.

Treatment: A complicated problem requiring careful medical supervision. Treatment is aimed at preventing joint deformity and keeping the child comfortable. Medications are given to reduce inflammation, with rest when joints are very inflamed and physcial therapy to keep joints functioning as well as possible. Heat may help if applied to the joints.

Prevention: None known.

Discussion: Disease can start as early as 2 years of age and is difficult to recognize. Girls are more commonly affected than boys. Children with juvenile rheumatoid arthritis, especially the type with only a few joints involved, need regular eye examinations to detect one of the complications, uveitis.

ARTHRITIS—RHEUMATOID

Chronic inflammatory disease of multiple joints, with many generalized body symptoms as well.

Symptoms: Generalized fever, loss of appetite, weight loss and fatigue. Begins with stiffness of joints, especially hands and feet, then joint swelling, redness and pain in the joints. Usually starts in the small joints of the hands and feet, then progresses to larger joints.

Cause: Generally unknown, although it has many features of a hereditary disease as well as a disease of the immune system. May appear related to infection in some people.

Severity of Problem: A general body disease with many possible complications. Can lead to severe disability with deformity of joints and limited movement and function, or it may "burn out" with little long-term damage.

Contagious? No.

Treatment: During times of active joint inflammation, rest and control of pain. Medications to reduce inflammation of joints (other than aspirin) require doctor's prescription. Heat to the joints, a physical therapy program and emotional support are also needed. Goal of treatment is to reduce both inflammation in joints and long-term joint deformity.

Prevention: None known.

Discussion: Usually begins in early adult life (between 20 and 40 years of age) and is more common in women than in men. Can have many general complications, including pericarditis, pleurisy and blood vessel inflammation. Can "burn out" with few long-term effects or continue with progressive joint inflammation and deformity.

ARTHRITIS—SEPTIC (INCLUDING GONOCOCCAL)

Acute infection of a joint.

Symptoms: Sudden pain, swelling, redness and excessive warmth in a joint. Fever, chills, generalized weakness, nausea, loss of appetite. Inability to move a joint because of pain and swelling. There may be an illness involving several weeks of joint pains, fever and chills, and unusual rash before joint swelling and inflammation are seen in gonococcal arthritis.

Cause: Infection of a joint resulting from injury to the joint, then settling of infection in it; spread of infection from another part of the body through the blood; spread of infection from bone. Can be caused by many different kinds of bacteria, but staphylococcus, gonococcus and hemophilus influenzae are the most common.

Severity of Problem: A serious infection that can cause destruction of a joint and spread of infection to nearby bone if not treated quickly.

Contagious? No. However, if the cause is gonorrhea and this infection has not been treated, it can be spread by sexual contact.

Treatment: Immediate medical care in a hospital. Intravenous antibiotics for several weeks. Rest of the joint, removal of joint fluid to keep pressure out of joint, pain relief. Heat to joint. Surgery may be needed if joint continues to accumulate pus or there is no response to antibiotics.

Prevention: No specific prevention, although prompt treatment of potentially infected injuries may be helpful.

Discussion: In gonococcal arthritis the person can be ill without being able to identify the cause for several days to weeks. There may be a rash. If treatment for any of the forms of septic arthritis is prompt and with the correct drug, recovery is usually very good.

ASCITES

A collection of fluid inside the abdominal cavity.

Symptoms: Full feeling in the abdomen; swelling of the abdomen; sometimes shortness of breath if there is a very large accumulation of fluid.

Cause: Most often caused by heart disease (heart failure), liver problems such as cirrhosis, and kidney disease. May result from tumors or inflammation inside the abdomen.

Severity of Problem: Depends on the cause. In some diseases ascites is a sign of worsening of the underlying problem.

Contagious? No.

Treatment: Involves vigorous treatment of the underlying disease. Rest, limitation of salt in the diet and removal of the fluid from the abdomen may be required.

Prevention: Careful control of the underlying disease may prevent ascites.

ASTIGMATISM

Unusual distortion or curvature of the shape of the eye and its lens, leading to abnormal or distorted focusing of the eye. Usually present in both eyes but may be to a different degree in each eye.

Symptoms: Blurred vision, headaches and eyestrain because of the tendency to try to correct for the distorted images seen.

Cause: Unknown, but the tendency to develop astigmatism as the eye matures is probably inherited. Sometimes injury to the eye will distort its shape.

Severity of Problem: Can vary but does not lead to blindness.

Contagious? No.

Treatment: Eyeglasses or contact lenses will correct the distorted vision and relieve the symptoms. There is no cure.

Prevention: None.

ATHEROSCLEROSIS

A part of the aging process for many people, atherosclerosis is the accumulation of fatty deposits inside the blood vessels, especially the large and medium-sized arteries.

Symptoms: May be silent, without symptoms in its early stages. Symptoms depend on the location of the deposits, called plaques. May cause high blood pressure, early kidney failure, narrowing of the coronary arteries with angina pectoris, cramps and severe pain in the legs after exercise, dizziness and headache or symptoms of stroke.

Cause: Fatty deposits build up inside the blood vessels as part of the aging process. Obesity, hereditary factors and diet (especially high in saturated fats and cholesterol) also contribute.

Severity of Problem: Can be mild to severe, depending on the location of the plaques and the length of time they have been developing. Ultimately the cause of death for many.

Contagious? No.

Treatment: Most treatment has to be directed at the results of the problem—angina pectoris and narrowing of the coronary arteries, stroke, kidney disease. General measures such as dietary discretion, salt limitation, control of hypertension, control of underlying disease, elimination of smoking, reduction of stress and an exercise program may be part of the treatment.

Prevention: Have a well-balanced nutritional plan, especially if there is a history of atherosclerosis in the family starting before middle age. Have a regular exercise program and control or eliminate obesity. Stop smoking if you smoke; never start if you don't. Control or eliminate excessive stress.

Discussion: Approximately 35 percent of all deaths in the United States are a result of atherosclerosis, which is an almost universal part of the aging process. Some families and individuals are more at risk and can be identified through medical evaluation. Males, especially those between 35 and 45 years of age, are much more likely to develop this problem than females, although there has been an increasing amount of atherosclerosis in women over the past decade.

BACKACHE

Common complaint of pain in the middle or lower back, with many possible causes.

Symptoms: Pain, varying from mild to severe, intermittent to steady, in the middle and lower back. Sometimes associated with pains that extend down the legs or into other areas. There is usually worsening of the pain with certain movements or positions, and the person may be stiff after prolonged periods of inactivity. The pattern of the pain helps the doctor determine the possible causes.

Cause: Many possible causes, including causes arising in the back itself or distant from the back. The most common are muscle strain or injury because of unusual activity or stress on the back; degenerative disc disease (called spondylosis); slipped or ruptured disc; and degenerative arthritis of the spine. Other possible causes are infection in the bone of the spine, unusual forms of arthritis, and tumor. Backache can be a sign of disease in the urinary tract or the digestive tract and can be a symptom of stress or anxiety.

Severity of Problem: Can vary from nagging and bothersome to completely disabling, usually depending on cause.

Contagious? No.

Treatment: Depends on cause, which must be investigated thoroughly. When the origin is muscular or in the spine, heat applied to the back, aspirin or aspirinlike anti-inflammatory medications and rest are most likely to be helpful. With degenerative joint disease and other forms of arthritis, physical therapy programs and exercise programs in order to prevent further stiffness are essential. Severe forms of backache may require strong medications, self-hypnosis techniques, nerve stimulation techniques and occasionally surgery, depending on the cause.

Prevention: To prevent muscle strain and ligament injury, learn to lift and move correctly; stay in shape and do not over-exert with new activities. With arthritis, avoid further injury and stress on the spine, while still continuing to move.

Discussion: Low back pain is one of the most common complaints of people who seek medical advice. It can be an uncomfortable, frustrating condition, which can interfere with work and everyday life to a great extent. Sometimes a specific cause is not found, and the person is left to learn techniques for dealing effectively with pain.

BAD BREATH (HALITOSIS)

A strong, unpleasant odor from the mouth.

Symptoms: Unpleasant, offensive or pungent mouth odor.

Cause: Inadequate or improper oral hygiene; dental caries (cavities); gum infections; chronic nasal and/or sinus problems; infected tonsils; fever; systemic diseases; chronic lung diseases; some gastrointestinal diseases. When the problem is not related to an illness or health condition, then it may be due to the production of strong-smelling metabolic end products. This can result from stagnated saliva in the mouth or improper diet. Certain foods (e.g., onions, garlic, other spicy foods) may, of course, cause temporary bad breath, as will tobacco smoking.

Severity of Problem: Essentially, bad breath is unpleasant and embarrassing for the person with it and those around him or her. A chronic problem may indicate an underlying disease and therefore needs evaluation.

Contagious? No.

Treatment: Proper oral hygiene (brushing and flossing the teeth) and the use of antiseptic rinses may be of help temporarily. For chronic bad breath, an evaluation by a physician can determine if there is an underlying disease that can be treated.

Prevention: Proper oral hygiene and dental care as well as avoidance of smoking and foods that cause bad breath.

BALANITIS

Inflammation of the glans penis (the tip of the penis) and the adjacent foreskin.

Symptoms: Pain and burning of the head of the penis. Red or bluish-red swelling, sometimes with small ulcers or crusting, of the tip of the penis. There may be discharge under the foreskin.

Cause: Can result from yeast infection (candidiasis) of the penis and is often associated with a tight foreskin. Most commonly a complication of a sexually transmitted infection (such as gonorrhea, chlamydia, other less common infections) and is seen several days after intercourse. Occasionally a result of sensitivity or allergy to vaginal secretions, spermicides or other hygiene products used by sexual partner.

Severity of Problem: Depends on cause but requires prompt medical evaluation for underlying infection. Uncomfortable.

Contagious? Yes, depending on cause.

Treatment: Frequent washing of the penis with a salt water solution or other soothing liquid (Burrow's solution is soothing). Treatment of the underlying infection, if present, with appropriate antibiotics. Cleansing under the foreskin to remove any debris and discharge. Avoidance of irritation (intercourse) while inflammation is severe.

Prevention: Avoid sexual contact with people with sexually transmitted infections. Carefully cleanse the penis and foreskin, especially if the foreskin is tight.

BEDSORE (DECUBITUS ULCER)

Type of skin ulcer caused by continuous pressure over bone, with loss of good circulation and blood supply.

Symptoms: Initially, small area of mild redness located over a bony protrusion (commonly the hip, buttocks, heels) in a person who is confined to one position. As the condition becomes more severe, tenderness, then breaks in the skin, with later development of an ulcer occur. If not treated, may become infected, and ulcer becomes progressively deeper, extending deep into the tissue.

Cause: Poor blood supply to the skin and tissue because of pressure. Most common in people who are paralyzed, old, unconscious, chronically ill or restrained (for example, in casts, splints, or a wheelchair) and are unable to change their own position.

Severity of Problem: Can potentially lead to serious tissue damage and large holes in tissue. May be chronically infected.

Contagious? No.

Treatment: Frequent turning and removal of all pressure at the earliest sign of redness or soreness. Avoiding wrinkles in sheets, moisture. Skin stimulation with back rubs, movement. If ulcers have developed, they require medical care and the use of antibiotic powder or ointment, removal of dead tissue.

Prevention: Should always be possible with good care. Turning and changing position of a person confined to bed at least every hour, powder to bony areas and use of foam or air mattresses are very helpful.

BIRTHMARK

Any of a number of skin marks or lesions present from or shortly after birth.

Symptoms: Appearance of any of several kinds of skin marks or lesions; some of them may change or enlarge. Some remain the same for life, while others change or disappear over years.

Cause: Unknown.

Severity of Problem: Depends on type of birthmark and its size. Most birthmarks improve over time, although some remain a cosmetic problem for life. A few types can potentially cause or be related to more serious problems.

Treatment: For nearly all types, no treatment is recommended. A few (to be discussed in separate entries) might require treatment. When a birthmark persists into adulthood, removal might be attempted, but often cosmetic cover-up is a better alternative.

Prevention: None.

Discussion: Birthmarks are a common cause of concern for many new parents. With the exception of those specifically mentioned in separate entries, most are temporary.

BIRTHMARK—HEMANGIOMA (STRAWBERRY, CAPILLARY)

Birthmark made up of abnormally arranged blood vessels (the smallest of which are capillaries). This type of birthmark may not be visible as such at birth but appears within a few weeks and gradually grows in size and red color over weeks to months.

The hemangioma appears as a pinkish-red, raised, soft swelling on the surface of the skin, with an appearance similar to a strawberry. When the hemangioma is pressed, the blood that is in the small capillaries can be squeezed out but quickly returns. These marks can occur as single or multiple and can appear on any part of the body. They can be very small or enlarge greatly, sometimes covering an entire body part.

Strawberry hemangiomas gradually increase in size and color over several months, then begin to fade away. When they fade away, the center of the mark becomes pale or gray (eventually the color of the normal skin). Over several months to years, the entire mark becomes the same color as the rest of the skin. The place where the birthmark was previously located may look like a wrinkled, soft scar.

Strawberry hemangiomas rarely cause problems with bleeding, but if they are large, they can form ulcers in the center because their blood supply is not enough to nourish all the tissue. Occasionally, very large ones (called cavernous hemangiomas) can lead to overgrowth of an extremity or bleeding problems because of trapping of blood inside the hemangioma. These large growths can also interfere with bodily function because of size or location (for example, if in the neck, may block breathing; if on the eyelid, may obstruct vision).

Treatment for the small hemangiomas is watchful waiting for the mark to disappear. For large hemangiomas that do or may interfere with function, laser treatment, surgery or cryosurgery (use of cold) may be necessary. Most forms of removal of hemangiomas leave greater scars than the mark itself.

BIRTHMARK—LYMPHANGIOMA

Birthmark formed of dilated vessels that drain lymph from the tissues. It appears as a soft, mushy swelling, perhaps with a faint bluish discoloration or no surface abnormality at all. This kind of birthmark may grow to be huge and interfere with function. Surgical removal is often the only choice when function is interfered with but is not very successful. There is a tendency for this form of birthmark not to disappear over time.

BIRTHMARK—MONGOLIAN SPOT

Bluish-black skin discoloration that occurs primarily in babies of dark-skinned racial origin. This birthmark most commonly is found over the buttocks or base of the spine but may occur on the arms or legs, and there can be many more than one mark. They fade over several months to years and disappear.

The greatest problem with Mongolian spots is that they look very much like bruises at first glance. They differ in that they have a uniform bluish color, with a distinct border between normal skin and the spot. In bruises the color is more variable, and there is usually not such a clear line of separation between normal and abnormal skin.

BIRTHMARK—PORT WINE STAIN

Deep reddish-purple mark, usually found on the face. This birthmark is often quite extensive and may be associated with mild swelling of the skin underneath it. It frequently extends over part or all of one side of the face and can be on the forehead or on the middle or lower portion of the face.

This birthmark usually does not disappear in time and persists as a deeply colored spot throughout life. It may also be associated with malformations of the blood vessels in the brain in an area underneath it. This condition is called Sturge-Weber syndrome and can be associated with seizures and brain hemorrhage. Removal of the birthmark itself is usually not possible, and cosmetics to cover it may be needed.

BIRTHMARK—"STORKBITE," "ANGEL KISS"

Flat, pinkish red, irregular-bordered spot that most commonly is seen on the nape of the neck (hence, "storkbite"). Such birthmarks, which are technically called "nevus flammeus," can also appear on the face in various areas, such as the center of the forehead, the eyelids, the upper lip and the chin. When they occur on the face, many people call them "angel kisses."

These very common birthmarks fade over several months, and those located on the face almost always disappear completely. A few children are left with a faint red mark on the forehead, which becomes brighter red when they are angry or upset. Those marks on the nape of the neck more commonly persist through life but are usually covered by hair.

BLACK STOOLS (MELENA)

Very black, almost tarry appearance to the bowel movement is often due to bleeding high in the intestinal tract. This can result from a bleeding ulcer, Meckel's diverticulum, varices of the esophagus and any other serious cause of intestinal bleeding. In order for the stool to be very black, there must be a large quantity of blood present. The bowel movement is usually loose.

While blood is the most serious and frequent cause of *tarry* stools, black color can be caused by several other common things: dyes or natural food colorings that were black or changed to black or a very dark green; Pepto Bismol®, which contains bismuth; iron treatment; and licorice.

See Section Three, "Bleeding," for more information.

BODY ODOR (BROMHIDROSIS)

Unpleasant odor to the body, usually originating from the armpits, but sometimes from the feet, the genital area or the clothing.

Symptoms: Disagreeable or unpleasant odor; sometimes excessive sweating as well.

Cause: The offensive body odor is usually caused by the action of bacteria on sweat. It may also emanate from the feet, when there is a difficult fungus infection of the skin.

Severity of Problem: Varies with the individual.

Contagious? No.

Treatment: Wash more frequently, using plain water and soap or a mild detergent with soap. Use of a mild antiperspirant may be preferred.

Discussion: Some people, usually those who perspire profusely, are more prone to develop body odor.

BOTULISM

Extremely deadly type of food poisoning.

Symptoms: Symptoms do not occur for 12 to 36 hours after eating the contaminated food. This often makes it difficult to put the cause (food) and effect (symptoms/illness) together. Initial symptoms include sudden fatigue, dizziness, blurred and double vision; swallowing and speaking become difficult; the person may complain of a very dry throat and mouth. As the poisonous effects progress, severe muscle weakness occurs; breathing difficulty begins; and collapse may result. Sometimes nausea, vomiting, cramps and diarrhea are present. As the situation worsens, the pupils of the eyes become fixed and dilated. Death can be sudden from respiratory and cardiac paralysis, since botulism strikes the central nervous system (not the gastrointestinal system).

Cause: Food contaminated by the Clostridium botulinum bacteria, which, by multiplying, produce a deadly toxin. This toxin is thought to be the most deadly poison presently known. Most cases of botulism are seen in those who have eaten home-canned vegetables, meats and fish (smoked as well as canned). Commercially canned foods can also be the culprits, but this is more rarely the case.

Severity of Problem: Botulism is extremely deadly and can kill rapidly. Any indication that botulism poisoning may have occurred requires an immediate trip to the nearest emergency facility. Prompt, intensive medical intervention and support are imperative. Depending on the type of botulism (there are six known types) the rate of death is anywhere from 30 percent to 70 percent if untreated.

Contagious? No. The contaminated food must be eaten.

Treatment: If a food is suspected of being contaminated with botulism, and it was just recently eaten, pumping the stomach may help remove some remaining, unabsorbed toxins. Most often, the person shows certain symptoms and the poisoning must first be diagnosed. Once identified, the botulism is treated with antitoxin (if the person is not sensitive to it). Oxygen is given, and often a respirator (a machine that breathes for the person) must be used, since respiratory paralysis is likely to occur. If respiratory obstruction has taken place, then a tracheostomy (incision into the windpipe to allow oxygen to reach the lungs) must be performed. Fluids are given intravenously (by vein).

Prevention: Those who home-can foods should use extreme care when doing so. Preparing, preserving, sealing and storing foods should be meticulously performed. Boiling foods for 20 minutes before eating inactivates botulism toxin as well. With commercial products, swollen or punctured cans should be thrown away. Home or commercial products in jars should be thrown away if the seal has been broken, is defective, loose or otherwise questionable.

Discussion: A newly recognized form of botulism should be noted. Called "infant botulism," it appears to affect infants in the first few months of life. The infant shows symptoms of weakness, poor feeding, muscle laxity (floppiness) and constipation. The botulism bacteria and toxin are found in the infant's stools, but not in the blood. This newly recognized problem is being investigated, and there seems to be some incrimination of honey fed to the infants who were diagnosed as having "infant botulism."

See also FOOD POISONING

BRADYCARDIA

Slow heartbeat.

Symptoms: Sensation of slow heartbeat. If profoundly slow, can cause fainting or death.

Cause: Normally seen in athletes. Also seen from various medications and with aging of the conducting system of the heart.

Severity of Problem: Not usually a problem in the young. Is a problem in the elderly.

Contagious? No.

Treatment: Medications that might slow heartbeat in the elderly are stopped. If the problem is more severe, a pacemaker may be needed. (See HEART BLOCK, "Treatment.")

Prevention: Unknown.

BREAST—FIBROCYSTIC DISEASE
(MAMMARY DYSPLASIA)

Chronic condition in which there is formation of multiple cysts in the breasts.

Symptoms: Initially, there may be no symptoms. Often, a woman discovers a lump in her breast, leading to the diagnosis. More often, there is breast discomfort or pain, worsened before menstruation and often associated with tender lumps in the breasts. Nipple discharge is common and may be clear, yellowish, greenish, brown or black in color. Lumps in the breast often vary in size over time, coming and going.

Cause: Unknown, but may be due to hormone fluctuations, since it is a problem primarily of mature women, before menopause.

Severity of Problem: Pain or discomfort can be quite bothersome. Cysts appear often, leading to frequent medical evaluation, and often either aspiration (removal of the cyst fluid with a needle) or surgical biopsy is done to be sure the lump in the breast is a cyst. The risk of cancer of the breast with this condition is about twice the risk of the regular population.

Contagious? No.

Treatment: One of the most important aspects of treatment is to first be sure of the diagnosis, either by aspiration of the cyst or by surgical biopsy. No specific treatment is recommended for this disease, but good support of the breasts and pain control will help with comfort. A hormone preparation has been tested in women with severe pain due to fibrocystic disease, with equivocal results. Rarely, mastectomy (removal of the breast) has been suggested for this problem, but this is quite drastic.

Prevention: There is no way to prevent fibrocystic disease. However, early detection of a mass can lead to early detection of a breast cancer, a very important part of the treatment of fibrocystic disease. Every woman should perform breast self-examination each month right after menstruation and report any concerns or problems to her physician.

Discussion: A very common problem among women. It is important as a problem that is likely to show up on a routine examination or to be detected accidentally.

BREAST—MASTITIS

Inflammation and infection of the breast, almost always in nursing mothers

Symptoms: Initially, the mother may feel slightly sick, not knowing what is bothering her. She has a slight fever, is tired and has generalized aches and pains. She will then notice a soreness or heaviness, engorgement or tenderness in one area of a breast. The spot on the breast may appear slightly reddened, warm and tender.

Cause: Infection of the tissues of the breast, not involving the actual ducts. This is most commonly caused by a staphylococcus organism that enters the breast through a nipple that is cracked.

Severity of Problem: If antibiotics are not started quickly, the breast may go on to form an abscess that needs to be drained.

Contagious? Not in its usual form. A more unusual form of mastitis occurs in epidemics in nurseries and can be spread from a healthy carrier to a human infant, then to the mother's breast.

Treatment: If mastitis is suspected or known, allow the baby to nurse frequently in order to empty the plugged milk duct. Applying warm compresses to the sore area is important. Antibiotic treatment is necessary for nearly all cases and is prescribed by a doctor.

Prevention: Knowledge and practice of good nursing technique is very important. Specifically, avoiding engorgement by encouraging the baby to take all he or she wants from the breast, as often as possible, will help.

Discussion: Mastitis is common in nursing mothers, especially those who are nursing for the first time. If you're nursing and have a symptom that is causing concern, call your doctor for reassurance. Teen-age boys, especially just at the start of puberty, usually have swelling and tenderness of small lumps under the nipple (hormone-stimulated breasts). They should be reassured that these are normal and not an infection, and will go away within the year.

BRONCHIECTASIS

Widening and infection of one or more areas within the bronchial tree, leaving pockets of pus within the airways.

Symptoms: Chronic cough, worse in the mornings, with coughing up of large amounts of sputum that contains pus. Coughing up blood is common and can result in loss of a large amount of blood. There are intermittent episodes of serious infection, with fever as well as the worsening cough. If it is not treated, signs of respiratory failure, with increasing respiratory difficulties, will occur.

Cause: The damage to the walls of the bronchi may occur as a result of infection in childhood (repeated pneumonia, for example) or as a result of pressure and damage from a foreign object in the bronchus. In some people the cause is unknown. It may result from a complicated pneumonia that was untreated, as a complication of cystic fibrosis or from tuberculosis.

Severity of Problem: A chronic problem that can progress if not treated promptly. Interferes with daily functioning because of the chronic cough and breathing difficulties. Bleeding in the lung can be a potentially life-threatening problem.

Contagious? Not as such, although some of the bacteria that can infect the abnormal tissue can be passed on to others via the cough.

Treatment: Careful medical supervision is necessary to keep this disease under control. Treatment measures include avoidance of all lung irritants, such as pollutants, smoke, dust and other particles; postural drainage (a technique used to move secretions from the deeper sections of the lungs, so they can be coughed up); inhalation of medications that loosen the sputum; control of infection with appropriate antibiotics; and consideration of surgical removal of the diseased sections of lung if the disease is severe or bleeding is hard to control.

Prevention: Prompt, vigorous treatment of respiratory infections, control of tuberculosis and cystic fibrosis. Avoid pollutants when possible; do not smoke.

Discussion: While this disease still occurs as a complication of serious underlying disease, it is much less common since antibiotics have been available to treat pneumonia.

BRONCHIOLITIS

Viral respiratory infection seen primarily in very young infants.

Symptoms: Mild cold symptoms in a young infant initially, followed by slight fever and increasing trouble with breathing. Breathing becomes fast and labored, and wheezing noises may be heard. Baby is often not able to suck because of the rapid breathing rate. Coughing may be a problem and may lead to vomiting. Baby usually looks pale and miserable.

Cause: Infection with the respiratory syncytial virus.

Severity of Problem: Usually a moderately severe disease that reaches its worst on the third or fourth day of illness and lasts about 7 to 10 days. Some infants become sick enough to need hospitalization, with oxygen and other intensive support.

Contagious? Yes, by contact with secretions from the respiratory tract. Infants under 1 year of age are particularly susceptible to this disease, and the infection spreads rapidly in settings where small babies are cared for in groups (for example, baby-sitting arrangements, day-care centers, hospital wards).

Treatment: General support, with moisture in the air (humidifier, vaporizer) for comfort. Sometimes doctors prescribe medications to control wheezing and cough, but these do not always help. It is important to make sure babies with this disease receive enough liquids to drink or are given fluids intravenously. When respiratory condition worsens, they may need oxygen and even a respirator. Antibiotics do not help this disease.

Prevention: Avoid contact between healthy babies and those with this kind of disease.

Discussion: This illness most often attacks infants a few months of age to 1 year and can be mild or severe. It looks very much like asthma. As many as half of babies who have this disease may go on to have asthma in the future. No one knows why this happens. Immunity to this virus can occur without apparent infection, and almost all older children and adults are immune.

BRONCHITIS—ACUTE

Acute inflammation of the tracheobronchial tube (air passages).

Symptoms: Cough that is initially hacking and dry, then gradually becomes loose, with production of mucus or yellowish sputum. There may be fever (if infection is present), generalized malaise and fatigue, sensation of tickling or tightness in chest, and sensation or sound of rattling in the chest. If the bronchitis follows a cold, there may also be congestion of the nose and postnasal drip. Coughing is often worse in the morning than at night.

Cause: Acute bronchitis may result from infection as a complication of a cold (upper respiratory infection) or as a result of irritation of the lining of the air passages by inhaling substances such as smoke, pollen, dust, fumes or fibers. The irritant type of bronchitis may progress to involve infection also.

Severity of Problem: Usually of mild to moderate severity and resolves with treatment. If cause is not corrected, may become chronic.

Contagious? Usually not, except if caused by a virus.

Treatment: Depends on cause but involves removing or avoiding any irritants (stopping smoking, avoiding dust, etc.), drinking much fluid and resting. Moisture in the air (inhaling steam) is sometimes soothing. If the cough is dry and irritating, or interferes with sleep, medication to suppress it might be recommended. Antibiotics may be prescribed by the doctor if bacterial infection is suspected or known.

Prevention: Avoid smoking, exposure to airborne dust or irritants.

Discussion: Mild acute bronchitis is almost always present temporarily with upper respiratory infection (common cold) and does not require antibiotic treatment unless high fever occurs, or sputum becomes yellow or greenish rather than white or clear.

BRONCHITIS—CHRONIC

Chronic inflammation of the linings of the air passages. The condition is usually defined by doctors as chronic when it occurs constantly for at least three months a year for two years.

Symptoms: Chronic cough, usually worse in the mornings, with production of mucus that is coughed up. There may be rattling sensation or sound in the chest and wheezing or unusual noises. If infection occurs, the mucus (sputum) changes from clear or white to yellow or green. As the disease progresses, there may be fatigue, difficulty breathing and weight loss.

Cause: Chronic irritation of the bronchial lining by exposure to irritants leads to inflammation of the mucous membranes and production of mucus. Cigarette smoking is the most common cause, and occupational exposure to dust, fibers, fumes and minerals is also a problem. The irritated, inflamed airways are susceptible to bacterial infection, which may be either acute or chronic.

Severity of Problem: Can vary from mild and bothersome to severe and disabling, depending on the individual and whether irritants can be avoided. May progress to emphysema or full-blown pneumoconiosis and lead to chronic respiratory failure and death. One of the common causes of disability in the United States. People with chronic bronchitis are at risk for serious problems with influenza.

Contagious? No.

Treatment: Avoid *all* lung irritants: Stop smoking, avoid smoke-filled rooms; avoid aerosolized sprays, dust pollutants; change jobs if origin of exposure is work-related. Infection must be treated with antibiotics, if appropriate. Other medications to ease breathing may also be prescribed.

Prevention: Do not smoke. Avoid exposure to dust, fibers, particles, fumes, pollutants.

Discussion: While chronic bronchitis is a real problem in adults, problems thought to be "chronic bronchitis" in infants and children are more likely to be asthma or other illnesses. "Bronchitis" where there is a lot of wheezing can be suspected of being asthma. People with moderate to severe chronic bronchitis should probably receive influenza vaccines ("flu shots").

BUNION (HALLUX VALGUS)

Enlargement and deformity of the joint at the base of the big toe.

Symptoms: At the start of the problem, only enlargement of the joint at the base of the big toe is noticed. As the enlargement increases, soreness or pain with walking and tenderness begins. Fitting of shoes becomes an increasing problem. The big toe joint then becomes deformed gradually, with turning of the big toe to the side so the joint protrudes, and the big toe overlaps the other toes or pushes them to the side.

Cause: Usually thought to result from poorly fitting shoes and/or heels that are too high. However, probably has a hereditary component, since the problem runs in families and may be seen when no abuse of the foot has occurred.

Severity of Problem: May be mild to severe, with much difficulty walking.

Contagious? No.

Treatment: At the beginning, properly fitting shoes, low heels and padding to protect the bunion from pressure from the shoes are the treatments. As the problem advances, surgical treatment may be necessary.

Prevention: Avoid tight shoes and high heels, especially if bunions run in the family. Prevention may be only partial.

Discussion: Bunions occur much more commonly in women than in men and can start early in life, even childhood, but most often reach the problem stage in the forties to sixties.

BURSITIS

Inflammation of a bursa, which is a protective structure between a muscle tendon and another tendon or a bone. Usually the bursa allows the tendon to slip over the bone easily without grating or irritation.

Symptoms: Pain, especially with movement, over a joint, along with a grating sensation. As the inflammation increases, fluid may accumulate in the bursa and be seen as swelling. Irritation and inflammation lead to the formation of calcium deposits in and around the tendons and bursa.

Cause: Trauma to or overuse of a muscle-tendon unit. For example, improper motions that put unusual stress on a muscle during a sport may lead to irritation and inflammation of a bursa. Sometimes the exact cause of the problem cannot be determined.

Severity of Problem: Ranges from mild and bothersome to severe and disabling. Tends to worsen with continued overuse or abuse.

Contagious? No.

Treatment: Rest of the injured body part is the key to recovery and prevention of long-term inflammation and disability. Heat or cold applied to the area and anti-inflammatory drugs (such as aspirin and related medications) can be helpful. Occasionally, removal of excessive amounts of fluid from a bursa (if present) or injection of steroid (cortisonelike) medication into the inflamed bursa might be recommended. Surgery to remove any calcium deposits may be recommended for severe cases.

Prevention: Avoidance of vigorous muscle activity without appropriate conditioning; avoidance of continued abuse of a part if symptoms appear.

CANCER

Each of us has a one in four chance of developing cancer in our lifetime. That means that approximately one of every four people will get cancer at some point in his or her life.

Cancer is actually a general name for an entire group of diseases. In reality there are presently 100 different cancers known to man, and each is unique. That is why it is so very difficult to find a cure for cancer, since that entails finding the answer to at least 100 diseases—not simply one disease. Progress, however, has been made in many cancers, and research continues in all cancers.

Since it would be impossible to cover all cancers in this book, the most frequently seen cancers are listed. These are in alphabetical order.

As an overview, cancer is the uncontrolled proliferation of abnormal cells (called cancer cells). These abnormal cells often form a mass or tumor (called a cancerous or malignant tumor). However, it should be noted that not all tumors found in the body are cancerous—they can be benign (noncancerous tumors). Cancerous cells are capable of multiplying rapidly; invading tissues and organs, destroying healthy cells and tissues; and spreading all over the body (to any organ, other tissues than the original cancer site, the blood and lymph nodes), a process called metastasis.

Today, the most widely used methods of cancer treatment include surgery (the cancer can be removed by cutting), chemotherapy (the use of potent drugs to destroy the cancer), and radiation therapy (the use of high doses of radiation to destroy cancerous cells).

CANCER—BLADDER

Cancer that invades the inner lining of the bladder (the reservoir for urine).

Symptoms: Blood in urine (either rusty in color or deep red); need to urinate more frequently than usual; possible discomfort during urination due to muscle spasm in bladder.

Cause: Unknown. More frequent in tobacco smokers, dye workers and some chemical industry workers.

Severity of Problem: Prognosis varies depending on the type of tumor and whether the cancer has spread to the lymph nodes or not. With low-malignancy polyps, nine out of ten people survive. When cancer is confined to lining of bladder, 60 percent survive five years after treatment. When it has broken through lining of bladder or penetrated muscle wall, 20 percent survive five years after treatment.

Contagious? No.

Treatment: Surgical removal of tumor in bladder, if possible; surgical removal of entire bladder; radiation therapy may also be recommended.

Prevention: Since bladder cancer is more frequent in tobacco smokers, dye workers and some chemical industry employees, care should be taken to avoid associated hazards.

Discussion: More frequently seen in people 55 to 69 years of age. Any blood in urine should be reported to physician for evaluation.

CANCER—BONE

Cancer of the skeletal structures of the body. Although there are more than 200 bones in the human body, bone cancer is most often seen in the arm, leg, rib or pelvis. Osteosarcoma is the most common primary bone cancer. Other primary bone cancers are lymphomas of the bone, Ewing's sarcoma and chondrosarcoma.

Symptoms: Usually no symptoms until disease is in advanced stages. Then symptoms may include pain and swelling in affected area: sometimes fever is experienced.

Cause: Unknown. Has been associated with exposure to radiation (atomic bomb explosions); working with radium dials; intense exposure to therapeutic low-voltage X rays.

Severity of Problem: Osteosarcoma: 15 percent to 20 percent survival five years after treatment (usually with amputation of limb). Chondrosarcoma: 50 percent survival five years after treatment. Ewing's sarcoma: 15 percent survival five years after treatment. Lymphomas (confined to bone): 50 percent survival five years after treatment.

Contagious? No.

Treatment: Depends on type of bone cancer. May include surgery, radiation therapy, chemotherapy or a combination of these. Amputation is often necessary if a limb is involved, but some experimental work is being done in removing diseased part of bone and replacing it with a transplant or artificial bone.

Prevention: None. Radium dial workers should take precautions; attempts should be made to avoid unnecessary exposure to radiation.

Discussion: Osteosarcoma: most common in persons 15 to 30 years old. Ewing's sarcoma: most common in those 15 to 25 years old. Chondrosarcoma: most common in those 30 to 50 years old. Any pain that seems persistent and swelling experienced in bone should be reported to a physician for evaluation.

CANCER—BRAIN

Cancer that invades any one of three of the major parts of the brain: cerebrum, cerebellum, or brain stem.

Symptoms: Depends on area of brain affected. In adults, may include headaches, seizures, speech impairment, decline in mental awareness, difficulty moving legs and arms, loss of recent memory and decrease in mental processes. In children, may include nausea, vomiting, eye disorders such as double vision, crossed eyes, drunken walk with frequent falling and, occasionally, blindness.

Cause: Unknown.

Severity of Problem: Most often incurable in adults. Most who are treated die within two years, and those who refuse treatment die sooner. In children, if tumor can be totally removed, the prognosis is more optimistic. Quality of life depends on the location of cancer in the brain and the functions affected.

Contagious? No.

Treatment: Depends on extent and location of tumor. May include surgical removal of tumor, where possible; radiation therapy; chemotherapy; or a combination of these.

Prevention: None.

Discussion: Persistent headaches or other symptoms noted previously require evaluation by a physician.

CANCER—BREAST

It is estimated that 1 of every 11 women will have breast cancer in her lifetime—approximately 90,000 new cases each year.

Symptoms: Usually a firm to hard lump (mass) that is non-tender; thickening of the skin; abnormal coloration; discharge from the nipple; nipple retraction; dimpling of the breast; swelling or other sudden changes in the breast.

Cause: Unknown. There is a higher incidence among women with a family history of breast cancer or a personal history of cancer; those who have not had children; those who experienced an early onset of menstruation or late menopause; and those who had a first child after the age of 30.

Severity of Problem: Any symptom requires immediate evaluation by a physician. Eighty-five percent cure rate if detected and treated early (before the lymph nodes are involved). However, presently breast cancer is the No. 1 cancer killer in women. It is estimated that 34,000 deaths per year in the United States are due to breast cancer. The greatest incidence is found in women 40 years of age and older.

Contagious? No.

Treatment: Depends on the extent of cancer spread. Includes: radical mastectomy—surgical removal of the breast, the muscles underlying the breast and the surrounding lymph nodes; modified radical mastectomy—surgical removal of the breast and underlying lymph nodes; simple mastectomy—surgical removal of the breast; and lumpectomy—surgical removal of the tumor only. Radiation therapy may also play a role. Chemotherapy may be included if the disease has spread to the lymph nodes.

Prevention: None. However, the emphasis today in breast cancer is on early detection, since cure rates are significantly increased when the cancer is detected and treated in its early stages.

Discussion: The vast majority of the time, a lump or other symptom suspicious of breast cancer proves not to be cancerous. Four out of five lumps are not cancerous. Also, although breast cancer is 100 times more frequent in women than men, men are not exempt from the disease. *For early detection:* Breast self-examination is recommended on a monthly basis; periodic professional evaluations based on a doctor's recommendation; and mammography and other more sophisticated testing as indicated and based on each woman's needs. The American Cancer Society has guidelines available, and a woman should check with her personal physician for individual recommendations.

CANCER—CERVICAL

Cancer of the cervix, the neck of the uterus that extends into the vagina. One of the few cancers that are 100 percent curable if diagnosed in its very early stages (before it can be seen or felt by examination).

Symptoms: Vaginal spotting or bleeding between menstrual periods; vaginal bleeding after intercourse; painful intercourse; abnormal menstrual flow. In very early stages, usually no symptoms.

Cause: Unknown. Investigations are being made into possible association with herpes simplex 2 (genital herpes). Also occurs more in women of low socioeconomic status (possibly because they seek fewer Pap smears for early detection). There is a higher rate among women who became sexually active early in life; those with many sexual partners; women with many pregnancies; women with uncircumcised partners.

Severity of Problem: Depends on extent of cancer spread when diagnosed and treated. Nearly 100 percent curable if detected very early in the disease.

When cancer is confined to the cervix, 70 percent to 90 percent survive five years after treatment. If surrounding tissue is invaded, 40 percent to 60 percent survive five years after treatment. If cancer has invaded bladder or rectum, 20 percent survive. If it has spread to lymph nodes, survival is markedly decreased.

Contagious? No.

Treatment: Two modes of therapy: surgical removal of cervix, uterus, Fallopian tubes and surrounding lymph nodes (ovaries may or may not be removed, depending on woman's age and extent of cancer); or radiation therapy (either by special X-ray machine or radioactive implants). Sometimes both modes of treatment are recommended.

Prevention: Unknown. However, a yearly Pap smear is the best insurance for detecting the disease in its earliest stages, when cure rates are near 100 percent (with prompt treatment).

Discussion: Occurs most frequently in women 40 to 55 years of age. In reality, there is no reason any woman should die from cervical cancer today, since the Pap smear is so effective in detecting the disease in its earliest stage.

CANCER—COLON AND RECTUM

Cancer of the muscular tube which forms the last part of the intestines.

Symptoms: Rectal bleeding is the major symptom, often in combination with abdominal or intestinal cramping and persistent or chronic diarrhea or constipation. Some people experience overall weakness, loss of appetite and/or weight loss, as well. However, any change in bowel habits (that persists) should signal the need for physician consultation.

Cause: Unknown. However, there appears to be a lower incidence of colon-rectal cancer among those who follow a diet high in fiber (vegetables, fruits and whole grains) than in those who follow a diet low in fiber and high in beef carbohydrates, fats and refined foods. Those with a family history of colon-rectal cancer, those with many polyps in the colon and others who have chronic ulcerative colitis appear to be at high risk for colon-rectal cancer and should be evaluated periodically for the disease.

Severity of Problem: If the cancer has not or does not spread to the lymph nodes, 70 percent of those will survive the cancer (with rigorous treatment). Approximately 50 percent of all those with colon or rectal cancer will be alive five years after treatment. Essentially, early diagnosis and treatment are keys to better cure rates.

Contagious? No.

Treatment: Surgical removal of the cancer and often surrounding lymph nodes. If the cancer is close to the anus, then the rectum (in total) must be removed and a colostomy is performed (a new opening constructed in the abdominal wall from which waste products can pass into a bag). Radiation therapy is sometimes used as adjunct therapy after surgery (to destroy any remaining cancer cells), but it has yet to be proved that this is beneficial. Chemotherapy may be used in some cases of colon or rectal cancer.

Prevention: If diagnosed and treated in its very early stages, colon and rectal cancers are curable the vast majority of the time. It is therefore recommended that those over 40 years of age, have routine proctosigmoidoscopy examinations (visual examination of the colon and rectum by means of a special, lighted instrument which is inserted through the anus into the colon). The age of 40 is chosen since the majority of colon and rectal cancers are seen after this age (and even more so after age 55).

CANCER—ESOPHAGUS

Cancer of the tube that connects the throat to the stomach.

Symptoms: Unfortunately, there are no reliable early warning signs. Pain,, difficulty swallowing, often a choking feeling when drinking liquids and gradual (but severe) weight loss are all later signs.

Cause: Heavy alcohol use and heavy tobacco use are associated with esophageal cancer. For those who use both alcohol and tobacco excessively,, the risk for the cancer is even greater.

Severity of Problem: Very poor survival rate. Only 4 percent survival rate five years after treatment. Many people live only six months, on the average, after symptoms appear.

Contagious? No.

Treatment: Radiation therapy may be used if early esophageal cancer is found. Surgical removal of the esophagus is often the only possible treatment. A combination of radiation therapy and surgery is sometimes recommended.

Prevention: Avoid the use of tobacco and excessive alcohol consumption.

Discussion: Besides those who use alcohol and tobacco excessively, those at greater risk for esophageal cancer include people with cancer of the throat and those who suffer from inflammation and/or scarring of the esophagus (sometimes as a result of having swallowed lye).

CANCER—HODGKIN'S DISEASE (HODGKIN'S LYMPHOMA)

Most often, cancer found in the lymph tissue (including lymph nodes) is secondary to a primary cancer somewhere else in the body. However, Hodgkin's disease (like all lymphomas) is a primary cancer of the lymphatic system, the body's immune or protective system. See CANCER—LYMPHOMAS (NON-HODGKIN'S) for more information on lymphomas.

Symptoms: Painless swelling of the lymph nodes(s); the node(s) are firm and not tender; recurring fever; fatigue; intense itching; excessive sweating; and unexplained weight loss.

Cause: Unknown. Investigators are now trying to determine if there is an association between Hodgkin's (and other lymphomas) and viruses. Those at high risk for Hodgkin's (and other lymphomas) are people who have been treated with drugs to suppress the immune system and people who have had an organ transplant.

Severity of Problem: Fifty percent of those with relatively localized disease diagnosed and treated will have no further manifestations five years after intense treatment. These people then have a 95 percent cure rate. Usually the other 50 percent of patients will have manifestations of the disease within two years of treatment. Therefore, the overall survival rate five years after treatment (for all Hodgkin's disease) is about 30 percent.

Contagious? No.

Treatment: Radiation therapy is generally used for stages I, II and III. In stages III and IV chemotherapy is utilized. Where deemed helpful, both radiation therapy and chemotherapy are recommended.

Prevention: Unknown.

Discussion: Great progress has been made over the years in treating Hodgkin's disease. Less than 20 years ago, little could be done, and few people survived more than two years. Today, the situation is much more promising.

CANCER—KIDNEY

Cancer can occur in the kidneys, those hard-working organs that filter potentially poisonous substances from the blood. They are able to cleanse the entire volume of blood every four or five minutes.

Symptoms: Blood in urine; pain; fever; changes in the body's hormones; pain in back or side, and lump can be felt in side in advanced cases. Greatly imitates other problems such as infection, anemia or polycythemia.

Cause: Unknown. However, there seems to be an association between the cancer and kidney stones and between kidney cancer and the pain-control drug phenacetin.

Severity of Problem: If detected and treated before the cancer has spread beyond the kidney, there is a 50 percent survival rate 10 years after treatment. Survival rates are much lower if the disease has spread to the lymph nodes, renal vein or membrane that covers the kidney.

Contagious? No.

Treatment: Removal of entire kidney, all surrounding tissue, ureter and a large portion of the renal vein. Radiation therapy may be included to destroy any remaining cancer cells. At times, radiation therapy is used to shrink the cancerous tumor before surgery is performed.

Prevention: Avoid the use of the pain-control drug phenacetin. Those with recurring kidney stones should be routinely evaluated for early signs of kidney cancer.

Discussion: Kidney cancer is more common in men than in women and occurs most often in adults 50 to 80 years of age. It is often a silent disease until it is well advanced. Blood in the urine should always be evaluated to determine its cause.

CANCER—LARYNX

Cancer of the larynx (the voice box with its vocal cords, found between the trachea and the pharynx) will kill approximately 13,000 people in the United States this year.

Symptoms: The earliest symptoms are persistent hoarseness and/or changes in the voice. Later symptoms include soreness in the throat; lump in the throat; difficulty swallowing; sometimes difficulty breathing; some people complain of earaches or a feeling of tenderness in the ears.

Cause: The risk for laryngeal cancer is five times greater in smokers compared to nonsmokers (includes cigarettes, cigars, pipes, etc.). Those who smoke heavily have laryngeal cancer mortality rates 15 to 30 times greater than nonsmokers.

Severity of Problem: Approximately 40,000 Americans will develop laryngeal and oral cancer this year alone, and 13,000 will die. Those who require removal of the larynx will need to learn esophageal speech or use an electrical or mechanical device in order to speak. For many this will be a major disability.

Contagious? No.

Treatment: Treatment varies depending on the extent of the cancer. Radiation therapy is used to treat small tumors that are confined to the vocal cords. Surgical removal of the larynx (laryngectomy) is usually necessary for large tumors. Radiation therapy is sometimes recommended after surgery to destroy any possible remaining cancer cells. Chemotherapy may be used to relieve some of the unpleasant symptoms when a cancer is considered incurable.

Prevention: Quit smoking if you smoke, and never start if you don't. Avoid other irritants to the larynx where possible. In some cases prevention is not possible.

Discussion: Eighty-five percent to 90 percent of those with small cancers of the larynx will be alive five years after treatment. If the cancer has spread to the lymph nodes, the five-year survival rate drops to 33 percent. It is therefore vital to detect the cancer early, before the tumor grows or the cancer spreads to the lymph nodes. Since hoarseness or changes in the voice are early symptoms, a physician should be seen if hoarseness or voice changes persist for two or three weeks.

CANCER—LEUKEMIA

A group of very complex cancers where abnormal white blood cell production occurs and crowds out normal white blood cells (which are vital components of our immune system), red blood cells (which carry oxygen to the tissues and organs of the body) and platelets (vital in control of bleeding).

Symptoms: The symptoms of all leukemias are essentially the same and unfortunately general in nature. Symptoms include fatigue and overall weakness; swelling of lymph nodes, spleen and liver; bruising and bleeding easily; low-grade fever; loss of weight and appetite; and frequent infections. Many people also experience bone and joint tenderness or pain. Most often the person is anemic and quite pale as well.

Cause: Many possible causes are now being investigated, and others have already been implicated. Since some animal studies have shown that viruses could produce leukemia (in animals), research is trying to determine if viruses could also cause leukemia in human beings. There appears to be a higher incidence of leukemias among children who survived the atomic bomb blasts of Hiroshima and Nagasaki and in children who have received high (therapeutic) doses of radiation (not diagnostic doses). Because of these two groups, it is believed that exposure to high doses of radiation may cause some cases of leukemia. Also, there appears to be a higher incidence of leukemia in children with genetic abnormalities (most specifically those with Down's syndrome). There seems to be a higher risk for leukemia in children whose mothers were exposed to very high doses of radiation during pregnancy.

Severity of Problem: The survival rate very much depends on the type of leukemia and the extent of the disease when diagnosed. Some people only divide leukemias into two general categories—acute leukemia and chronic leukemia. However, these are subdivided further here. The specific type of leukemia is determined by the type of white blood cell affected. *Acute lymphocytic leukemia* (also called acute lymphoblastic leukemia): more frequent during childhood; for those under 20 years of age (when diagnosed) who are treated vigorously, more than 90 percent will experience a remission of the disease. The average duration of remission is 1 to 3 years. Fifty percent of those with "ALL" will experience a 5-year survival rate. *Acute myelocytic leukemia* (also called granulocytic leukemia): most often seen in adults; survival can be as low as a few months to several years (for some). *Chronic myelocytic leukemia* (also called chronic granulocytic leukemia, chronic myeloid leukemia, chronic myelogenous leukemia): 50 percent of those with the disease will survive for 3 years and 10 percent will experience a 5-year survival rate. *Chronic lymphocytic leukemia*: Temporary remission is experienced by 90 percent of those afflicted, with 40 percent to 50 percent experiencing a 5-year survival rate. For 30 percent of those with the disease, a 10-year survival rate will be achieved.

Contagious? No.

Treatment: Chemotherapy (with a combination of drugs) is the usual primary means of treatment. Radiation therapy is sometimes used in conjunction with a vigorous chemotherapy regimen. Blood and platelet transfusions are also part of treatment, as is the administration of antibiotics in an attempt to control infection when it occurs. Bone marrow transplantation (although quite rare) may be considered in very specific cases.

Prevention: Presently, little is known about preventing all leukemias. However, radiation exposure should be avoided unless absolutely necessary.

CANCER—LIP

Cancer of the lip is seen most often in those over 50 years of age and more frequently in men.

Symptoms: Symptoms are easily ignored or overlooked. They include an irritated area, blister or sore (most often on the lower lip) that does not heal; an irritated area,, blister or sore that bleeds easily or chronically; chronic scabbing of an area of the lip; ulceratin on the lip; or at times a raised nodule may signal cancer of the lip.

Cause: Excessive exposure to sunlight may result in lip cancer. Pipe, cigar and cigarette smoking may be associated with cancer of the lip.

Severity of Problem: Cancer of the lip has a very high cure rate, since it is more easily treated (because of its location). However, prompt recognition and treatment are vital to continued high cure rates.

Contagious? No.

Treatment: Surgical removal of the cancer is the mainstay of treatment. Radiation therapy may be used as an alternative to surgery in some specific cases. At times surgery and radiation therapy are used in combination to treat the lip cancer.

Prevention: Avoidance of excessive exposure to sunlight. Avoidance of pipe, cigar and cigarette smoking. Early detection and treatment are the cornratones for successfully eradicating the cancer.

CANCER—LIVER

Cancer of the liver is fairly rare in Western countries but is almost always fatal.

Symptoms: Like cancer of the stomach, liver cancer has few early warning signs, and the symptoms tend to be those of general gastrointestinal disturbances: stomach upset; sensitive stomach; overall weakness; nausea, vomiting; and constipation. Later symptoms include jaundice; rapid weight loss; anemia; and sometimes discomfort, pain or sensation of fullness in the abdomen.

Cause: There appears to be an increased incidence of liver cancer among those who have cirrhosis of the liver and those who have experienced certain parasitic infections that attach to the liver.

Severity of Problem: Almost always fatal—only 50 percent of those with liver cancer will be alive three months after diagnosis. Although rare, cures have been reported when the cancer has been confined to a tumor of the liver, with surgical removal of all the cancer then possible.

Contagious? No.

Treatment: If detected early enough, surgical resection of the liver (removal of as much of the cancer as possible but not total removal of the liver) may be effective. Most liver cancers, however, are too far advanced at the time of diagnosis for surgical intervention. Chemotherapy and radiation therapy may also be used to treat the cancer.

Prevention: Since alcoholics (who have a greater incidence of cirrhosis of the liver) have a higher rate of liver cancer, chronic alcohol consumption should be avoided. Care should be taken to control the spread of parasites, as well, which is a matter of public health.

CANCER—LUNG

Cancer of the lungs, the organs that process oxygen for the body and release carbon dioxide from the blood, accounts for 25 percent of all cancer deaths in the United States.

Symptoms: Chronic cough in early stages. Shortness of breath, pneumonia and bloody sputum are possible signs of moderately advanced lung cancer. In late stages there is chest pain, weight loss, severe shortness of breath, hoarseness, swallowing difficulty and accumulation of fluid in the chest cavity.

Cause: There appears to be an absolute cause-and-effect relationship between cigarette smoking and lung cancer. Estimates indicate that 85 percent of lung cancer deaths are the result of cigarette smoking. At least 111,000 people will die each year as a result of lung cancer. Those who smoke more than two packs of cigarettes a day run a risk of dying from lung cancer 30 times higher than that of nonsmokers. Other causes of lung cancer include asbestos, coal tar fumes, petroleum oil mists, arsenic, chromium, nickel, iron, isopropyl oil, radioactive substances and air pollution.

Severity of Problem: The survival rate for lung cancer is very poor. Less than 10 percent survive five years after treatment. In 15 years the survival rate has not markedly changed, making it one of the most devastating cancers.

Contagious? No.

Treatment: Unfortunately, 75 percent of lung cancers are usually detected too late for surgical intervention. If the cancer is found before it spreads to other areas of the body, then it can be surgically removed. Radiation therapy and chemotherapy are used, depending on the type of lung cancer involved. Sometimes radiation therapy is used to help relieve the painful symptoms the disease can cause.

Prevention: The best prevention is to quit smoking if you smoke cigarettes and never start if you don't presently smoke. Also, avoid those chemicals associated with causing lung cancer.

Discussion: Lung cancer is most often found in adults between the ages of 40 and 70. Each year, the number of cases of lung cancer increases. One important note: The incidence of lung cancer is rising rapidly in women. This reflects the increasing number of women smoking today.

CANCER—LYMPHOMAS (NON-HODGKIN'S)

Cancer can originate within lymph tissue (usually within a lymph node). The lymph nodes are part of the body's immune (protective) system. There are many kinds of lymphomas, and these are divided into two major groups: the non-Hodgkin's lymphomas and the Hodgkin's lymphoma (Hodgkin's disease). See CANCER—HODGKIN'S DISEASE for additional information.

Symptoms: Generally, painless swelling of a lymph node (usually stays enlarged for three or more weeks); unusual fatigue; sometimes intense itching; recurring fever; and unexplained weight loss.

Cause: Unknown. However, investigations are now taking place into the association between lymphomas and viruses. Those at high risk include people who have had an organ transplant or others who have undergone treatment with drugs to suppress the immune system.

Severity of Problem: Survival rate depends on the type of lymphoma involved. However, when cancer is confined to the lymph nodes, there is a 20 percent to 70 percent survival rate five years after treatment. When the disease has gone beyond the lymph nodes, the survival rate drops to a zero to 20 percent five-year survival rate after treatment. With non-Hodgkin's lymphomas that occur in the lymph tissue of the small intestine, stomach or bone that are treated before spreading to the lymph nodes, there is a 40 percent to 50 percent survival rate five years after treatment.

Contagious? No.

Treatment: Often a combination of surgery, radiation therapy and chemotherapy is utilized to treat lymphomas.

Prevention: Unknown.

Discussion: Lymphomas can occur in all age groups. Most often, cancer in the lymph nodes is secondary to a primary cancer somewhere else in the body. However, a lymphoma is a primary cancer of the lymphatic system.

CANCER—MALIGNANT MELANOMA

A type of skin cancer, it is most often a fast-growing cancer that can be quite devastating.

Symptoms: More than 50 percent of malignant melanomas occur in preexisting moles on the body. Symptoms include an often sudden increase in a mole's size; the mole may suddenly darken; the mole may bleed, ulcerate or become inflamed.

Cause: Unknown. However, there may be some association with excessive exposure to sunlight.

Severity of Problem: There is an 80 percent cure rate if malignant melanoma is detected and treated in its earliest stages (before there is spread to surrounding lymph nodes). The five-year survival rate after treatment drops to 20 percent and the ten-year survival rate drops to 12 percent when the cancer is detected and treated after it has already spread to the lymph nodes.

Contagious? No.

Treatment: Surgical removal of the cancerous mole and surrounding tissue. If the lymph nodes are involved, they may be removed as well. Radiation therapy is often used for malignant melanoma of the face (in an attempt to avoid disfiguring the face). Often chemotherapy and radiation therapy are used in combination with surgery.

Prevention: Since malignant melanoma is a rapid and often deadly cancer, any change in a mole should signal the need for an immediate medical evaluation so that the cancer can be detected in its earliest stages. Avoid excessive sunlight where possible.

CANCER—MOUTH (ORAL CAVITY)

Cancer of the mouth (oral cavity) is most often seen on the lip, tongue or soft tissue directly under the tongue, although it can occur in the salivary glands, the gums, the lining of the cheek or the palate.

Symptoms: A white or red, hard, fibrous sore seen in the mouth; may or may not be painful; sore does not heal; sometimes pain when chewing; toothache may occur; some complain of swallowing or speaking difficulty; and earaches may accompany other symptoms.

Cause: There is at least a fivefold relative risk for those who use tobacco. Recent information shows that the use of chewing tobacco is a factor in the development of cancer of the mouth, as well. Excessive alcohol consumption has also been associated with this cancer. Those who both smoke and drink heavily are at greatest risk. Factors that increase the risk for mouth cancer include those with chronic oral injuries from jagged teeth, fillings or improperly fitted dentures; and those with leukoplakia.

Severity of Problem: Sixty percent to 70 percent survival five years after treatment when tumor(s) are small. Forty-five percent to 55 percent survival five years after treatment when tumor(s) are of moderate size. Approximately 20 percent five-year survival rate where an advanced cancer is diagnosed and treated. Once the mouth cancer has spread to the lymph nodes (usually in the neck), the cure rates decrease substantially.

Contagious? No.

Treatment: Surgery or radiation therapy may be used, or with some cancers these will be combined in treatment.

Prevention: Avoid the use of tobacco products and excessive alcohol consumption. Poorly fitted dentures, jagged fillings and teeth should be properly repaired. Routine dental evluation may detect cancer of the mouth early. Any sore that does not heal within two to three weeks should be evaluated.

CANCER—MULTIPLE MYELOMA

Cancer of the bone marrow (the center of the bone where blood cells are produced)—one of the worst fatal cancers.

Symptoms: For some, anemia is the only symptom experienced; constant or sharp bone pain; bone pain or tenderness with motion or exercise; spontaneous fractures (most often of the upper arms, hips, ribs and pelvis); severe or rapid weight loss; and sometimes swelling of the skull. Bone pain can become so severe that the person simply collapses or is rendered unconscious by the pain.

Cause: Unknown. Bone cancers, in general, are more frequent in those who have experienced excessive exposure to radiation (such as atomic bomb blasts) or high doses of X rays.

Severity of Problem: The overall average survival time after diagnosis is 1½ to 2 years. However, in some cases the cancer is so deadly that the survival time is only a few months after diagnosis.

Contagious? No.

Treatment: Radiation therapy and chemotherapy are the usual modes of treatment. Blood transfusions may be included to fight the anemia, and medication may be prescribed for pain control.

Prevention: Unknown. However, although no cause and effect relationship has been proved, it is always prudent to avoid excessive radiation exposure and any unnecessary X rays.

CANCER—OVARY

Cancer of the ovaries (part of the female reproductive system), the two structures that produce and house the ova (eggs) and produce sex hormones.

Symptoms: No early warning signs in almost all cases. Later symptoms may include abdominal swelling; low back pain; abdominal pain; abnormal vaginal bleeding; a mass that can be felt in the pelvis; sometimes changes in bladder or bowel habits. Sometimes a mass is detected during a routine physical examination when the doctor is feeling the ovaries for enlargement or tumor. Unfortunately, 50 percent of the time the tumor is not detected until it is so advanced and has spread so extensively that surgery cannot be performed.

Cause: Unknown.

Severity of Problem: Depends on the type and extent of the cancer. Seventy percent five-year survival rate after surgical treatment if the cancer is on the outside of the ovary and confined to the ovary. Twenty percent to 50 percent five-year survival rate after treatment if the cancer began on the outside of the ovary and has spread beyond the pelvic area. Only a 10 percent survival rate if the cancer has spread to the upper abdomen. For some ovarian cancers survival times are less than a year and a half.

Contagious? No.

Treatment: Surgical treatment is most often recommended. This usually includes removal of both ovaries, the uterus, Fallopian tubes, the omentum (layer of tissue that supports and protects the pelvic organs and intestines) and surrounding lymph nodes (if indicated). Radiation therapy and/or chemotherapy may also be used in an effort to destroy any remaining cancer cells.

Prevention: None. However, it is always wise to avoid unnecessary X rays to the pelvis or abdomen. Also, when X-ray studies are being performed, the pelvis and abdomen (if at all possible) should be covered with a protective shield that does not allow radiation exposure to the area. This is not to imply a cause- and-effect relationship but is simply prudent.

CANCER—PANCREAS

Cancer of the pancreas (which produces and secretes hormones and digestive juices) is one of the most deadly cancers known today.

Symptoms: Persistent abdominal discomfort or pain; yellow color to the skin (jaundice); often weight loss; dark-colored urine; constipation; indigestion; overall weakness.

Cause: Unknown. However, investigations into alcohol, caffeine and tobacco as possible causes are now underway.

Severity of Problem: Fifty percent of those with pancreatic cancer die in less than three months from the time of diagnosis. Two percent or less survive for three years. Usually the cancer is so well advanced when detected that little can be done to fight it.

Contagious? No.

Treatment: Radical surgery seems to be the only potentially effective treatment if the cancer has not spread to organs and blood vessels vital to life. Radical surgery involves removal of the pancreas, stomach, parts of the intestines, bile duct and sometimes the spleen. However, of every 100 people who have radical surgery for pancreatic cancer, 32 will die from the operation itself, and only 8 will survive for five years. Approximately 15 percent to 30 percent of those who undergo the surgery will die from abdominal complications or serious infection. The surgery is essentially the last-hope effort in many cases. Experiments are presently going on in combining surgery, radiation therapy and chemotherapy in the treatment of pancreatic cancer.

Prevention: Unknown.

Discussion: Finding a means of early detection of pancreatic cancer may make a marked difference in the survival rates. This continues to be investigated. This cancer occurs most frequently between the ages of 35 and 70. However, approximately 50 percent of cases occur in those over 70 years old.

CANCER—PROSTATE

Cancer of the prostate (the gland in males that produces the milky white fluid that, when mixed with sperm, forms semen) is second only to lung cancer as the most common cancer seen in men (in the United States).

Symptoms: Unfortunately, the symptoms of prostate cancer mimic other problems, and therefore, the disease often goes unattended. Although most often a silent disease, some men experience difficulty or pain when starting to urinate; need for frequent urination; weak urine flow, often interrupted or difficult to stop; blood in the urine; sometimes back pain or discomfort; and later in the disease, pain in the pelvic area and impotence.

Cause: Unknown. Investigations are underway to determine if a hormone imbalance may cause prostate cancer or if certain types of sexual behavior have any association with an increased incidence of the cancer. Some think that it may be due to old age.

Severity of Problem: Approximately 50 percent of those who develop the cancer and are over 60 years old at the time of diagnosis will beat the cancer and die from other causes. For those diagnosed with prostate cancer who are under 60 years old, 50 percent will experience a five-year or greater survival rate.

Contagious? No.

Treatment: Radiation therapy is most often used to eradicate the cancer in both the prostate gland and in the surrounding lymph nodes. Radiation implants are sometimes used as well. Surgery may be recommended for a select few men when the disease is diagnosed early and they are able (physically fit) to tolerate extensive surgery. When cure is not possible, the cancer can many times be controlled by hormone (estrogen) therapy.

Prevention: Unknown. Early detection and treatment are emphasized today as a means of curing or controlling the cancer.

Discussion: Since 80 percent of prostate cancers are seen in men over 60 years of age, all men should have a rectal examination every year, starting at age 50 (since many prostate cancers are diagnosed by rectal examination). Hormone therapy causes impotence, as does surgical removal of the prostate.

CANCER—SKIN (BASAL CELL AND SQUAMOUS CELL CARCINOMA)

Skin cancers can be divided into two types: basal and squamous cell carcinoma; and malignant melanomas (see CANCER—MALIGNANT MELANOMA for more specific information on that type of skin cancer). Basal cell and squamous cell carcinoma are the most common and most treatable human cancers. These two cancers are usually called "skin" cancers, while malignant melanoma is very much a different disease (although it is a type of skin cancer).

Symptoms: May include a lump in the skin that enlarges; a change in color, size or overall appearance of a pigmentated area of skin present for many years; any change in an area of the skin that does not disappear or heal rapidly; a reddened, hard or raised area of the skin. None of these may prove to be a skin cancer, but a physician should be seen to determine whether or not a skin cancer is present.

Cause: Possible causes include excessive exposure to sunlight and/or radiation; exposure to coal tars, arsenic, pitch, nitrate, nickel, beryllium, creosote, a variety of oils and more than 500 other chemical compounds. Also more prevalent in those people with keratosis (a problem where there is scaly thickening in small areas of the skin) and those with xeroderma pigmentosum (a rare skin disease).

Severity of Problem: One hundred percent cure rate when the basal or squamous cell cancer is confined to less than one inch in size (in total). Basal cell has the highest cure rate because it rarely spreads (metastasizes). Squamous cell cancer acts a little differently and more often metastasizes. However, with prompt detection and treatment, cure rates for these types of skin cancer are quite high. These are truly the more hopeful cancers.

Contagious? No.

Treatment: Surgical removal of the skin cancer and some of the surrounding tissue. Radiation therapy is often used for skin cancers of the face, eyelids, ears, lip or nose. Chemotherapy (often in lotion form) is sometimes used on the skin cancer. In some situations cryosurgery (use of cold to remove tissue) or electrocautery (use of heat to remove tissue) may be used to treat it.

Prevention: Avoidance of excessive exposure and/or chronic exposure to sunlight and/or radiation. Where possible, avoidance of other chemical compounds and agents known to cause or be associated with skin cancers.

CANCER—STOMACH

There are many very different types of stomach cancers, and these more often occur more in men (over 40 years of age) than in women.

Symptoms: Most often stomach cancer is detected late in the disease because early symptoms are rare, and they often mimic chronic touchy stomach, digestive problems or ulcers (which most people attempt to treat themselves for some time). Symptoms include upper gastrointestinal problems, such as heartburn; belching; upset stomach; indigestion; a feeling of heaviness (most often after eating); and a feeling of being full even with little food intake. More advanced symptoms include gradual weight loss; anemia; sudden fatigue; and lack of appetite and a particular sudden dislike for meats. If vomiting of blood, severe stomach pain or bloody bowel movements occur, then the disease is usually tremendously advanced.

Cause: Unknown. However, there seems to be some association of an increased incidence of stomach cancer in those with pernicious anemia, chronic gastritis, gastric ulcer and achlorhydria (a lack of hydrochloric acid in the stomach's gastric juices).

Severity of Problem: In those situations where the cancer has not spread beyond the stomach and surgery has been successful, five-year survival rates reach 30 percent. However, most often the cancer is already far advanced. In these situations 50 percent of those with stomach cancer live more than six months after diagnosis. Only about 10 percent of all those with stomach cancer will be cured.

Contagious? No.

Treatment: In very advanced disease surgical intervention is usually not a part of treatment, since it would not significantly change the situation (the cancer has spread to too many other vital organs and tissues). However, when indicated, the stomach or a portion of the stomach is removed (called gastrectomy), as well as other tissues and lymph nodes, as indicated. Radiation therapy and chemotherapy may also be utilized as part of treatment.

Prevention: A diet high in fiber, fresh fruits and vegetables, and milk, and low in meats, fats, oils and sugars may have some preventive effect. Diet may be the reason stomach cancer is seen more often in those in low socioeconomic groups. It is also seen more often in Japanese and blacks.

CANCER—TESTICLE

Malignant tumor of the testicle.

Symptoms: Lump in one of the testicles, usually without pain. In some men, enlargement of one or both breasts is a symptom, since some tumors secrete hormones.

Cause: Unknown. However, there is an increased risk of developing cancer in a testicle that was not descended during fetal development (cryptorchidism). This risk persists, even if the testicle is brought down into the scrotum by surgery early in life (but if it has been brought down, the chances of finding the lump are much greater than if the testicle was left inside the abdomen).

Severity of Problem: Cancerous tumors of the testicle are all very malignant and metastasize (spread) to the lymph nodes of the abdomen, as well as the chest and neck, and to the lung. Some tumors secrete hormones, such as those which produce breast enlargement and other signs of feminization. Certain types (especially a tumor called seminoma) are easily treated if they are detected and treated early. This type of tumor has as much as an 85 percent survival rate after five-years, while the other types of tumors have five-year survival rates of 40 percent to 70 percent.

Contagious? No.

Treatment: The mainstay of treatment of testicular cancer is surgical removal of the involved testicle and the lymph nodes of the abdomen. Certain tumors also respond to radiation therapy very well. When there has been spread to the lymph nodes and lungs, chemotherapy (drugs) and radiation are used.

Prevention: None known. However, careful examination of a testicle that was not descended before birth will allow early detection and treatment of some of these tumors.

CANCER—THYROID

Cancer of the thyroid, the gland that controls the body's metabolic rate.

Symptoms: Enlargement of the thyroid is the earliest symptom (but does not always mean cancer is present). Later symptoms include hoarseness, difficulty swallowing; sometimes difficulty breathing; choking; and swollen lymph nodes in the neck.

Cause: There is a higher rate of thyroid cancer among adults who have had X-ray treatments to the neck or head during childhood (for example, to shrink the thymus gland or to fight ear and tonsil infections). There is also a higher rate among survivors of the atomic bomb blasts at Nagasaki and Hiroshima.

Severity of Problem: Tumors that are undifferentiated and have spread to the lymph nodes are rarely curable. However, for those with tumors that are well-differentiated and confined to the thyroid gland and the lymph nodes in the neck, 80 percent are alive 15 years after treatment.

Contagious? No.

Treatment: Most often requires surgical removal of almost all of the thyroid gland and, where indicated, the surrounding lymph nodes. If the tumor has spread to the throat tissues, radiation therapy is often used as well.

Prevention: Avoidance of unnecessary X-ray exposure, particularly to the neck or head. Avoidance of radiation exposure when possible.

CANCER—UTERUS (AND ENDOMETRIUM)

Cancer that occurs in the mucous lining of the uterus (endometrium) or in the muscle tissue of the uterus itself. It is seen most often in women between 40 and 70 years of age.

Symptoms: *For menstruating women*: spotting between menstrual periods; vaginal bleeding after sexual intercourse; abnormal menstrual flow (most often includes unusually heavy and/or lengthy periods).

For postmenopausal women: Vaginal bleeding is the most frequently experienced symptom. Some women also note abdominal cramping or pain.

Cause: Unknown. However, there appear to be more endometrial and uterine cancers among women who are obese; those who have hypertension; women with diabetes; those who have never had children; and the disease appears to be more prevalent among whites than blacks.

Severity of Problem: If the cancer is contained in the lining of the uterus (endometrium), the five-year survival rate is 85 percent. When the cancer has spread to the deep muscle layers of the uterus itself, 60 percent to 70 percent of women will be alive five years after treatment. However, once uterine cancer has spread to surrounding lymph nodes, the cure rate is extremely low.

Contagious? No.

Treatment: Depends on the location and extent of the cancer. Most often surgical removal of the uterus, Fallopian tubes, ovaries and surrounding lymph nodes (where indicated) is recommended. Radiation therapy may be included if the cancer is advanced. In some cases radiation therapy or radiation implants are the sole therapy or are used as adjunct therapy. Sometimes hormones are also used if the cancer has spread to other areas of the body.

Prevention: Unknown. There are those who have suggested an association between uterine and endometrial cancer and the long-term use of estrogen.

CANDIDIASIS (YEAST INFECTION, THRUSH)

An infection caused by yeast organism.

Symptoms: In adult women, infection is usually vaginal: itching; pain; redness and swelling of the vulva and vagina; cottage cheese-like discharge. Urinary burning, sense of urgency and frequency. Pain and discomfort can be very intense. In men, if symptoms occur, they are usually mild: soreness of the foreskin and tip of the penis, especially after intercourse; rarely a discharge. In infants, infection is of mouth and diaper area: white patches in the mouth (inside cheeks, on tongue); very raw, red diaper rash that spreads quickly, with tiny blisters that open and merge together.

Cause: Infection with the yeast Candida albicans, which thrives in warm, moist areas. In adults, can be spread by sexual contact, although the yeast is commonly found in the body without causing infection. Infants may get infected from their mothers, in passage through the birth canal.

Severity of Problem: Bothersome problem that can be chronic. Life-threatening in people with abnormal immunity (they are at risk for a generalized, very serious candida infection of the blood and deep organs and ultimately death as a result).

Contagious? Yes, as a sexually transmitted disease. However, these organisms can normally be found in the intestine.

Treatment: For adults, use of prescribed medication given as a vaginal tablet or suppository is usually successful. Vinegar and water douches or sitz bath can be soothing and somewhat helpful. Infants with candidiasis of the mouth (thrush) need treatment with medicine put into the mouth. Diaper rash is treated with medicated cream or ointment. Infection can be stubborn, especially if underlying reason for infection is not corrected.

Discussion: Infection can follow prolonged use of certain antibiotics (e.g., ampicillin, tetracycline) in both children and adults. Hormone changes increase susceptibility (pregnancy, birth control pills). Persistent or recurrent infection may be a sign of diabetes mellitus.

CARDIAC ARRHYTHMIA

An irregularity of heart rhythm, possibly originating from either the upper chambers (the atria) or the lower chambers (the ventricles) of the heart.

Symptoms: Feeling of heart jumping out of chest; beating rapidly or slowly, irregularly or extra forcefully. Can be associated with signs of heart failure, weakness, fainting and even death.

Cause: Usually unknown. Often associated with poor blood supply from coronary arteries. Can be related to metabolic disturbances, hormonal abnormalities, valvular disease and aging.

Severity of Problem: Can vary from not noticeable (asymptomatic) to all of the above symptoms.

Contagious? No.

Treatment: Varies with the type of irregularity. See a doctor to determine the underlying cause and treat it. Often treated with medications. If asymptomatic, is not treated.

Prevention: Control the causes. Otherwise, none.

Discussion: Cardiac arrhythmias may come and go. Only certain ones need definite treatment.

CARDIAC ARRHYTHMIA—ATRIAL FIBRILLATION

Abnormal heart rhythm in which the upper chambers (the atria) quiver and beat extremely rapidly rather than at the usual slow rates. This results in a very irregular heartbeat, because not all the beats result in contraction (beating) of the heart.

Symptoms: Palpitations, accompanied by feelings of irregular, fast pulse, with fluttering in the chest. There may or may not be symptoms or signs of underlying heart disease. Episodes might last for several hours or continue on indefinitely.

Cause: There are many possible causes, but the most common are rheumatic heart disease and coronary artery disease. It may be seen in bursts in thyrotoxicosis (hyperthyroidism) and may be seen in normal people after surgery, trauma, poisoning or excessive alcohol intake.

Severity of Problem: A very common problem in the elderly. Usually it is possible to correct the fast heart rate with medication, but the person will in almost all cases need to be on medication indefinitely.

Contagious? No.

Treatment: Requires medical evaluation and treatment. At the start the purpose is to slow down the rate of the heart, so the stress on the heart is not any greater than it needs to be. After the rate is slowed with medication, and if the atrial fibrillation persists, medication or electroshock can be used to permanently return the rhythm to normal. Digitalis is the most commonly used drug for atrial fibrillation, although others have been effective and continue to be investigated.

Prevention: A combination of drugs can be used to prevent attacks of atrial fibrillation in people who have had previous episodes.

Discussion: Atrial fibrillation is the most common of the arrhythmias. It is most often found in people with underlying heart disease, especially rheumatic heart disease and arteriosclerosis.

CARDIAC ARRHYTHMIA—PAROXYSMAL SUPRAVENTRICULAR (ATRIAL) TACHYCARDIA (PAT)

Very rapid but organized contraction of the heart with effective ejecting of blood to the tissues.

Symptoms: Rapid heartbeat; pounding in chest; sometimes faintness or weakness.

Cause: Usually unknown. Sometimes unusual conduction pathways that allow very rapid passage of the impulses and result in rapid contraction.

Severity of Problem: Episodes are usually self-limiting and recurrent. Can be bothersome during the episodes. Congestive heart failure can occur if episode lasts for a prolonged time. Requires physician evaluation and management.

Contagious? No.

Treatment: Medications to slow heartbeat. Rarely, electric shock must be used.

Prevention: None.

CARDIAC ARRHYTHMIA—VENTRICULAR FIBRILLATION

A life-threatening abnormality of heart rhythm in which the ventricles (lower chambers) do not effectively beat and circulate blood.

Symptoms: Feeling of faintness and fluttering in chest followed by unconsciousness and collapse within seconds to minutes. No pulses are able to be felt.

Cause: Many possible causes, including coronary artery disease, with sudden lack of blood flow to an area of heart muscle (heart attack); disturbance of heart conduction for no apparent reason; unknown or known congenital heart defects; shock; lack of oxygen from any cause.

Severity of Problem: Leads to death almost immediately if not corrected or the blood is not circulated by cardiopulmonary resuscitation (CPR).

Contagious? No.

Treatment: If suspected and no pulses are present, start CPR immediately and call for help. Electrical shock (cardioversion) is the treatment to correct the arrhythmia, followed by general support, drug treatment and intensive medical care afterward, with identification and treatment of the underlying cause.

Prevention: Depends on underlying cause and is usually not possible. However, if fibrillation occurs, early treatment is imperative to prevent death.

Discussion: Ventricular fibrillation is the most serious complication of a heart attack in the first few hours or days after the attack and is the leading cause of sudden death with heart attack. Also seen in apparently healthy athletes, leading to sudden collapse and death during exercise. (Most of these individuals in fact have underlying problems that were undetected.)

CARIES (DENTAL CAVITIES, DENTAL DECAY)

Decay, first of the tooth enamel, then of the underlying structures of the tooth.

Symptoms: At first slight yellow or brown discoloration of the surface of a tooth, often in a natural crevice. As the process continues, softening and added discoloration, then a visible hole or cavity appears. Unless there is penetration of the decay to the pulp, or infection, there is no pain, but teeth may be sensitive to hot and cold or to sweets.

Cause: Not completely understood, but a combination of poor tooth cleaning, with buildup of residue (called plaque) on the tooth; sugars in the mouth; normal mouth bacteria; and perhaps the acidity of the mouth are all factors.

Severity of Problem: Can vary from minor to very severe. In the severe form can lead to dental abscess and loss of teeth.

Contagious? No.

Treatment: Prompt care by a dentist for caries at the earliest possible stage. Includes cleaning out the decayed area, then filling the tooth with a protective substance.

Prevention: Dental decay can be prevented or lessened by the following program: regular tooth and gum care, including rinsing the mouth after eating and brushing the teeth regularly; reducing the amount of sugar in the diet (especially sticky foods and snacks that will stick to and between the teeth); use of fluoride in the water supply or as a supplement by infants and children (to age 12), while the teeth are forming; application of fluoride treatments to the surface of the teeth in growing children; and regular dental checkups and care throughout life.

Discussion: Dental caries are one of the most common health problems in both children and adults. The problem can be prevented or controlled through good dental hygiene and care. It is important not to ignore decay in baby teeth, since these teeth can become abscessed, and early loss of them can lead to malocclusion and crooked teeth. A very severe form of dental caries is found in toddlers and young children who drink from a bottle constantly.

CARIES (DENTAL CAVITIES, DENTAL DECAY)— NURSING BOTTLE CARIES (NURSING BOTTLE MOUTH)

Particularly severe form of dental decay seen in toddlers and young children who have constantly sucked on a bottle after their teeth have come in.

Symptoms: Yellow or brown discoloration of the upper front teeth in a toddler or young child. As the problem gets worse, the teeth get more discolored and begin to rot away, leaving pegs and broken areas. The gums underneath are usually inflamed and sore. With further advance, other teeth besides the upper front teeth will begin to show signs of decay.

Cause: Continual contact of sugary liquids with the teeth. The use of a baby bottle containing milk, fruit juice or other sweet liquid, especially overnight or at nap time, allows the liquids to be in constant contact with the upper front teeth. The other teeth are partially protected by the tongue. Some liquids (such as apple juice and other acid, sweet liquids) are especially likely to cause this. Lack of fluoride, family tendency to decay and poor toothbrushing also contribute.

Severity of Problem: Progresses to complete decay and loss of the front teeth during the first few years of life if not promptly treated. Can be associated with serious gum disease (gingivitis, periodontitis) and infection.

Contagious? No.

Treatment: Vigorous dental treatment of the caries, with fillings and temporary caps if needed. Elimination of drinking from a bottle, reduction of sugar intake, use of fluoride and good toothbrushing can stop the progression. If tooth loss is impossible to prevent, use of temporary spacers is important.

Prevention: Elimination of drinking from a bottle for prolonged periods of time as soon as the teeth have come in is very important, as are reduction of sugar intake, use of fluoride, good tooth hygiene and regular dental care.

Discussion: In addition to being an uncomfortable and disfiguring problem, nursing bottle caries can lead to early loss of the front teeth and decay of the others. Early loss of baby teeth leads to crooked secondary teeth and poor development of the jaw.

CARPAL TUNNEL SYNDROME

Group of symptoms occurring because a nerve of the arm is entrapped.

Symptoms: Pain and numbness of the part of the hand served by the ulnar nerve (the fourth and fifth fingers). Usually happens at night to start with, then may increase so it is present all the time. As the problem worsens, there is weakness of the muscles of the hand, followed by a characteristic deformity called a "claw hand."

Cause: Chronic trapping of the involved nerve, with pressure on the nerve damaging it. This pressure usually is found at the underside of the wrist but may also be found at the elbow.

Severity of Problem: Progresses from a nuisance to potentially deforming. The hand may become weak. These changes can be permanent.

Contagious? No.

Treatment: The problem can be cured in its early stages by surgery to remove the pressure on the affected nerve. With mild cases reduction of obesity, if a factor, is useful.

Prevention: Avoid trauma or constant pressure to the wrists and elbows. Avoid or treat obesity if that is a problem. Prompt, careful treatment of certain types of arm fractures is also important.

Discussion: Condition is more common in women than in men. Acute trauma to the wrist or elbow, with a fracture that deforms the arm; chronic damage due to repeated trauma (for example, jackhammer use); severe obesity, with buildup of fat tissue around the tendons.

CATARACT

Clouding of the normally crystal-clear lens of the eye, which lies just behind the colored iris. This clouding of the lens blocks or distorts the passage of light that is needed for vision.

Symptoms: Most obvious symptom is degrees of blurry vision. Some people say they see fuzziness, spots or ghost images. Some experience double vision and notice that lights never seem bright enough to read by. As the lens of the eye becomes more opaque, vision worsens. Total vision loss can eventually occur without treatment.

Cause: Unknown. Some feel that cataracts may somehow be part of the natural aging process. A cataract is not a growth on or in the eye but a clouding of lens of the eye. A person with a cataract cannot actually see the cataract.

Severity of Problem: Cataracts may involve one or both eyes. Some cataracts develop very slowly, never reaching the stage where surgery is necessary. The process of others, however, is much more rapid. A hypermature cataract means the lens is totally opaque, and no light is coming through the lens. At this point the person is blind. The best timing for removal of a cataract must be determined by the person in consultation with his or her doctor. Usually, when vision is so poor that it disrupts one's everyday life (and vision cannot be upgraded any further by corrective glasses), the cataract needs to be removed.

Contagious? No.

Treatment: Surgery is the only way to remove a cataract. Although a cataract may be removed at any time, it is best to wait until the person's vision is bad enough to warrant removal. Removal requires that the entire lens of the eye be removed. After removal, an intraocular lens may be placed into the eye to replace the lens of the eye; a contact lens or special glasses can also replace the removed lens. Ninety-five out of 100 persons who undergo cataract surgery enjoy full recovery of their vision.

Prevention: None.

CELLULITIS

Inflammation of the skin and subcutaneous tissue due to infection. Spreads rapidly without formation of pus.

Symptoms: Gradual or sudden start of deep redness, warmth, swelling and tenderness of the skin and tissue below it in one area of the body. May spread rapidly. There may be a general feeling of tiredness, aching, fever, poor appetite and chills. Red streaking along the skin may be seen in the most severe forms. Severe skin swelling and blister development are seen, but rarely.

Cause: Bacterial infection of the skin, usually caused by a streptococcus organism, rarely by other bacteria. May follow a cut or other skin injury that is infected.

Severity of Problem: Usually minor to moderately severe and without serious complications. May lead to overwhelming infection (sepsis) in the very young or very old, or in people with poor immunity.

Contagious? The bacteria that cause it may be mildly contagious and are usually carried in the nose and throat, as well as in the infected skin area.

Treatment: Must be treated by a physician with antibiotics. Hot packs placed on the skin and aspirin or aspirin substitutes for fever and pain can be helpful.

Prevention: Careful washing of any skin wound to prevent invasion by bacteria.

CEREBRAL PALSY

term used to refer to a large group of movement disorders that result from brain injury. These disorders involve a combination of weakness of muscles and spasticity (increased tightness of muscles).

Symptoms: In early infancy slow development of motor (movement) skills, with floppiness and general weakness. With advancing age some muscles may become tighter, and controlled movements are difficult or impossible. The extreme muscle tightness (spasticity) leads to unusual postures and stiffness. Some children have unusual movements (writhing, jerking) along with wekness. The spasticity may lead to deformity. The weakness ans spasticity amy involve only a few muscle groups or areas of the body or may involve all or nearly all of the body.

Cause: Brain injury just before, during or shortly after birth. This injoury often results from lack of oxygen for a variable period of time but can occur as a result of hypoglycemia (low blood sugar), generalized infection or brain infection. One form of cerebral palsy, in which there are continuous, bizarre writhing and twisting movements (called choreo-athetosis), is caused by excessive jaundice in newborn life, with deposit of the yellow bilirubin pigment in a certain area of the brain. (This condition is called kernicterus).

Severity of Problem: Can range from almost imperceptible weakness that does not interfere with function significantly to severe and debilitating. May be associated with intellectual deficits.

Contagious? No.

Treatment: There is no cure for cerebral palsy once it occurs. Intensive physical and occupational therapy, especially in a group, is ideal. There is usually a need to surgically repair any correctable problem that is likely to get worse or interfere with rehabilitation.

Prevention: Improved techniques for resuscitation of the newborn infant and further advances in intensive care may help. Careful monitoring of the serum bilirubin (the yellow pigment that cuases jaundice), especially in very tiny or very sick infants, with early treatment of the jauntice, reduce the effects of bilirubin encephalopahty, as it is called. Recent control and prevention of serious Rh disease have been very effective in reducing kjernicterus and the number of children with this particualr form of cerebral palsy.

Discussion: While many people assume that children and adults with cerebral palsy are retarded, this is not necessarily true. Intellectual function may remain normal, with damage limited to areas of the brain that control motor functions.

CERVICITIS

Inflammation and usually infection of the cervix, the neck of the uterus.

Symptoms: White vaginal discharge, pain or discomfort with intercourse (dyspareunia,), discomfort and difficulty with urination, frequency of urination. Low back pain, pelvic discomfort, dysmenorrhea and spotting between menstrual periods may also occur.

Cause: Acute or chronic infection and inflammation of the lining of the cervix. The cervix develops an ulcer at its opening, then changes its appearance in response to the inflammation. The original infection may be caused by gonococcus or by a combination of bacteria.

Severity of Problem: Chronic cervicitis is one of the major causative factors in infertility, habitual spontaneous abortion and infections around the time of delivery.

Contagious? Yes, depending on the cause of the infection. (Gonorrhea is contagious as a sexually transmitted disease; other mixed infections can also be passed by sexual contact.)

Treatment: Requires close observation and treatment by a physician. For acute infections antibiotic treatment is necessary. For chronic inflammation the treatment is more complex and includes surface treatment of the ulcer on the cervix with silver nitrate to cause it to heal; antibiotic treatment, with or without hormone therapy; cautery (burning), cryosurgery (cold surgery) or laser treatment are all possible.

Prevention: Avoid contact with individuals who have suspected or known sexually transmitted disease.

Discussion: Cervicitis is a common problem experienced by as many as 75 percent of the adult female population; over 60 percent of women who have had children have had one episode of cervicitis as a result.

CHICKENPOX (VARICELLA)

A childhood disease that produces small blisters that crust over quickly.

Symptoms: At first, child may seem mildly ill with fever and listlessness, or have no fever and begin with a rash. Rash starts as small "spots," which quickly develop tiny blisters on the top. Blisters crust over in a few hours. Pox appear in clusters, with new ones appearing several times a day for four to six days. Itching of the rash is severe.

Cause: Infection with the varicella-zoster virus.

Severity of Problem: A mild but bothersome and uncomfortable disease in most infants and children. Can be a life-threatening infection to those whose immune system is not normal. Complications include pneumonia, which is a difficult problem, and encephalitis. The pox can become infected if scratched.

Contagious? Yes. One of the most contagious of the childhood diseases, it can be spread by contact with nasal secretions just before the rash appears and from contact with the blister fluid until all the spots have crusted over.

Treatment: No cure. The disease runs its course in 10 to 14 days. Treatment is aimed at making the person comfortable. Cool baths and dressing lightly will reduce itching, which can also be helped by putting soothing lotions on the skin and taking aspirin substitute.

Discussion: Infants under 6 months are usually partly immune to chickenpox because of immunity from their mothers. If they are exposed then, they may only develop partial immunity and be susceptible to having shingles later in life. Chickenpox is a more serious disease with advancing age.

CHLAMYDIA INFECTION

Sexually transmitted disease that causes inflammation of the urethra in men and vaginal inflammation in women. Can cause eye infection and/or pneumonia in young infants.

Symptoms: *Symptoms in men*: difficulty in urination caused by pain in the urethra and pain in the head of the penis and the testicles. There may be burning during urination and itching in the urethra; discharge from the urethra, which varies from very thin and watery to heavy pus. *Symptoms in women*: a white vaginal discharge accompanied by itching; there may be pain during sexual intercourse. *Symptoms in infants*: eye inflammation with discharge of pus and much tearing during the first six to eight weeks of life. If pneumonia develops, infant will have severe cough, ending with vomiting at times, and mild difficulty breathing.

Cause: Chlamydia organisms, between bacteria and viruses in size, are transmitted sexually from one person to another. Infants may get the infection during delivery through the infected birth canal.

Severity of Problem: Very irritating and extremely uncomfortable for both men and women. A common result of chlamydia infection for the newborn is an eye infection that appears about 5 to 14 days after delivery. Another manifestation is a combination of pneumonia and eye infection occuring within the first two months of life.

Contagious? Yes. Chlamydia infection is sexually transmitted. Any person infected should refrain from sexual intercourse until the disease is eradicated.

Treatment: Requires doctor's evaluation and a laboratory test to diagnose. Such infections can be treated with an antibiotic when recognized. This is not a reportable venereal disease at this time, although it is best to advise any and all sexual partners that they may have the infection.

Prevention: Because the infection is sexually transmitted and difficult to identify, avoid sexual activity with people with symptoms that suggest this disease.

Discussion: May be the most common sexually transmitted disease in the United States, more prevalent than gonorrhea. One of the causes of the problems called "nonspecific urethritis" and "nonspecific vaginitis."

CHOLECYSTITIS—ACUTE

Sudden, severe inflammation and infection of the gallbladder.

Symptoms: Sudden onset of fever, chills and pain in the right upper part of the abdomen under the rib cage. Pain may be felt in the right shoulder as well as in the abdomen. Nausea and vomiting may be present, and there might be slight jaundice (yellow color to the skin). The abdomen is distended and tender to the touch.

Cause: Inflammation and infection of the gallbladder, associated with gallstones in about 90 percent of cases. Stones probably block the drainage of the bile, and bacteria enter the gallbladder from the intestine. A few cases are caused by injury to the abdomen or previous surgery.

Severity of Problem: Intense pain and illness. Can result in generalized infection (sepsis), gangrene of the gallbladder and cholangitis.

Contagious? No.

Treatment: Hospitalization is usually needed. Antibiotics, intravenous fluids, pain control and stomach rest until the symptoms are improved. Surgery to remove the gallbladder (cholecystectomy) is usually recommended after the acute attack has subsided.

Prevention: Removal of gallbladder if gallstones are present. Otherwise, none.

CHOLERA

Infection of the intestine that leads to profound diarrhea.

Symptoms: Sudden onset of explosure, massive diarrhea, which leads to profound dehydration within hours. Diarrhea is watery, grayish and does not smell like stool. There is mucus, but no blood (has been described as "rice water stool"). Collapse from electrolyte imbalance and dehydration can occur within hours or days of the start of diarrhea if it is not treated. Little if any fever; rarely vomiting.

Cause: Infection of the intestine (usually the small intestine) with an organism called Vibrio cholerae. This is contracted through food and water contaminated with waste of people with the disease. The organism produces a toxin that causes the bowel to pour out massive amounts of water and salt into the stool.

Severity of Problem: Somewhat variable, but leads to death in 20 percent of 80 percent of victims if not treated promptly. With good treatment, death rate is reduced to around 1 in 100.

Contagious?: Yes, by eating food or drinking liquids contaminated by infected feces. The disease is found in many areas of the world at the present time.

Treatment: Prompt replacement of the water and electrolytes (salt, potassium) lost in the massive diarrhea. In many countries in which cholera is common, this is effectively done with a specially made solution drunk by the infected person. Sometimes fluids must be given intravenuously. The bacteria can be controlled by administering an antibiotic, tetracycline. The disease usually lasts about three to five days.

Prevention: Although there is a vaccine available against cholera, it is not very effective. Best prevention is avoiding possibly contaminated food and water as boiling all water and other liquids, foods and eating utensils in areas with known cholera.

CIRRHOSIS OF THE LIVER

Chronic, permanent scarring of the liver that eventually leads to liver failure and death.

Symptoms: At the beginning the symptoms are subtle and consist of loss of appetite, fatigue, weakness and weight loss. With time there might be nausea, vomiting, abdominal discomfort and pallor (anemia). Peculiar skin changes (appearance of small red spots called spider angiomas, red palms of the hands and dilated capillaries on the skin) occur, and jaundice appears later. There are also changes related to sex hormones—disappearance of menstrual periods in women and enlargement of the breasts with impotence in men. Loss of sexual desire and sterility occur in both men and women. There may be fever and progressive sleepiness and ultimately coma.

Cause: Severe damage to the cells of the liver result in their attempt to heal themselves. This scarring is not successful, and as the damage continues, progressive liver failure develops. Alcohol abuse is the most common underlying cause, although viral hepatitis and certain forms of gallbladder and biliary disease also cause a type of cirrhosis.

Severity of Problem: The problem is irreversible but may progress either rapidly or slowly. People with advanced cirrhosis are at particular risk for overwhelming infection (septicemia) and massive bleeding from varices of the esophagus.

Contagious? No.

Treatment: There is no specific treatment. Prompt recognition and treatment of the complications of cirrhosis (infection and bleeding) are important. Maintaining good nutrition and avoiding anything that could be injurious to the liver are important. Avoidance of alcohol may slow the progression of the disease.

Prevention: Some types (especially that caused by alcohol abuse) are preventable by removing the cause. Otherwise, no prevention possible.

Discussion: While alcohol abuse is the most common cause of cirrhosis of the liver, it is important to remember that there are other causes.

COLIC—BILIARY

Severe abdominal pain due to acute obstruction within the biliary system (gallbladder, bile ducts).

Symptoms: Sudden onset of severe abdominal pain, usually in the right upper side, under the rib cage. Pain increases in severity over minutes and may last for minutes to hours. It may come and go, depending on the cause. There might be nausea, vomiting of clear or green-stained liquid (bilious material) and movement of the pain to the shoulder area. The abdomen may be tender or sore to the touch.

Cause: Most commonly caused by sudden blockage of one of the bile ducts by a gallstone or spasm of the duct. If the blockage is severe and persistent, inflammation and infection of the gallbladder and sometimes the liver itself can follow. Meals that make the gallbladder excrete bile (fatty meals, spicy foods) tend to lead to biliary colic in people with gallstones.

Severity of Problem: Can be mild and occasional or frequent and severe. If obstruction is persistent, can lead to inflammation and infection of the gallbladder (cholocystitis, acute or chronic).

Contagious? No.

Treatment: Rest, pain relief, refraining from eating during the acute attack. It is important to find and treat the underlying cause.

Prevention: Avoiding fatty foods may help prevent the problem in some people with gallstones, but most often attacks cannot be prevented except by removing the gallbladder.

Discussion: While symptoms that look like biliary colic are most often due to gallstones, some people with this kind of problem do not appear to have gallstones. It is important to have such symptoms evaluated by a doctor before assuming gallbladder disease is the problem.

COLIC—INFANTILE

Pattern of behavior seen in young infants involving repeated, cyclic crying.

Symptoms: Repeated bouts of inconsolable crying in an infant between about 3 weeks and 3 months of age. The crying tends to happen about the same time of the day, and nothing that is done for the baby consoles it. With prolonged crying the baby develops a slightly enlarged abdomen and may have increased gas. Some babies act hungry and will suck repeatedly. There is no significant vomiting or changes in bowel habits, but some babies may spit up more than usual.

Cause: Has always been thought to be caused by intestinal gas and cramping in the past, although there is no proof. Babies who get colic tend to have a personality or temperament that makes them more sensitive to changes in their environment and perhaps to gas. Rarely due to food intolerance when it occurs at only one time of the day or only periodically. Prolonged crying leads to air swallowing, which increases the amount of gas in the stomach and intestines.

Severity of Problem: Can be a severe problem, with bouts of crying for as long as an hour or more a day, every day, for several months, or can occur less often. Most babies have a few fussy periods during early infancy.

Contagious? No.

Treatment: Most often, the goal is to reduce the crying spells and comfort the baby. Commonsense measures often do not work, and parents must resort to more drastic creative steps. Most babies with colic will calm down somewhat with constant motion: riding in an automobile, an infant swing or being carried in an infant carrier close to the body. However, sometimes nothing works, and the infant must be left to cry until the spell ends (this will cause no harm).

There is almost never any benefit from changing feedings from breast to formula; and there is rarely benefit, other than temporary, from switching formulas, unless the crying is constant (around the clock) and there are also other symptoms (vomiting, diarrhea or poor weight gain). Likewise, medications that supposedly treat intestinal gas and cramping are not usually helpful and may be harmful. When symptoms are severe, a mild sedative might be prescribed by your doctor.

Prevention: None. However, bouts of colicky behavior can sometimes be lessened by avoiding over-feeding. (Babies who have a colicky personality tend to overeat and gulp their feedings, swallowing much air in the process.) Frequent burping may help them.

Discussion: Colic is a common source of frustration and worry for new parents. It rarely results from poor techniques of baby care but rather is a result of the baby's personality. Colicky behavior tends to start about 3 weeks of age and end between 3 and 4 months. Frustration with infants with this problem often leads parents to lose control and hurt their babies. If the frustration level is approaching, call for help or put the baby in its own room to cry and leave the room. Crying will *not* harm the baby.

COLITIS—IRRITABLE COLON SYMDROME (IRRITABLE BOWEL SYNDROME, SPASTIC COLITIS, MUCOUS COLITIS)

Groups of symptoms that occur together in people bothered by some variety of chronic or recurrent diarrhea.

Symptoms: Intermittent bouts of diarrhea or loose bowel movements, usually containing mucus; crampy abdominal pain and increased gas; some nausea and loss of appetite; and a certain amount of emotional tension or stress.

Cause: Exact cause is not completely understood. However, people with this problem have a tendency to have overactive intestines, which increase in activity in response to a variety of factors, including stress and dietary indiscretion. There is a tendency in certain families to react with bowel symptoms.

Severity of Problem: Can be mild and very tolerable or severe and bothersome.

Contagious? No.

Treatment: Probably the most important aspect of treatment is to control or alleviate the stress and anxiety that are likely to be at the bottom of the symptoms. This includes adequate rest, exercise and a regular schedule, as well as dealing with any particular problems present. Some people do well with emotional counseling or techniques to control stress. Diet changes that reduce the amount of fiber and irritating foods (spices, milk products for some) are helpful for certain people, while use of bulk-forming agents help others. Cigarette smoking and alcohol intake should be reduced or eliminated. Medications from a doctor that slow the movement of the intestines may be tried.

Discussion: Irritable colon syndrome is a very common reaction to stress. In fact, most people normally react to stress and anxiety with some change in bowel habits. When this becomes extreme, a true irritable colon syndrome is present.

COLITIS—ULCERATIVE

Chronic inflammatory disease of the lower bowel (colon).

Symptoms: Severe, profuse watery diarrhea, with mucus and blood. There is severe cramping of the abdomen and a feeling of constant pressure on the rectum, as well as involuntary passage of stool. Weight loss, severe prostration and illness occur, and the abdomen may be swollen and sore. The rectal area becomes very sore and irritated, sometimes with formation of fissures and fistulas. If blood tests are done, the person is anemic.

Cause: Unknown, although it seems to be related to certain of the generalized diseases of the connective tissue and blood vessels (rheumatoid arthritis, arthritis).

Severity of Problem: A very serious, debilitating disease until under control. Complications can include fistula to the outside of the body because of the ulcers in the colon; arthritis that behaves in a way similar to rheumatoid arthritis; inflammation of the eye, including uveitis; infection with staphylococcus, which produces great dilation of the colon and serious illness (toxic megacolon); growth disturbances when it affects children; scarring and narrowing of the rectal opening.

Contagious? No.

Treatment: This disease requires immediate medical attention, and often hospitalization is needed. Complete rest of the bowel, with feeding through an venous catheter after the person's fluid status is stable; antibiotic treatment to prevent or control the development of staphylococcal infection. As the disease improves, starting a diet that is low in residue (everything must be cooked) and eliminating milk products. Sulfa drugs are given, and prednisone, a cortisone relative, can be given for the cramping and colitis. In severe cases with widespread disease, surgery to remove the diseased colon may be done in order to minimize cancer risk.

Prevention: None known for the disease.

Discussion: This disease usually affects women more often than men and tends to start between the ages of 20 and 40. Inflammation of the lowest part of the colon leads to the formation of ulcers on the surface of the bowel lining. There is a higher incidence of colon cancer among people who have ulcerative colitis.

COLOR BLINDNESS

Inability to distinguish certain colors, most commonly red and green.

Symptoms: Usually none to the person with color blindness. Other people may notice an unawareness of color differences by a person (often a child) with the problem.

Cause: Most often an inherited lack of nerve cells in the retina of the eye that detect colors. The condition may skip generations and most commonly affects males, who are likely to have problems with red and green colors. Less commonly, can result from excessive use of alcohol and/or excessive smoking of cigarettes.

Severity of Problem: Varies widely, from a mild difficulty in differentiating green from red (both of which are seen as shades of gray), to severe inability to differentiate any colors (essentially seeing the world like a black-and-white photograph).

Contagious? No.

Treatment: None for the hereditary type. Elimination of smoking and alcohol ingestion for the acquired kind.

Prevention: None for the inherited variety. Avoidance of heavy smoking or drinking for the acquired type.

Discussion: One of the more worrisome potential problems is the inability of the affected person to tell the difference between red and green lights (for example, traffic lights). This requires teaching children the position of the safe lights. The same type of problem, as a bothersome handicap, can occur with the use of other equipment that employs colored lights as a means of communication.

CONCUSSION

Temporary alteration in the brain that results from the soft brain tissue's being jolted inside the skull.

Symptoms: Total or partial loss of consciousness; dazed or "spacy" feeling; episode of confusion; varying amounts of memory loss; headache; dizziness; a "fuzzy" feeling; nausea; and possibly vomiting.

Cause: A blow to the head that causes the brain to be jolted against the skull. This causes mild to severe swelling of the brain tissue (either localized, where blow occurred, or it can involve much of the brain).

Severity of Problem: Requires medical evaluation and attention to ensure that greater damage did not occur (contusion, intracranial bleeding or skull fracture). Head injuries with loss of consciousness are always potentially serious, and medical evaluation should not be delayed.

Contagious? No.

Treatment: If there are no complications, person usually requires adequate rest, fluid intake and nutrition. Care is taken to "follow" someone with a concussion to make sure that recovery is complete (the brain swelling has resolved) and all functions are normal.

Prevention: When possible, avoid situations where head injuries are more frequent, or take safety precautions; use protective helmets when involved in athletics; wear special hats when working on certain jobs where head injury is a risk (e.g., construction).

CONGENITAL HIP DISLOCATION (DYSPLASIA)

Abnormal development (dysplasia) of the hip socket during fetal life, which allows the hip bone to slide out of joint (dislocate).

Symptoms: At the time of birth, one or both hips may be out of the socket, or the baby may be loose-jointed enough to allow the hip to slide partially or completely out of joint during the doctor's examination. The baby is usually not uncomfortable during this procedure. There may be some subtle abnormalities of the legs as well. If the problem is undetected until later, there may be tightness of the muscles around the hip, widening of the hips and later a waddling or limping gait.

Cause: Abnormal or incomplete development of the hip socket before birth allows the hip bone to slide upward and backward, partially or completely out of the socket. If this dislocation (if complete) or subluxation (if partial) continues, further deformity of the hip joint results.

Severity of Problem: If detected and treated within weeks or months of birth, the outlook is good for complete recovery of normal hip joints. The longer the condition goes undetected and untreated, the more likely it is that there will be permanent damage to the hip joint.

Contagious? No.

Treatment: The goal of treatment in this condition is to make sure the hip joints stay in alignment while the socket and hip bone develop during infancy. This is done by holding the baby's hips in a frog-leg position continuosly. This can be done using several kinds of braces or harnesses, or with body casts. Splinting is usually needed for at least three or four months, sometimes longer. The earlier the problem is detected, the shorter the treatment. Treatment is usually supervised by a specialist in orthopedics.

If the problem is not detected until later in the first year, traction to align the hips, then a body cast kept in place for at least six months, is needed. If detected after walking has started, the treatment is much more complicated and usually requires one or more surgical operations.

Prevention: There is probably no way to prevent the abnormal intrauterine development of the hips, but worsening of the problem can be prevented by prompt diagnosis and treatment in early infancy.

Discussion: While no one is sure exactly why congenital hip dysplasia occurs, it is much more common in girls than in boys and can occur in either one or both hips. Abnormal or unusual positions before birth may play a role by putting unusual pressure on the legs and hips during development. For example, hip dysplasia is more common in breech babies (babies born bottom first) than in cephalic (head-down) babies.

A careful look for this problem is part of the earliest examinations of newborn and young infants during regular checkups.

CONJUNCTIVITIS
Inflammation of the membrane of the eyes, noticed as redness and irritation of the white parts of the eyes.

Symptoms: Pain and irritated feeling of the eyes; feeling of something in the eye; redness of the eye membranes, especially the white part; swelling of the eyelids if severe; excessive tearing; sensitivity of the eyes to light. There may be mucus or pus discharge.

Cause: Many possible causes. Infection and allergy or irritation are the most common.

Severity of Problem: Uncomfortable but not usually serious. Exception is herpes infection with keratitis (inflammation of the cornea), which can lead to scarring and blindness.

Contagious? With infectious forms only.

Treatment: Depends on the cause. See entries for the various types of conjunctivitis.

Prevention: Avoid contact with persons who have infectious forms of conjunctivitis. Avoid contact with substances that are known to cause eye irritation or allergic conjunctivitis.

CONJUNCTIVITIS—ALLERGIC (VERNAL CONJUNCTIVITIS)

Inflammation of the membranes of the eye caused by an allergic reaction.

Symptoms: Itching, swelling and redness of the eyes; excessive watering; feeling of something in the eyes. Usually affects both eyes and may have a mucous discharge in addition to the tearing. There may also be other allergic problems, such as allergic rhinitis, asthma and eczema.

Cause: Direct contact with a material to which the person is allergic. Most often pollens, dust, pollutants, animal dander and fungus spores.

Severity of Problem: Usually a relatively minor problem. However, certain people can have severe enough allergy to leave them with permanent irritation and scarring of the eye membranes.

Contagious? No.

Treatment: Eliminate contact with the offending allergen(s) as soon as possible. Cold compresses on the eyes and forehead may relieve itching and discomfort. See a doctor for severe or frequent problems. Sometimes an antihistamine medication taken by mouth will help reduce symptoms.

Prevention: Avoid contact with the offending allergen(s). Sometimes allergy desensitization injections can reduce or prevent the problem.

Discussion: Most allergic conjunctivitis is mild and goes away without specific treatment. Very common as a spring and summer problem (therefore the name *vernal conjunctivitis*). A few people have a more severe form of the disease, with growth of small, irritating lumps on the undersurface of the eyelids and constant, severe inflammation.

CONJUNCTIVITIS—INFECTIOUS (BACTERIAL, VIRAL, CHLAMYDIA)

Inflammation of the membranes of the eye caused by an infection. Viruses, bacteria or fungi can be responsible.

Symptoms: Discomfort and redness of the membranes of the eyes. Usually considerable swelling of the eyelids and production of large amounts of pus or mucus discharge. May affect only one eye at a time.

Cause: Infection with a particular microorganism. Common bacteria that cause this inflammation are staphylococcus aureus, hemophilus influenzae and chlamydia. Many viruses are also implicated. Fungus infection of the eyes is rare, but occurs.

Severity of Problem: Some forms are particularly severe and require vigorous treatment under a doctor's care. Others are minor problems and go away with little or no treatment. In small infants and those with poor immunity, the risk for overwhelming infection (sepsis) is quite high.

Contagious? Most forms are contagious, by touching the secretions of the eye. Some forms spread rapidly as epidemics.

Treatment: In general, keep the eye clean of discharge and as comfortable as possible. See a doctor if swelling or redness is a problem, or for any other related problems. Various antibacterial eye ointments are available and effective for bacterial inflammation.

Prevention: Avoid contact with a person who has conjunctivitis if infection is known or suspected. Avoid rubbing eyes and spreading infection.

Discussion: Staphylococcal conjunctivitis is very contagious and can occur in epidemics, as can several forms of viral inflammation. In fact, viral conjunctivitis can be more severe and long-lasting than bacterial disease. Sometimes there is enough inflammation that there is bleeding under the membranes of the eyes, especially with viral infections. Conjunctivitis caused by the chlamydia organism affects small infants and can be associated with pneumonia. (See CHLAMYDIA INFECTION.)

CONSTIPATION

Unexplained delayed and difficult passage of stools.

Symptoms: Days since last bowel movement; stools unusually dry and hard; and difficulty, discomfort and/or pain when trying to have a bowel movement.

Cause: Rectal lesion; slow metabolism; psychological stresses; change in dietary habits; insufficient liquid consumption; refined low-residue foods; inactivity (lack of exercise or long-term bed rest); use of certain drugs (narcotics, diuretics, belladonna and its derivatives, iron and calcium); structural or functional problems; and some cultural factors.

Severity of Problem: Usually causes mild discomfort. If the problem becomes chronic, bothersome or painful, or if there appears to be blood in the stool, a doctor should be consulted.

Contagious? No.

Treatment: Adequate intake of fluids; diet should include bulk and residue (high-fiber foods such as bran, raw fruits and vegetables); adequate and routine exercise; and the use of mild laxatives as a temporary measure (these should not be used on a continual basis and should be stopped once the constipation improves). Enemas actually interfere with the normal bowel reflex, so they should be used only when the stool is impacted or the constipation is very severe. A physician should be consulted if constipation becomes chronic, troublesome and painful.

Prevention: Follow a proper diet, exercise adequately and consume a sufficient amount of liquids.

CORNEAL ABRASION

Scratch or scrape on the surface of the cornea, the thin, transparent membrane that covers the pupil of the eye.

Symptoms: Severe, sudden pain in the eye, with severe redness and a sensation of something in the eye. Spasm of the eyelids and sensitivity to light make it almost impossible to open the eye. Blurred vision. Headache is quite common.

Cause: A mechanical injury to the surface of the cornea. Commonly caused by a contact lens injury, a scratch from a foreign object that has gotten into the eye or a scratch from a fingernail or another object brushing the eye.

Severity of Problem: Very painful, but usually heals quickly and completely. More serious if the abrasion becomes infected.

Contagious? No.

Treatment: Requires evaluation and follow-up by a physician. Most often, the eye is patched closed after an antibacterial ointment has been applied. The patch is removed after the abrasion is healed, usually in 24 to 48 hours. Pain is relieved with aspirin, aspirin substitute or stronger pain reliever. Rest and cold compresses to the forehead may help.

Discussion: One of the most painful of eye problems, corneal abrasions are amazing in their tendency to heal rapidly and without complications. In people who wear contact lenses, abrasions can occur if lenses are worn for too long a time, or if the lenses are irregular or fit poorly.

CORONARY ARTERY DISEASE

Disease of the arteries that supply blood to the heart muscle.

Symptoms: There may be chest pain associated with exercise, which resolves when exercise is stopped. Shortness of breath may be associated. Pain may radiate down left arm or to the jaw. This pain is called angina pectoris. More severe pain associated with nausea, vomiting, sweating and feeling faint are symptoms of "heart attack." Pain of heart attack may be confused with pain of upset stomach or gas.

Cause: Deprivation of oxygen-carrying blood to the heart muscle because of narrowing of the coronary arteries by plaque formation on the walls. The plaque contains cholesterol and cellular debris and may block the entire channel of flow. As a result, the deprived tissue creates the sensation of pain and may die.

Severity of Problem: Depends on the severity of blockage of the arteries, the suddenness of the problem and, in the setting of a heart attack, if ventricular fibrillation occurs. (See CARDIAC ARRHYTHMIA—VENTRICULAR FIBRILLA- TION.) Chronic chest pain should be evaluated by a physician. If chest pain is severe, call the paramedics.

Contagious? No.

Treatment: In the case of chronic recurrent chest pain, the treatment involves diagnosis, diet, medication and prescribed exercise in a controlled setting. If good control is not possible, surgery is considered.

In the setting of a heart attack, the treatment involves immediate hospitalization and administration of medicines for pain and to prevent ventricular fibrillation. If pain recurs after a heart attack, medical treatment and surgery are usually recommended.

Prevention: Diet low in cholesterol and saturated fats; no smoking; maintain weight within 10 percent of ideal weight; a routine exercise program; control of stress; periodic physical examinations for early detection of problems.

Discussion: Coronary artery disease is a major killer in this country. Risk factors that strongly increase the likelihood of coronary artery disease occurring are cigarette smoking, high blood pressure and diabetes. These should be controlled or avoided where possible. Coronary artery disease does run in families. In recent years dietary changes, exercise, early treatment and the training and use of paramedics have reduced the mortality from coronary artery disease.

CRAMPS—LEG

Sudden, involuntary, persistent contraction of a muscle or series of muscles; occasionally associated with severe, immobilizing pain.

Symptoms: Sudden involuntary contraction (almost like a spasm) of a leg muscle; mild, moderate or severe pain in cramped area. Cramping muscles feel like hard knots.

Cause: Leg cramps have many possible causes: muscle fatigue; poor flexibility due to lack of stretching exercises; incomplete conditioning (inability of the heart and lungs to sustain the desired level of muscle activity); binding clothing around the muscles; increased nerve irritability; disturbance in salt concentration in the blood may be involved.

Severity of Problem: Usually temporary pain and discomfort; soreness of the leg muscle when severe cramping has occurred.

Contagious? No.

Treatment: Pain can usually be alleviated very quickly. The discomfort will subside by simply grabbing the front part of the foot (including the toes) and pulling the foot toward the body. This procedure pulls the shortened muscle in the direction opposite to that of the muscle concentration, relieving the cramps. Do not shorten the muscle further. If recurrences of cramping persist or worsen, the cramping muscle should be rested.

Prevention: Proper muscle conditioning; proper stretching of leg muscles before physical activity; avoid over-exercising of leg muscles; free muscle area of binding clothing.

CROHN'S DISEASE (REGIONAL ENTERITIS)

Chronic inflammatory disease of the intestine that can cause inflammation, ulceration and formation of small masses and scar tissue anywhere along the intestine. The disease most often involves the area where the small intestine joins the colon, but the colon can also be involved.

Symptoms: Symptoms of this disease come and go, because the amount of inflammation varies with time. Crampy abdominal pain, usually in the lower right side, is common during an acute attack. Diarrhea, with mucus and blood, is usually part of the acute episode, but bowel habits may be normal between attacks. There is usually mild fever, fatigue, weight loss, loss of appetite and developing malnutrition.

Cause: Unknown, although the disease shares some features of the connective tissue diseases and runs in families. There does not appear to be an infection as the cause.

Severity of Problem: Crohn's disease is a chronic progressive illness that has many potential complications: ulceration and perforation of the intestine; malnutrition; generalized infection; development of fistulas connecting the bowel and the rectal area or bladder; and a greater incidence of colon cancer than among the general population.

Contagious? No.

Treatment: When the disease is acute, intensive support using antibiotics, rest of the bowel and intravenous feeding, and sometimes administration of cortisonelike medications to reduce inflammation of the bowel. Long-term use of certain antibiotics has been helpful in many people with this disease, as has good nutritional support. Surgery to repair fistulas or remove badly diseased bowel may be needed in severe cases.

Prevention: None known.

Discussion: Crohn's disease can affect people of all ages but usually begins in adolescence or early adulthood.

CROUP (LARYNGOTRACHEOBRONCHITIS

Acute inflammation and swelling of the area of the vocal cords and upper airways, causing a barking cough and a harsh, loud noise on breathing in because of obstruction of air flow. Usually a problem of infants and children between 6 months and 3 years of age.

Symptoms: In infectious croup, runny nose and congestion, mild cough for several days, then sudden trouble breathing in, usually starting at night. Harsh noise called stridor, barking cough and abnormal movement of the chest. There may or may not be fever. Hoarse voice.

Cause: Most often a viral infection, with many possible viruses as cause. Can also be allergic or as a result of irritation of the airway.

Severity of Problem: Usually of mild to moderate severity, although severe airway obstruction can occur and require placement of a plastic tube into the windpipe to aid breathing.

Contagious?: Yes, for the viral form, by contact with secretions.

Treatment: No specific treatment to cure the infection. Moisture in the air—by vaporizer, shower steam or a "croup tent"—helps with comfort and easing breathing. Rest and keeping the child calm help by not further irritating the inflamed vocal cords. If breathing difficulty is severe or increases, get immediate emergency medical care. Antibiotic treatment is not helpful for viral croup.

Prevention: None for viral problem. Allergic and irritant croup (also called spasmodic croup) can sometimes be prevented by avoiding contact with substances that trigger it.

CURVATURE OF THE SPINE—KYPHOSIS

Abnormal increase in the usual curvature of the spine at the chest area, causing a humpback deformity.

Symptoms: Increase in the appearance of humpback, usually without other symptoms. There may be mild backache associated or other bone or joint symptoms, depending on the cause.

Cause: Often caused by degeneration or collapse of one or more of the vertebrae of the upper spine, because of either injury (fracture) or infection of the bone. In decades past tuberculosis of the spine was the most common cause of this deformity. Paget's disease of the bone is commonly associated with this problem in the older individual. Kyphosis can be a part of certain congenital malformations and can run in families.

Severity of Problem: The curvature can vary between individuals. Usually the problem is more cosmetic than painful.

Contagious? No.

Treatment: No treatment known, except for that of the underlying problem.

Prevention: Only as is possible for the underlying problem.

CURVATURE OF THE SPINE—SCOLIOSIS

Curvature of the spine to the side, so the spine looks like and S.

Symptoms: Usually there are no symptoms unless the curvature is very pronounced and advanced. As the abnormal curvature develops, the person notices difficulty in fitting clothing, an elevation of one shoulder or a prominence of one shoulder blade. Later the definite curvature may be noticed. With severe scoliosis, there is also deformity of the rib cage and reduction in lung capacity.

Cause: There are several possible causes, including congenital deformities of the vertebrae; neurofibromatosis (a disease of the nervous system); diseases such as polio and muscular dystrophy, in which some of the muscles of the spine are paralyzed or weak; and unequal length of the legs. The most common form, however, is called "idiopathic"—no definite cause is known. This type appears in adolescence and usually affects girls much more often than boys.

Severity of Problem: Can vary from a mild, almost unnoticeable curvature to a very pronounced deformity with limitation of lung function.

Contagious? No.

Treatment: Depends on the cause, to some extent. With idiopathic scoliosis, the goal of treatment is to prevent further curvature during growing. This can be accomplished by specific exercises to strengthen back muscles, bracing the back and sometimes plaster casts to prevent further deformity. With severe curvature, surgery to straighten the spine may be needed.

Prevention: No prevention known, but early detection and treatment can limit the progression of the problem. Early detection programs are particularly effective if screening sessions are set up in schools during junior high and high school and screening of all girls takes place.

CYST

Fluid-filled lump.

Symptoms: Appearance of a lump. Varies in size and can occur in almost any part of the body, either near the skin surface or deep in an organ. Usually not red or sore unless infected.

Cause: Unknown. In some cases may result from irritation.

Severity of Problem: Usually minor, although it can be problematic in some locations because of pressure on existing organs or structures, or interference with function.

Contagious? No.

Treatment: Surgical removal if cyst is bothersome or unsightly. Can be allowed to remain and be observed for unusual changes.

Prevention: None known.

Discussion: Common locations for cysts are under the skin, in the breast, in ovaries and over tendons.

CYSTOCELE
Herniation or rupture of the bladder wall into the vagina.

Symptoms: A feeling of fullness in the vagina; frequent urination; the need to urinate again just after urinating; stress incontinence (release of urine when exercising, laughing, coughing, sneezing, etc.); chronic or frequent urinary infections.

Cause: Greater likelihood of cystocele with many cesarean births or the birth of large babies; sometimes many pregnancies weaken the pelvic structures; at times happens as part of the aging process, where weakness of the pelvic structures occurs; there may also be a congenital weakness of the pelvic structures.

Severity of Problem: Most often a nagging, uncomfortable and embarrassing problem. However, recurrent or chronic infections are always potentially dangerous in that they can eventually cause permanent damage to the kidneys and/or bladder. Acute urinary retention or overfilling may occur as well.

Contagious? No.

Treatment: A pessary (a device inserted into the vagina) may be used to help support the pelvic structures for those who could not tolerate surgery, those whose surgical risks are too great or where temporary treatment is warranted. Surgical repair of the bladder and other pelvic structures involved (as indicated) is usually recommended. If urinary infections are chronic or frequent, intensive antibiotic therapy is initiated. If urinary retention or overfilling have occurred, catheterization (insertion of a thin tube into the bladder through the urethra) may be necessary.

Prevention: None.

CYTOMEGALOVIRUS INFECTION
Very common viral infection that is often not even apparent to the person who has it. Causes three different types of disease: an acute illness in otherwise normal people, congenital infection and a very serious pneumonia in people with abnormal immunity.

Symptoms: *For the acute infection:* fever; generalized tiredness and weakness, cough, swollen lymph nodes, aches and pains, enlarged and tender liver, and slight sore throat. Can be very similar to the symptoms of infectious mononucleosis.

For congenital infection: sudden onset of jaundice, enlarged liver and spleen, bleeding disorder and lethargy. Infants look very critically ill.

For immunologically abnormal people: a picture of severe infection, usually a very bad pneumonia, with fever, difficulty breathing and generalized weakness.

Cause: Infection with the cytomegalovirus, which is related to the virus that causes infectious mononucleosis. Congenital infection is contracted during fetal development when the mother is infected (although her infection may appear to a very mild, flulike illness or be unrecognized altogether). The other types of infection can be contracted from another person, but a common cause is receiving massive blood transfusions.

Severity of Problem: A very serious problem in infants and in people with poor immunity. In others, usually a mild but lengthy disease that goes away without complication. Congenital disease can lead to long-term brain damage, with mental retardation and seizures, and sometimes liver damage. Can lead to death in infants and immune-suppressed persons.

Contagious? Yes, probably by direct contact with infected person and by receiving blood from someone who has the infection (usually without symptoms).

Treatment: No treatment except for support of the person and treatment of symptoms and complications. Control of fever and discomfort, support of breathing and nutrition, transfusion of infants with bleeding problems.

Prevention: Ideally, avoidance of transfusions of blood received from people with this infection (currently it is not practical to screen blood for this infection). Also, avoidance of contact with people with flulike illness, especially for pregnant women and those with immune problems.

Discussion: This virus is extremely common, with as many as 10 percent to 25 percent of the normal population carrying it in their salivary glands (in the mouth). Most have no knowledge of any illness. May also be found in the cervix of as many as 10 percent of healthy women and 1 percent of healthy infants. Infection with this virus is one of the common complications of any illness or surgery that requires massive transfusions, such as open-heart surgery, serious injury or kidney failure with dialysis (use of the "artificial kidney").

DACRYOCYSTITIS

Inflammation and infection of the tear duct, with partial or complete blockage of the duct.

Symptoms: Watery eye, followed by discharge of mucus or pus in the eye. There may be some redness also. Pain, tenderness and swelling over the tear duct, which is located over the upper part of the nose, near the inside corner of the eye. Symptoms may come and go. One or both tear ducts may be involved.

Cause: Infection of the tear duct with a number of possible types of bacteria. Underlying cause is partial or complete blockage of the tear duct. This can be caused by injury in the older person, or perhaps as a result of inflammation of the duct following use of silver nitrate drops after birth.

Severity of Problem: Usually a minor smoldering infection. Occasionally leads to abscess formation over the tear duct. In young infants it may rarely lead to generalized infection (sepsis), which can be very serious.

Contagious? Not as such, although the bacteria that cause the infection may be spread to another susceptible person.

Treatment: Treatment of the infection with eye drops or ointment prescribed by a doctor. Warm compresses to eye and tear duct if very inflamed. In young infants or with severe infection, antibiotics given by mouth or injection may be needed. Relief of the blockage of the tear duct after the acute infection (may require minor surgery).

Prevention: Relief of blocked tear duct, if known. Early treatment of infection may prevent development of an abscess.

DEVIL'S GRIPPE (BORNHOLM DISEASE, PLEURODYNIA)

Viral infection with inflammation of the pleura (membranes that cover the lungs and line the chest).

Symptoms: Severe, incapacitating chest pain, usually starting in one spot but extending around the chest to be general. Pain is worse with deep breathing, cough; it may be present with each breath, but there are often separate shooting pains or sudden, unexpected stabbing episodes. Mild fever; cough may be present.

Cause: Virus infection with a specific type of virus in the Coxsackie family. Usually seen in late summer and early fall; may be seen in epidemics.

Severity of Problem: The pain can be very incapacitating.

Contagious? Yes, although not all people who get infected with the same virus will have Devil's grippe. (They may have other symptoms of viral infection.)

Treatment: No cure available. Pain relief, sometimes with very strong medications; heat applied to the chest.

Prevention: None.

Discussion: Pain is very severe and causes fear of serious disease. Person should be seen by a doctor to make sure there is no pneumonia or pneumothorax (collapsed lung). Disease may last several weeks.

DEAFNESS

Partial or total loss of hearing either due to obstruction of sound (conductive hearing loss) or as a result of mechanical failure, nerve damage or brain transmission problems (perceptive hearing loss).

Symptoms: *Conductive hearing loss*: Person may suddenly talk quietly because his or her voice sounds very loud (it is amplified by the skull bones); seems to hear fine on the telephone (because the receiver against the ear and head results in bone conduction of sound); does not respond to loud noises; does not respond when someone is talking but not facing him or her; frequently misunderstands what is being said or asks that something be repeated.

Perceptive hearing loss: Person talks very loudly; often says others are whispering or mumbling; cannot hear well on the telephone; loud sounds cause even greater distortion; frequently asks that things be repeated or does not respond when spoken to; misunderstands what is being said; and the sounds *g, k, p* and *t* are not in his or her hearing range, so the person hears the wrong words.

In children: May not respond to sounds; may not startle when someone approaches from behind; may not be awakened by very loud noises; doesn't respond, sing or dance to music or to a toy that plays music unless he or she sees it; and may not look to see where a voice or noise is coming from. As baby grows older, he or she may not respond to "no, no"; seems to ignore people who are talking to him or her if people can't be seen; seems preoccupied or distant; doesn't seem to be able to talk clearly or knows only very basic words and sounds for his or her maturation level. In school the child may be seen as unable to concentrate; rude because he or she ignores other children; may be seen as a "problem child" by teachers unaware of a hearing difficulty; doesn't seem to be progressing in communication skills (speech and vocabulary) for his or her maturation level.

Cause: *Conductive hearing loss*: wax or water in the ears (temporary or chronic); boils or growths in the ear; eardrum damage; result of deseases such as mastoiditis, otitis media and even due to eustachian tube blockage from the common cold.

Perceptive hearing loss: A severe blow to the ear or head or persistent loud noises (or a sudden blasting sound) can cause injury to the ear and permanent damage; Ménière's disease (tumors of the brain); German measles (rubella) contracted by the mother during the first three months of pregnancy often leads to congenital deafness (the baby is deaf at birth); congenital deafness may also be due to mechanical or structural problems or nerve damage; complication from diseases such as mumps, meningitis, measles, syphilis, anemia, strep infections and leukemia; problems of the arteries that reduce blood flow to the acoustic nerve (particularly seen in the elderly);

overdoses of aspirin (and other salicylates) can sometimes result in hearing loss or noises in the ear; alcoholism has been associated with hearing loss; and certain drugs (quinine) may cause hearing loss.

Severity of Problem: Complete hearing loss is a disability and requires the teaching of alternative methods of communication. The severity of the problem depends on the cause and degree of hearing loss and whether or not there is the possibility of correction.

Contagious? No.

Treatment: Children should be seen by a physician as soon as possible if hearing loss is suspected. Wax and water in the ears and boils and growths must be treated by a physician. Ear infections should be diagnosed as early as possible so that complications, such as hearing loss, do not occur. Hearing aids (prescribed and fitted by an audiologist or otologist) resolve some hearing problems. Surgery may be required to repair damage or structural problems. And in some cases, little can be done to restore or promote hearing, and the person must then learn lip reading and sign language.

Prevention: Ear infections should be diagnosed and treated promptly; loud, booming noises or constant loud noises should be avoided; trauma to the head or ears should be avoided, if possible; and any indication of hearing loss should be a signal for a professional evaluation.

DERMATITIS—NEURODERMATITIS

Chronic skin inflammation that is localized to one area of the body, usually a small area.

Symptoms: Dry, very itchy, scaly patch of skin that becomes thickened and pigmented. Area is well demarcated and flares up with stress and continued scratching.

Cause: Unknown. Initial irritation leads to skin inflammation, then itching and scratching causes further damage and skin thickening.

Severity of Problem: Relatively minor, but bothersome and uncomfortable.

Contagious? No.

Treatment: Avoid scratching. Use soothing lotions and creams to prevent drying. Steroid creams provide some relief. Antihistamine medications may help to relieve itching.

Prevention: None known.

DIABETES MELLITUS ("SUGAR DIABETES")

Disease in which the body is unable to correctly metabolize glucose for energy. In *insulin-dependent diabetes mellitus*, the body does not produce enough insulin to help with the utilization of glucose. In *non-insulin-dependent diabetes mellitus*, the body produces enough or nearly enough insulin, but the cells are unable to effectively use it.

Symptoms: Both forms of diabetes are often made known because a person has intense thirst and increased urine output, both day and night. There is usually fatigue as well, and blurred vision is common. When there is little or no insulin, there is increased appetite with weight loss. Women with either kind of diabetes tend to have candidiasis of the vagina. Insulin-dependent diabetics may become very ill with ketoacidosis, become very dehydrated and go into coma (ketoacidosis results when fat is burned improperly, leading to the buildup of substances called ketones and extra acids in the blood; this results from lack of insulin). This does not occur in non-insulin-dependent diabetics.

Cause: The basic problem is either absolute lack of insulin or inability to use the insulin that is present. There is increasing evidence that insulin-dependent diabetes occurs in people who are genetically at risk, after such insults as infections with certain viruses or exposure to certain toxins. Non-insulin-dependent diabetes occurs often in obese people and in certain others who have a strong family tendency toward diabetes.

Severity of Problem: Insulin-dependent diabetes is a more serious disease, with a risk of coma and serious illness if the disease is not under control, coupled with risk for complications of premature arteriosclerosis, kidney disease, cataracts, peripheral artery disease and retinopathy. These same complications can occur in non-insulin-dependent diabetes but tend not to be as severe. The length of time a person has had the disease, as well as how well controlled it is, both influence the final outcome. In insulin-dependent people, effects of too much insulin represent a risk, too—coma from hypoglycemia.

Contagious? No.

Treatment: *Insulin-dependent diabetics*: carefully controlled insulin dose, usually given as one shot a day, but can require two or more or the use of an insulin pump; a well-balanced, controlled diet; regular exercise; frequent evaluation for presence of complications; and a thorough education program regarding the disease, its treatment and its complications. *Non-insulin-dependent diabetics*: controlled weight loss for those who are obese; carefully controlled diet; regular exercise; use of oral medications that reduce blood sugar in a select group of people; careful medical follow-up regarding progress and complications; and a thorough education program regarding the disease, its treatment and its potential complications.

Prevention: Prevention may be possible by avoiding obesity for people who are at risk for non-insulin-dependent diabetes. Otherwise, prevention is limited to possible lessening of complications by careful control of diabetes.

Discussion: Diabetes can occur at any stage of life, from infancy through old age. Infants and children are usually insulin-dependent, and most adults who acquire the disease after middle age are not insulin-dependent. Complications can appear at any time and contribute to shorter-than-usual life expectancy. However, the outlook can be quite good if there are no serious complications after 10 to 20 years with the disease.

DIPHTHERIA

Infection that usually starts as a throat or respiratory infection, but with serious, life-threatening consequences.

Symptoms: Usually begins in throat and respiratory tract with sore throat, swelling of the throat. A very thick membrane forms on the tonsils, in the nose and along the windpipe, leading to breathing difficulty and airway obstruction. Later, weakness, heart failure, delirium and progressive nervous system deterioration can occur.

Cause: Infection with the bacteria Corynebacterium diphtheriae.

Severity of Problem: Life-threatening both from airway obstruction and from effects on the heart and nervous system.

Contagious? Yes, by contact with contaminated respiratory secretions.

Treatment: Requires vigorous medical treatment in a hospital intensive care unit. Penicillin must be administered along with antitoxin to halt the disease. Recovery is slow.

Prevention: Can be totally prevented by immunization. Children are immunized in early infancy and should receive booster injections. Adults should receive booster immunizations every 10 years (they can be given along with tetanus booster).

Discussion: Initial illness with diphtheria is the respiratory infection. When the bacteria multiply in the throat and respiratory tract, they produce a toxin that causes local paralysis of nerves (and swallowing problems), as well as damage to distant organs, especially the heart muscle, the kidneys and the nervous system. Antitoxin can be given to halt the poisonous effects of the toxin, and penicillin can kill the bacteria. Both must be administered early in the disease to be effective. Diphtheria is still found and has not been eliminated with vaccine.

DISC, RUPTURED (ALSO CALLED SLIPPED DISC)

Injury to an intervertebral disc (made of cartilage and separating the vertebrae of the back).

Symptoms: Mild to severe low back pain that intensifies with certain movements; stiffness in the lower back or spine; muscle spasms in the lower back (near or below the waist); pain may radiate down buttocks and/or legs. Pain and stiffness can occur suddenly or may gradually build in intensity over a period of time.

Cause: Can result from strain or shock sustained during athletic activity, physical accident or injury (lifting something too heavy or falling); tumor; disc degeneration; or everyday wear and use.

Severity of Problem: The vast majority of those with this problem will recover totally. However, the injury is painful and often incapacitating until recovery is complete. For some, back pain and ruptured discs become chronic problems. Sometimes surgical intervention, which may include fusion of the involved intervertebrae, is necessary. If bladder function is impaired (due to the back pain experienced when attempting to urinate) immediate surgery is often recommended.

Contagious? No.

Treatment: Conservative measures are usually attempted first. Depending on the degree of pain and damage, complete bed rest may be required for days to weeks. Physical therapy and sedatives may be indicated for some. Hospitalization may be necessary in more severe cases where traction is required or where the person is totally incapacitated from injury. Surgery may be recommended for severe or chronic injury.

Prevention: Exercise is the best preventive measure. Stretching exercises are particularly beneficial, as is swimming. Care should also be taken when lifting objects. Proper body mechanics are essential (bending the knees and not twisting when bending or lifting anything).

Discussion: Intervertebral discs work like shock absorbers for the spine. Made of cartilage and found between the vertebrae, the discs take the stress and strain put on the spine by everyday activities. If a disc experiences unusual strain or is strained as a result of the muscles' being weak, the disc may bulge (rupture or slip) out of its place. If it presses or pinches a nerve, pain will not only be experienced in the lower back but also in the area the nerve serves (the legs, buttocks, etc.). Great care should be taken to prevent back injuries, since they can become chronic or debilitating.

DIVERTICULAR DISEASE—DIVERTICULITIS

Inflammation and infection of the diverticula (outpouchings of the colon).

Symptoms: Cramping abdominal pain, usually in the lower left side, with chills, fever, tenderness in the lower left side, blockage of the colon and evidence of septicemia (generalized infection). Rectal bleeding is common.

Cause: Inflammation and infection of the diverticula lead to perforation or rupture of the little pouches, with leakage of infected material into the abdominal cavity. These perforations are usually tiny but can lead to severe infection. Abscesses develop, and tracts may form between the bowel and the bladder. Infection with the many bacteria that normally reside in the colon spreads throughout the abdomen and sometimes through the blood.

Severity of Problem: Usually diverticulitis is a relatively mild infection that can be managed without serious complications. However, when abscesses form, fistulas develop or obstruction occurs, the problem is more serious and may require vigorous medical intervention.

Contagious? No.

Treatment: Intravenous antibiotic treatment is needed when diverticula become infected. When the inflammation calms down, dietary management that emphasizes increased bulk or residue in the diet, as well as stool softeners, are important. If there are repeated episodes of diverticulitis or formation of fistulas or abscesses, surgical removal of the diseased portion of the colon may be needed.

Prevention: Treatment of diverticulosis with a high-residue diet and avoiding constipation or irritation of the diverticula may help prevent acute infection of the diverticula.

DIVERTICULAR DISEASE—DIVERTICULOSIS OF THE COLON

Presence of diverticula, which are small outpouchings of the wall of the colon.

Symptoms: There may be no symptoms unless inflammation and infection of the outpouchings (diverticulitis) occur, or there may be alternating constipation and diarrhea, as well as mild cramping abdominal pain in the lower left abdomen. Rectal bleeding is common and may be in large amounts or unnoticed except by laboratory testing of the bowel movement.

Cause: Probably a feature of aging, but exact cause is not known for certain. There may be a pressure component, since the outpouchings usually occur in areas of the colon (the lower sigmoid area) where the pressure is normally highest.

Severity of Problem: In many people the condition is totally silent and undetected. In about 20 percent to 25 percent of people with diverticulosis, inflammation of the little sacs, with other possible complications, occurs.

Contagious? No.

Treatment: Diet that is high in bulk and residue. Stool softeners to reduce straining and pressure on the sigmoid colon area. If there are recurring attacks of acute inflammation or other complications such as hemorrhage, surgery to remove the diverticula may be recommended.

Prevention: Diet that is high in residue may play a role, but this is not certain.

Discussion: Diverticulosis is a common disease that is usually seen in people over 40. Its symptoms and findings must be distinguished from those of cancer of the colon.

DIVERTICULAR DISEASE—DIVERTICULOSIS OF THE ESOPHAGUS

Outpouching of the esophagus.

Symptoms: Difficulty swallowing, associated with discomfort or a feeling of fullness or pain in the chest. Regurgitation and bad breath are common. There may be night cough and recurrent pneumonia because of aspiration (inhalation of food caught in the pouch).

Cause: Outpouching of the esophagus may be congenital (present from birth) and increase in size with age, or it may develop because of resistance to food passing into the stomach (for example, because of achalasia, or narrowing of the esophagus). Most times, no cause is known. As the pouch fills with food and debris, it enlarges, further increasing the difficulty swallowing. In certain types of diverticula located high in the neck, a swelling in the neck may be noticed.

Severity of Problem: May range from producing no symptoms to complete blockage of swallowing and malnutrition. Usually increases in size gradually over a period of years.

Contagious? No.

Treatment: Depends on location and size or severity of the problem. There may be no treatment recommended, or surgery to remove the diverticulum may be needed.

Prevention: None.

Discussion: There are several types of esophageal diverticula, with differing locations and severity. Those located high in the neck (Zenker's diverticulum) usually produce the biggest problem. Those in the middle of the esophagus and those down near the stomach usually are not as such a problem.

DYSENTERY—AMEBIC (AMEBIASIS)

Infection of the large bowel with small organisms called amebae. The infection may produce no symptoms, or very severe diarrhea.

Symptoms: When there are symptoms, they include severe diarrhea with mucus and blood, mild fever and severe abdominal cramps. The watery diarrhea can lead to severe weakness and dehydration.

Cause: Invasion of the lining of the colon with the tiny ameba parasites.

Severity of Problem: The illness can be very severe or totally without symptoms. Dehydration is the major complication. Abscess in the liver can result from this infection.

Contagious? Yes, by direct contact with someone who carries the organisms or by eating contaminated food. The organisms are found in the bowel movements of the infected person or on contaminated food, especially vegetables that have been improperly washed or washed with contaminated water.

Treatment: Prevent or treat dehydration by being sure liquid is taken in adequate amounts. Diet should be bland or consist only of liquids. Sometimes hospitalization is needed for treatment and intravenous fluid therapy. Drug treatment is successful both for the infection with no symptoms and for that with severe diarrhea. It must be supervised by a physician. (Infection without symptoms may be discovered during evaluation for another problem, or it may go undetected.)

Prevention: Avoid eating contaminated food or food that is questionable in areas where amebiasis is common. Wash hands well at all times and be sure water supply is safe.

Discussion: Amebic dysentery is most often found in tropical areas and is frequently acquired during travel. It can be diagnosed by identifying the small characteristic microorganisms in the diarrhea fluid.

DYSENTERY—BACILLARY (SHIGELLOSIS)

Severe form of diarrhea due to infection of the bowel with shigella bacteria.

Symptoms: Differ in children and adults. In infants and children there is sudden fever, drowsiness, loss of appetite, abdominal pain and profuse, watery diarrhea with blood and mucus. Abdomen is distended and passage of stool explosive and uncontrollable. There may be a feeling of having to pass stool continuously. Children may have convulsions at the start of the disease. In adults the disease is more mild, with abdominal pain, little if any fever and less diarrhea.

Cause: Infection of the large bowel with the microorganism Shigella flexneri. Produces severe inflammation of the lining of the bowel, leading to the bloody diarrhea.

Severity of Problem: In children the disease can be serious. Leads to severe dehydration, convulsions and malnutrition. In adults the disease is more minor.

Contagious? Yes. Passed from one person to another (bacteria are carried in the stool) or by contaminated food or water.

Treatment: Careful replacement of fluids by mouth if possible, or intravenously in a hospital. Antibiotic treatment may be necessary for severe illness in children but is often avoided in adults. When diarrhea is severe, feeding may make the problem worse.

Prevention: Wash hands carefully after contact with people with diarrhea. Avoid suspicious or contaminated food and water. Wash contaminated clothing and linens in very hot water.

Discussion: One of the most contagious forms of diarrhea. Diarrhea begins about three days after infection with the bacteria and may last up to two weeks. A person may continue to harbor the germs in the bowel even without diarrhea for as long as six months, and this "carrier state" may be lengthened if antibiotics are given. Stools should be cultured every month or two after diarrhea has stopped until the germ has disappeared, and preventive precautions taken until the germ has disappeared.

DYSMENORRHEA

Discomfort or pain with menstrual periods.

Symptoms: Discomfort or pain in the lower abdomen and pelvis just before and during the menstrual period, often cramping in nature.

Cause: Dysmenorrhea and pelvic congestion is thought to be caused by the release of a substance called prostaglandin from the lining of the uterus during menstruation. So-called *primary dysmenorrhea* starts during adolescence and has no apparent cause other than this. *Secondary dysmenorrhea* is caused by an underlying abnormality in the pelvis, such as endometriosis, uterine tumor, fibroid tumors or pelvic inflammatory disease. It can also be associated with uterine prolapse. Secondary dysmenorrhea usually begins later in life than the primary form.

Severity of Problem: Cramping usually lasts for several hours to several days. It can be mild and easily controlled with medications or limit a woman's activity severely.

Contagious? No.

Treatment: For primary dysmenorrhea relief of discomfort is often possible by using aspirin, which has a specific effect against prostaglandins as well as pain-relieving effects. More powerful pain relievers are not usually needed. Temporary use of birth control pills to prevent ovulation for several months is frequently effective, and a pregnancy often relieves the problem significantly. In secondary dysmenorrhea these measures plus treatment of the underlying cause can provide relief.

Prevention: None known, except prevention of ovulation (usually with the birth control pill).

DYSPAREUNIA

Pain or discomfort during sexual intercourse.

Symptoms: Pain or severe discomfort during sexual intercourse, specifically vaginal penetration. This discomfort may be described as originating near the introitus (the opening of the vagina); in the vagina itself; or on deep penetration, with cervical and uterine contact.

Cause: There are many possible causes, including endometriosis, pelvic inflammatory disease, abnormal uterine position, uterine or pelvic tumors, vaginitis, genital herpes infection, imperforate or tight hymen, and cysts and infections of the genitals. Purely emotional causes, such as fear of intercourse or fear of pregnancy, while possible, are less common than many of the problems listed.

Severity of Problem: Can vary from mild and annoying to severe and incapacitating enough to prevent intercourse.

Contagious? Not as such. (Untreated gonorrhea, herpes simplex type 2 infection and other sexually transmitted diseases that can cause dyspareunia are contagious.)

Treatment: Depends on identifying and treating the underlying cause.

Prevention: Depends on the the underlying cause.

Discussion: There is a tendency for people to believe that pelvic pain with intercourse is psychologically based most of the time. It is important that a woman have a thorough medical evaluation if this problem exists, in order to identify other problems that may be hidden. If there are none, psychological treatment is warranted.

EDEMA

Swelling of body tissues (in the ankles or in whatever is the body's lowest point with respect to gravity) due to accumulation of fluid.

Symptoms: Swelling, tightness of skin, usually of legs and feet. If fluid accumulation is severe in the whole body, edema in the lungs might cause shortness of breath.

Cause: Many possible causes, including heart failure; poor tissue constitution; low protein in the blood because of malnutrition or other cause; incompetent leg veins; water retention for an unknown reason. Some women retain fluid before menstrual periods (see PREMENSTRUAL SYNDROME).

Severity of Problem: Depends on cause more than on the amount of water retained.

Contagious? No.

Treatment: Depends on cause. With many causes, restriction of salt intake is helpful in addition to measures that treat the specific cause.

Prevention: Again, depends on cause.

EJACULATION, PREMATURE

One of the forms of sexual dysfunction in which there is release of semen before penetration during sexual excitation.

Symptoms: Inability of the male to maintain an erection long enough to complete penetration during intercourse. Semen is released suddenly before the height of excitation. There may be other manifestations of sexual dysfunction as well, and symptoms of prostatism (difficult urination, frequent urination at night, inability to start the urinary stream, dribbling, burning on urination) are frequent.

Cause: Most often, premature ejaculation is a symptom of emotional upset or stress, or a marital or relationship problem, especially in young men. It can be a sign of other illness, such as prostatism, spinal cord problems or use of medications (including alcohol) that interfere with normal function, especially in older men.

Severity of Problem: If persistent, leads to serious problems with relationships and self-esteem. If there is a physical basis for the problem, its control may lead to resolution of the sexual dysfunction.

Contagious? No.

Treatment: Depends on the underlying cause. Physical causes need to be identified and treated. Sexual therapy or psychological therapy are often successful in improving sexual function.

Prevention: Avoidance of stress where possible, open communications in relationships.

EMBOLISM

Movement of a broken-off piece of blood clot, fat or debris from one part of the body to another through the bloodstream.

Symptoms: Depends on the size of the embolus and the location where it lodges. If it lodges in a large blood vessel and completely blocks it, symptoms of failure or malfunction of that part will occur. For example, if an embolus lodges in a large artery to the brain, the person will have severe symptoms of a stroke and may even die. On the other hand, if the embolus is small and lodges in a small vessel, there may be no symptoms at all and no aftereffects.

Cause: Disruption of a blood clot or fat or plaque and its movement in the bloodstream.

Severity of Problem: If the embolism is small and does not completely block the vessel it lodges in, it may be a minor problem. If the blood vessel is completely blocked and the blood cannot make a channel through it, the tissue supplied by that blood vessel will die.

Contagious? No.

Treatment: Depends on location, size of embolus and cause.

Prevention: Again, may or may not be possible, depending on the cause.

EMPHYSEMA (CHRONIC OBSTRUCTIVE PULMONARY DISEASE, COPD)

Chronic lung disease in which there is progressive loss of lung elasticity. There are areas of over-expansion and areas of collapse in the lung.

Symptoms: Shortness of breath, difficulty in exhaling; dry, raspy cough or wet-sounding cough; barrel-shaped chest. Later, weakness, weight loss, cyanosis with exertion.

Cause: Smoking, environmental gases, fumes and bronchial irritants, aggravated by bronchitis and asthma. Seems to be a combination of irritation and an individual susceptibility to this kind of damage.

Severity of Problem: An incurable, usually progressive disease that can lead to chronic disability and death. Severe emphysema is a major problem in the United States, ranked only behind coronary disease as a disabling illness.

Contagious? No.

Treatment: No curative treatments available. Breathing exercises, oxygen if needed, antibiotics when infection occurs. Medication to relieve airway spasms might help.

Prevention: Stop smoking, or don't start; avoid irritating and contaminating atmosphere when possible.

ENCEPHALITIS

Inflammation of the brain.

Symptoms: Fever, headache, general aches and pains, and often a stiff neck. Irritability and lethargy initially, then progressive loss of awareness and progression into coma. There may be convulsions and varying degrees of weakness or paralysis.

Cause: Most often, encephalitis is caused by a virus infection of the brain, and that infection sometimes also affects the meninges (producing meningitis). Some of the viruses are acquired by being bitten by an infected mosquito. Other forms of encephalitis result from other virus infections (measles, chickenpox, infectious mononucleosis, for example); immunizations (for example, pertussis, rabies); and toxins related to other infections (such as bacillary dysentery).

Severity of Problem: A potentially life-threatening problem that can leave permanent residual brain damage.

Contagious? Some forms are directly contagious, but most must be spread via a mosquito.

Treatment: There is no specific treatment for encephalitis. Often the symptoms arise because of increased pressure around the brain. It is now possible to reduce that pressure successfully and perhaps reduce the risk of permanent damage. Intensive medical care is needed.

Prevention: For many types of encephalitis, control of mosquitos is the primary goal. For others, there is no known prevention.

ENDOCARDITIS

Inflammation and infection of the lining and usually the valves of the heart by bacteria. The infection may be very acute, "subacute" (developing steadily over time) or chronic.

Symptoms: For the acute variety, sudden onset of high fever, chills and signs and symptoms of heart failure. For subacute or chronic endocarditis, the symptoms are more subtle: low-grade fevers, generalized fatigue, aches and pains, weight loss, poor appetite, night sweating, often without any indication that the infection is in the heart.

Cause: Infection of the heart lining or valve(s) with bacteria that reach the heart through the bloodstream and attach themselves to the lining or valves. There is almost always an underlying problem with the heart lining or valves (roughened surface, narrowing, congenital heart defect, arteriosclerosis). The bacteria usually originate in another part of the body and are introduced to the bloodstream through trauma: dental procedures and cleaning of teeth; introducing a catheter into an infected bladder; surgery on the bowel; procedures that involve inserting instruments into the rectum, infected bladder or esophagus; manipulating a site of skin or soft tissue infection (boil, pimple, etc.). People who have artificial heart valves are at special risk for this problem.

Severity of Problem: Always serious, often life-threatening if the infection is not promptly recognized and treated. Even with vigorous treatment, further damage to the heart may occur.

Contagious? No.

Treatment: Recognizing the problem and identifying the infecting bacteria is one of the most important aspects of treatment, because it enables the correct antibiotic to be used. Antibiotic treatment is required for weeks (six or more) and must be given intravenously. General support, treatment of heart failure and good nutrition are important. If there is an artificial heart valve in place, it may need to be removed or repaired to control the infection.

Prevention: People with known heart defects or valve problems should take antibiotics (usually penicillin) by mouth before, during and after dental work and other procedures that may lead to showering of bacteria into the blood. These people need ongoing medical treatment and supervision.

ENDOMETRIOSIS

Disorder in which endometrial tissue (the lining of the uterus) is found outside the uterus, growing on other organs and tissues. In a related disorder, called adenomyosis, endometrial tissue grows down into the muscles of the wall of the uterus.

Symptoms: Increasing problems with pain before and during menstrual periods and abnormal uterine bleeding, usually excessive menstrual flow. Pain with intercourse, especially for up to a week before and during periods, is common. Pain with bowel movements, especially around menstruation, may also occur.

Cause: Endometrial tissue moves from inside the uterus and attaches to other organs and tissues for no apparent reason. Normal hormone changes are responsible for the relationship of symptoms to menstrual cycles: The aberrant tissue swells in response to hormones, as if it were in the uterus.

Severity of Problem: The disease is progressive in most women and leads to infertility in many. Pain and bleeding can be severe.

Contagious? No.

Treatment: Pregnancy often reduces the symptoms and slows the progress of the condition, as can hormone therapy. When the disease is extensive, surgical removal of the abnormal tissue is effective, but it tends to recur. When the disease is very advanced or the woman is past the childbearing years, removal of the uterus, fallopian tubes and ovaries may be recommended. Radiation therapy can be successful when surgery is not possible but results in sterility.

Prevention: None known.

Discussion: Endometriosis usually affects women in their twenties and thirties and worsens over the reproductive years. It causes infertility in a considerable number of the women it affects, so many of them are advised to become pregnant as early as possible if they wish to have children.

EPIDIDYMITIS

Inflammation of the tube (epididymis) where sperm mature. This tube rises from the testis (protected by the scrotum) and directs the sperm into the vas deferens (where the sperm are stored).

Symptoms: Swelling, tenderness and often severe pain in the testis; the spermatic cord (at the underside of each testicle inside the scrotum) also becomes warm, tender and swollen; fever, chills and nausea may occur.

Cause: Usually bacterial infection and often secondary to a primary infection of the prostate gland.

Severity of Problem: Can be painfully disabling until treatment has been effective. Infection is always potentially serious, so prompt attention could avoid complications or any permanent damage.

Contagious? It is thought that some infections are transmitted through sexual contact.

Treatment: Intensive and rapid antibiotic therapy is vital to prompt recovery. Bed rest, scrotal elevation and support; application of ice packs to affected area; the use of pain medications, as needed.

Prevention: The use of a condom will prevent those cases due to sexual transmission of infection.

ESOPHAGITIS (PEPTIC OR REFLUX ESOPHAGITIS)

Inflammation of the esophagus, usually in its lower portion near the stomach, because of irritation by gastric acids and juices.

Symptoms: Heartburn, sensation of regurgitation of food and acid into the esophagus, especially after a heavy meal or when lying down. There may be episodes of regurgitation with choking and gasping during the night or while lying down. Later, pain on swallowing, especially with hot or cold foods, may appear.

Cause: Regurgitation of stomach contents into the esophagus because of increased pressure in the abdomen. This is likely to occur after heavy meals, in pregnancy or in those who are obese. It can also occur when the muscle between the esophagus and stomach (the sphincter muscle) is not as efficient as it should be. Smoking tends to make the situation worse, because it allows the sphincter muscle to be lax.

Severity of Problem: Can be a mild, occasional problem or chronic. Repeated episodes of inflammation and irritation of the lining of the esophagus lead to scarring of the lower esophagus. Sometimes, reflux (the regurgitation of the acid) during the night leads to chronic pneumonia if the regurgitated material is aspirated (inhaled).

Contagious? No.

Treatment: Staying in an upright position, especially after eating, will often prevent the regurgitation and heartburn. Eating small meals, using antacids is also helpful. Stop smoking; lose weight if obesity is a problem. Sometimes lying on the right side will help prevent regurgitation.

Prevention: Treatment or avoidance of regurgitation will prevent the irritation and inflammation of the esophagus.

Discussion: While heartburn is most often caused by reflux esophagitis or dietary indiscretion, repeated pain in the upper abdomen, even if related only to meals, should warrant a medical evaluation.

FAINTING (SYNCOPE)

State where a person nearly or totally loses consciousness. Fainting takes place when the blood supply to the brain is reduced. This can be due to many minor to major problems. True fainting lasts only a few seconds to a few minutes.

Symptoms: Sometimes person is white or pale and has cool, moist skin right before fainting. May also include nausea; dizziness; sense of weakness; sweating; giddiness; impaired vision; a feeling of faintness; and possible vomiting.

Cause: Many possible causes: emotional shock; tense situation; exhaustion; hyperventilation; severe pain; heat exhaustion; hypothermia (drop in body temperature due to severe cold); blood loss; head injury; exposure to noxious fumes; change in heart rhythm; middle-ear infection; breath-holding in children; anemia; cardiovascular disease; lung problems; hypoxia.

Severity of Problem: Depends on reason for fainting. If attacks repeat, medical evaluation should take place. Bodily injury may occur if person faints while standing and/or falls over sharp or dangerous object upon fainting.

Contagious? No.

Treatment: If person feels faint: Have him or her lie down and elevate feet 8 to 10 inches or sit down and place head between legs. If person has already fainted: Make sure he or she is in comfortable position and keep lying down until fully alert and feeling all right. If episode repeats: Seek medical evaluation so proper treatment can be given.

Prevention: Depends on underlying reason for fainting.

FARSIGHTEDNESS (HYPEROPIA)

Inability to clearly see things up close (reading, writing or objects close at hand).

Symptoms: Blurred, fuzzy vision or difficulty seeing objects up close. Distant and mid-distant vision is clear. Headaches, blinking, squinting, rubbing eyes and holding things at a distance may also be signals that an eye examination is necessary. This problem may appear in childhood. Some degree of farsightedness (called presbyopia) is a normal feature of aging.

Cause: The eyeball is too short, which results in difficulties in close (or near) vision.

Severity of Problem: Visual difficulty may be mild to severe and requires a professional examination.

Contagious? No.

Treatment: Corrective glasses remedy the visual difficulty.

Prevention: None. Each person is born with a certain eye shape and structure.

FIBROID TUMOR—UTERUS

So-called fibroid tumors of the uterus are actually myomas—benign (noncancerous) growths made up of muscle and supportive tissue. They can be found anywhere in the uterus (in the wall, on the outside, on the inside or on the cervix) or occasionally outside the uterus attached to another organ.

Symptoms: Many cause no symptoms and are found on routine examination because of enlargement of the uterus. Fibroids can cause excessive uterine bleeding during or between menstrual periods. Some are large enough to cause pelvic pain, discomfort with periods, dysmenorrhea, pain or discomfort with intercourse, or vaginal discharge, depending on their location. During pregnancy they can lead to miscarriage (spontaneous abortion) and difficulties with delivery because of abnormal position of the fetus or interference with the birth canal. They can also be associated with bleeding after delivery.

Cause: Unknown

Severity of Problem: Many fibroids cause no difficulty except enlargement of the uterus. Others may be large and multiple, with severe pain or bleeding. Infertility or repeated spontaneous abortions are possible.

Contagious? No.

Treatment: Surgery is the only effective treatment and is recommended when symptoms are severe. Removal of the tumors is very effective and does not usually interfere with future pregnancies. Hysterectomy (removal of the uterus) may be needed if the tumors are very large, or when women are beyond the childbearing years.

Prevention: None.

Discussion: The fibroid is the most common tumor of the female reproductive organs. Most women who have them have more than one. The size can vary from very small to massive.

FISSURE—ANAL

Break or crack in the skin around the anal opening.

Symptoms: Burning or pain around the anal opening with a bowel movement; spotty bright red bleeding with or after bowel movement. Constipation is common, both as a cause of the problem and as a result of the pain with bowel movements. A hemorrhoid may be present before or after the bleeding or pain.

Cause: Constipation with passage of large stools that tear the skin at the anus; diarrhea; hemorrhoids; tearing during childbirth.

Severity of Problem: Annoying but not serious. Blood loss is usually very slight, and infection is not common. However, anemia can worsen if constipation is not controlled.

Contagious? No.

Treatment: For pain relief, sitz baths and use of soothing or anesthetic ointments. Avoid further irritation from scratching. Develop regular bowel habits and avoid constipation. Softening of bowel movements by adding liquid to the diet, use of mineral oil or temporary use of glycerin suppositories if recommended by a doctor. Use of petroleum jelly or other lubricant may also be helpful. Surgery may be helpful if hemorrhoids are the problem.

Prevention: Avoid constipation and irritation of the anus.

Discussion: This problem is common at any age and is the most frequent cause of rectal bleeding in infants and young children. Fear of pain often leads to further constipation because of avoidance of having a bowel movement. In such cases, careful use of stool softeners and laxatives for a short period of time may be needed.

FLAT FOOT

Condition in which the arch of the foot at the instep is flattened, so the entire sole of the foot rests on the ground.

Symptoms: Most often there are no symptoms, except that a parent notices from infancy that a child's foot (or feet) is flat. With certain types of flat feet, there can be leg pains and cramps associated, because of muscle imbalance. Abnormal shoe wear and pressure marks on the feet from shoes can also be a problem.

Cause: The most common form of flat foot is a flexible or relaxed foot, in which all the structures are normal, but the foot is excessively relaxed. Therefore, the arch is visible when the person is sitting, but completely or partially collapses when he or she stands. Less commonly, there is a structural problem with the bones of the arch, so the foot never has a normal arch. Usually in this non-flexible kind of flat foot, there is pain as well as limited movement of the foot both up and down.

Severity of Problem: The amount of flatness is variable, with the normal baby having a flat foot until walking is well established. The foot can rest completely on the floor, or there can be a small arch. The non-flexible flat foot is usually painful and requires correction. This condition usually involves both feet, but the amount of flatness can vary.

Contagious? No.

Treatment: The flexible flat foot of the infant needs no correction except walking, preferably with soft, nonrestraining shoes. Later, if there is foot pain or leg cramping, a wedge on the sole of the shoe (called a Thomas heel) might be helpful. Arch supports inside the shoe for children are not usually helpful, except to make the foot look better. In adulthood arch supports may be helpful for a few people. If the flat foot is caused by a deformity in the bone structure of the foot itself, surgical correction is often needed.

Prevention: None. Walking early (for infants) does not increase either flat foot or bowlegs.

Discussion: Many people who have flat feet have no problems with them at all. There is no reason to spend excessive amounts of money on shoes for children in order to correct flat feet, unless recommended by a physician who knows your child.

FLATULENCE

Real or perceived increase in the amount of intestinal gas.

Symptoms: Feeling of bloating or needing to belch; passing much gas by rectum; intestinal discomfort, gurgling and occasional cramping pain. These may or may not be associated with an obvious cause.

Cause: Many possible causes, including air swallowing (very common);

ulcer disease; inflammation of the stomach, the intestine or the colon; abnormal movement of the intestines; anxiety; dietary indiscretion; food intolerance; and many others.

Severity of Problem: Can vary from mild and occasional to severe and constant, depending on the underlying cause.

Contagious? No.

Treatment: Depends on the cause, but might include treatment of underlying anxiety; calling the person's attention to air swallowing or sighing; correction of things that make a person mouth-breathe; adjustment of eating habits; decreasing liquids drunk with meals; and altering the diet to avoid foods that increase gas production. Medications, unless prescribed to treat an underlying disease, are usually not helpful.

Prevention: Depends on the cause. Often, attention to eating and swallowing habits, with slowing of eating and drinking, is all that is needed. In other people prevention can be more complex.

Discussion: A common cause of worry, increased gas is usually not indicative of a serious problem but rather is uncomfortable and embarrassing.

FLOATERS

Name given to dark spots seen moving in front of the eyes.

Symptoms: Black spots are seen, especially when a person looks at a light or white background. They move in position, seeming to "float" around in the eye.

Cause: Tiny particles normally found in the jellylike fluid inside the eye. These are seen as solid specks.

Severity of Problem: A normal, common finding.

Contagious? No.

Treatment: None needed.

Prevention: None.

Discussion: Sudden appearance of spots that are accompanied by blurry vision or pain in the eye require evaluation by an ophthalmologist. Likewise, a spot that does not move (stays in one place), affects only one part of the vision or seems to move in an orderly way across the eye requires immediate evaluation. (These are symptoms of hemorrhage in the eye or detachment of the retina and require care.)

FOOD POISONING (STAPHYLOCOCCUS GASTROENTERITIS)

Acute illness caused by contaminated food.

Symptoms: Inflammation of the stomach and small intestines results in stomach and intestinal pain and cramps, nausea, vomiting and diarrhea. Some people complain of profuse sweating or chills and overproduction of saliva. In more serious cases shock can even occur. The first symptoms appear 2 to 4 hours after eating the contaminated food. Symptoms generally begin abruptly and subside 4 to 24 hours later.

Cause: When staphylococcus (staph) bacteria infest food, they are capable of multiplying rapidly. The by-product of this multiplication of staph bacteria is a colorless, odorless and tasteless toxin. Once in the food, the toxin is there to stay. Cooking, boiling or reheating the food can destroy the staph bacteria, but not the toxin. Food is usually contaminated by a food handler who is a carrier of the staph bacteria or possibly has a staph skin infection.

Severity of Problem: Staph food poisoning rarely kills, but those with chronic illnesses, the very young and the elderly are more at risk for serious problems or even death. However, most people get fairly sick and feel weak and shaky for a while after the attack of food poisoning is over. A physician should be consulted in all cases of possible food poisoning. Dehydration and shock are always potentially dangerous, and it would be imperative to manage the food poisoning if it appears to be getting out of control. Other problems also mimic food poisoning; therefore, a diagnosis should be reached.

Contagious? No. The contaminated food must be eaten.

Treatment: As long as vomiting and nausea continue, food and liquids should be withheld. The person should be made as comfortable as possible: Lying on the side or on the stomach is usually best, and once the nausea and vomiting end, bland liquids help replenish the body fluids lost and assist in settling the stomach. Hospitalization and intravenous therapy may be required if the food poisoning is severe and dehydration is occurring.

Prevention: Care should always be taken when handling and preparing food. Foods should never sit out for long periods of time but should be refrigerated instead. It doesn't take much time for the staph bacteria to multiply and produce enough toxin to poison the food. Careful hand washing (soap and hot water) is also imperative when preparing and handling food.

Discussion: There are certain foods that are more easily contaminated by staph, and special care should be taken with them. These include mayonnaise (and anything with mayonnaise in it); cheeses and other dairy products, including sour cream; cream pies; and processed meats. Often food poisoning occurs at picnics or other large gatherings where food is not refrigerated for long periods of time. Sometimes, dinner leftovers can also be the culprits, because they were not put away right after dinner was completed. Upon eating the food later, someone experiences food poisoning. (Establishing the cause and effect is often difficult, since the original dinner did not make anyone sick because it was not contaminated—only the leftovers became infested.) If someone experiences a bout of food poisoning after eating in a restaurant,

the restaurant should be notified and the food eaten described.
See also BOTULISM.

FOREIGN BODY—ESOPHAGUS

Foreign body that is caught in the esophagus (the passage between mouth and stomach), usually high up near the throat.

Symptoms: Sudden onset of gagging and choking, with pain in the neck or throat and a sensation of something caught in the throat. If the object becomes lodged in the esophagus, continued difficulty with swallowing and inability to swallow solids may persist. Sometimes in children there are no particular symptoms other than the child's inability or unwillingness to eat solids. Vomiting or regurgitation may also occur.

Cause: Accidental swallowing of an object that is too large to fit through the esophagus or was not meant to be swallowed. This can happen if a person laughs or is surprised while carrying something in the mouth, or when eating carelessly or too fast. Adults most often swallow overly large pieces of food or bones, while children often swallow toys, coins and other objects.

Severity of Problem: Very uncomfortable, prevents swallowing of food. Occasionally a sharp object may penetrate the wall of the esophagus, causing inflammation and serious infection of the tissues of the chest.

Contagious? No.

Treatment: If there is no breathing difficulty and the sensation of something in the esophagus is present, trying to swallow a piece of soft bread or liquid may dislodge the foreign body. If there is no success, see a doctor. An X ray may help to locate an object, if the object is of a kind that can be seen on X ray. Removal of a foreign body usually requires a procedure called esophagoscopy, during which the doctor looks down the esophagus with a lighted tube and retrieves whatever has been swallowed.

Prevention: Avoidance of chewing and swallowing too fast or while preoccupied; keeping small objects out of the reach of small children.

Discussion: Most foreign objects in the esophagus become lodged in the neck region, which is the narrowest part of the gastrointestinal tract. If they pass this area, they will usually progress to the outside via the rectum in time.

FOREIGN BODY—IN THE AIRWAY (LARYNX, TRACHEA, BRONCHUS)

Accidental lodging of an object in the voicebox (larynx) or windpipe (trachea or bronchus).

Symptoms: Sudden choking, with varying degrees of difficulty breathing. Type of symptoms depends on the size of the foreign object and where it became lodged. For an object at the *larynx*: choking, harsh coughing, hoarseness, loud and harsh noise with breathing, and varying degrees of difficulty breathing. A large object caught at the voicebox may completely obstruct the airway, leading to total inability to breathe, cyanosis and collapse. Symptoms are similar for objects stuck in the *trachea*.

A smaller object is able to pass down the airway and may lodge in the *bronchus*, producing a different set of symptoms. At first, after the initial choking period, there may be no symptoms at all or the presence of a persistent, mild cough and wheezing. The object may go completely undetected, especially in children, for months, until an episode of pneumonia occurs, or the lung partially collapses. Recurrent pneumonia, especially in infants and children, can be due to a foreign body.

Cause: Fright, surprise or laughing while eating or drinking may all produce inhalation at the same time as swallowing. Material can then slip down the airway rather than down the esophagus. Infants and children, who constantly put things into their mouths, are particularly at risk. Adults who have been drinking alcohol or are weak or have problems with swallowing incoordination are also at risk and most often inhale large pieces of food.

Severity of Problem: Always potentially life-threatening. Foreign bodies in the larynx area are particularly likely to produce complete airway blockage if not removed. Objects caught in the bronchus are more likely to produce recurring pneumonia, especially if made of an irritating substance, such as plant products (seeds, nuts).

Contagious? No.

Treatment: If there is complete blockage of the larynx, with no air moving and the person turning blue, use the Heimlich maneuver or back blows and chest thumps (the techniques should be learned at a formal training class in CPR) until the obstruction is relieved. If airway obstruction is not complete and the person is having difficulty breathing, get emergency care immediately.

All foreign bodies in the airway must be removed promptly. This can usually be done through an instrument called a bronchoscope, which allows the doctor to look down the windpipe and grasp the foreign body. Removal of a nut or similar foreign body that has been in a bronchus for a long time can be very difficult.

Prevention: Avoid laughing and swallowing at the same time; take small bites of food. Do not hold small objects in the mouth. Avoid giving small children nuts and similar foods, as well as small toys that might be inhaled.

Discussion: Aspiration of a large foreign body with complete obstruction of the larynx or trachea is a potentially lethal accident. Since the development of the Heimlich maneuver and the widespread training of lay people in CPR and techniques of relieving airway obstruction, the death rate has decreased markedly. All teen-agers and adults should have formal training in CPR.

FROSTBITE

Form of cold injury known to cause tissue loss or damage.

Symptoms: Initial symptoms include pain, redness and tingling of the affected area. Area then becomes white and numb, and the pain disappears. Next the area becomes difficult to move and looks whiter and waxy (ice crystals are developing in the tissues—the skin, blood vessels, muscles and then in the bones).

Cause: Prolonged exposure to extremely cold temperatures. When an area of the body becomes very cold, the body tries to increase the blood flow to the endangered cold area to increase its temperature. As this fails, ice crystals form, reducing or stopping blood flow to the area. Without adequate oxygenation, tissues (cells) become endangered and eventually die. Alcohol consumption, fatigue, windchill and lack of good nutrition increase the possibility of injury. The very young and the elderly also tend to be more susceptible to frostbite.

Severity of Problem: Can be mild to very serious and usually depends on the length of exposure, the area affected and the extent of permanent tissue damage. Serious cases can result in loss of function or even amputation. All cases of frostbite should be seen and evaluated by a doctor.

Contagious? No.

Treatment: Rapid rewarming of the affected part or area (this is done indoors where heat and cold can be regulated). Warm water (between 100° F and 110° F) is used to immerse the area. Once defrosted, it must not be allowed to become cold again. Rewarming may cause pain and redness, and blisters may form over the few weeks following the frostbite.

Prevention: Much of the time, frostbite can be prevented by using good sense and preparing for the cold. Proper protection is the key to prevention: Wear warm clothing on all parts of body, including a warm hat; all small parts (toes and fingers) need added protection, such as warm mittens and waterproof gloves, warm socks and shoes resistant to wetness.

FUNGUS INFECTION—ATHLETE'S FOOT

Fungus infection of the skin of the feet.

Symptoms: Itching and burning of the skin of the feet, especially between the toes. Cracking, peeling and bleeding. May cause distortion of a toenail, with lifting of the nail if the infection is located under the nail.

Cause: Infection of the skin with one of several fungi. (A fungus is a microscopic plant that thrives in a warm, moist place on and under the skin.) Poor foot care and hygiene as well as excessive moisture also make the problem more severe.

Severity of Problem: A chronic, annoying and uncomfortable condition, but not serious.

Contagious? Slightly. May be acquired by contact with an infected person or by contact with towels, socks, etc., used by that person. Passage from one person to another in a shower or locker room, for example, is probably not significant.

Treatment: Keep the feet clean and dry. Wash and rinse the feet well, then dry well, especially between the toes. Use clean, dry socks, preferably cotton, and change them often. Change shoes often and allow them to dry between uses. Use an over-the-counter antifungal powder or cream as directed for mild to moderate athlete's foot. See your physician for severe cases. (A strong antifungal medication that is given orally may be needed but can only be taken under a doctor's supervision.)

Prevention: Keep feet clean and dry. Treat irritated, itchy areas between the toes as soon as they are noticed.

FUNGUS INFECTION—RINGWORM OF THE SCALP

Fungus infection of the scalp, usually seen in children before puberty.

Symptoms: Round patches on the scalp that are scaly and "bald." These patches may appear gray and, if looked at closely, are not actually bald but have broken hairs in them. There might be mild itching of the scalp.

Cause: Infection of the scalp and hairs with any of a number of surface fungi. The disease is acquired from other children (by sharing hats, etc.) or from infected household pets.

Severity of Problem: The infection can be very persistent, even in spite of treatment, but disappears at puberty. It can lead to an unusual reaction called a kerion, which is a large abscess with multiple areas that drain pus, located on the scalp. (This reaction is thought to be a sensitivity reaction to the fungus, not a sign of worse infection.)

Contagious? Yes, from person to person (by sharing hats, etc.) and from infected household pets.

Treatment: The infection needs to be treated with an antifungal medication taken by mouth for two weeks. Sometimes an antifungal cream or lotion is also helpful. See a doctor if ringworm of the scalp is suspected.

Prevention: Avoid contact with infected persons or animals. Teach children not to share hats. Inspect household pets regularly, especially when there are small children in the house, for signs of ringworm.

Discussion: Ringworm must be distinguished from other causes of patchy baldness, but this is not usually difficult, because the hairs are broken in ringworm rather than missing.

FUNGUS INFECTION—RINGWORM OF THE SKIN

Fungus infection of the skin, also called tinea corporis.

Symptoms: Appearance of round, scaling patches on the skin. The centers initially have tiny blisters, which clear, then the blisters spread in a ring from the center. Itching is usually very severe. There may be only a few or many patches, which usually appear on the arms and legs (the exposed areas of the body).

Cause: Skin infection with one of several fungi.

Severity of Problem: Usually not a serious problem but can spread to involve the scalp or the nails.

Contagious? The infection is often gotten from a household pet that is infected but can be passed from person to person by direct contact.

Treatment: The infection can be easily controlled and cured by taking a (prescription) medication, griseofulvin, by mouth and/or by using skin creams or lotions that are effective against the fungus.

Prevention: Avoid contact with infected pets or people.

Discussion: There are several types of rashes that produce circular skin lesions. See a doctor to help make the diagnosis and to obtain recommendations for treatment. Do not assume that a rash is ringworm. Household pets should be carefully checked for signs of skin infections and fungi and treated if necessary, particularly if there are young children in the house.

GALLSTONES (CHOLELITHIASIS)

Occurrence of hard, stonelike masses in the gallbladder.

Symptoms: In the early stages of formation, there are usually no symptoms. Abdominal discomfort, especially after eating a fatty meal, with occasional episodes of gassiness associated with pain in the right side of the abdomen under the ribs may occur. There may be one or more attacks of fever and chills, with jaundice along with these symptoms.

Cause: In most people the cause is not known. However, gall-stones are found more often in women who are middle-aged and older, certain groups of people (such as certain Indian tribes) and with certain diseases (such as diabetes, sickle-cell anemia and several other forms of hereditary anemia, inflammatory bowel diseases). For whatever reason the cholesterol and other substances found in the bile crystallize to form hard stones of varying sizes.

Severity of Problem: For some people there are no apparent problems, and they do not know they have gallstones. For others the effects can range from one mild episode of acute cholecystitis to severe chronic cholecystitis. If the stones move out of the gallbladder and block the common bile duct between the liver and intestine, serious problems can result.

Contagious? No.

Treatment: Surgery to remove the gallbladder and its stones is currently the only proven treatment. Sometimes medical treatment without surgery (diet control, certain medications that are thought to dissolve gallstones over a long period of time) can be tried.

Discussion: As many as 10 percent of men and 20 percent of women who are between 55 and 65 years of age have gallstones, which are a common problem of aging. There is controversy about whether all people with gallstones should have the gallbladder removed.

GASTRITIS

Inflammation of the stomach lining, which can be either acute or chronic.

Symptoms: Sensation of fullness in the upper abdomen, loss of appetite. In acute gastritis there may be fever, nausea and vomiting, as well as diarrhea and general aches and pains, depending on the cause. In chronic gastritis there may be intermittent burning pain, nausea and vomiting, intolerances to certain foods and anemia, or no symptoms at all.

Cause: *Acute gastritis* may be caused by dietary indiscretion, specific food intolerances, chemical irritants (especially aspirin and alcohol), food poisoning, or many types of viral or bacterial infections. *Chronic gastritis* is probably not very common (other diseases or conditions are often called gastritis, however) but can be associated with gastric ulcer, gastric carcinoma and pernicious anemia.

Severity of Problem: Usually bothersome and temporary.

Contagious? No.

Treatment: For acute gastritis removal of any irritants and rest of the stomach is usually all that is needed. Changing the diet to bland liquids and increasing what is eaten are usually curative. For chronic gastritis removal of any potential irritants (caffeine, alcohol, aspirin, tobacco, spices, specific foods that are not tolerated) and small, frequent meals may be of help. If there are underlying conditions (for example, pernicious anemia), these should be treated.

Prevention: Possible only when the cause is dietary indiscretion or indiscriminate use of alcohol, tobacco or caffeine.

Discussion: Probably many problems that are labeled chronic gastritis are actually due to such conditions as peptic ulcer disease and reflux esophagitis. Chronic or recurrent abdominal distress warrants a medical evaluation.

GASTROENTERITIS, ACUTE (INTESTINAL FLU)

Acute inflammation or infection of the intestinal tract, usually characterized by vomiting and/or diarrhea.

Symptoms: Sudden onset of abdominal pain or discomfort, which is usually mild to crampy; vomiting and nausea; diarrhea. There may or may not be fever. Symptoms are usually more severe in infants and children.

Cause: Usually thought to be due to a virus infection of the intestine, and many viruses that cause this kind of illness have been identified. However, it may be seen with infections of other parts of the body (for example, otitis media, urinary tract infection), especially in infants and children. If there is no fever, dietary indiscretion and/or poisoning (in children) must be considered.

Severity of Problem: Usually mild to moderate illness that resolves on its own. In infants, children and the elderly, can lead to dehydration if severe.

Contagious? Yes, the viral form is.

Treatment: Home treatment includes allowing the stomach and intestines to rest by avoiding solid food and irritating liquids. Water, dilute fruit juices, carbonated drinks and dilute punches in small amounts, given often, are usually tolerated. Bland foods in small amounts may also work well. If vomiting persists, or signs of dehydration occur, prompt medical help is required. Fluids may need to be given intravenously. (Signs of dehydration include reduction in or cessation of urination; dry, sticky lips and mouth; dry, sunken, listless eyes; doughy skin; listlessness and irritability.)

Prevention: When possible, avoid contact with persons who have gastroenteritis.

Discussion: Gastroenteritis usually involves both vomiting and diarrhea, although every person differs in how much of each is involved. When symptoms are particularly severe or persistent, other causes (such as bacillary dysentery or parasites) must be considered.

GIARDIASIS

Intestinal infection with a parasitic protozoan organism (a small, one-celled animal).

Symptoms: Although an infection may be completely without symptoms, many people with this problem have intestinal symptoms of abdominal pain and bloating, nausea, lack of appetite; diarrhea, either profuse and watery, or bulky, loose, greasy stools without blood or mucus; and general listlessness and feeling poorly. Diarrhea may last for a short time or become chronic. Malabsorption of food occurs in some people and can lead to weight loss and malnutrition.

Cause: Infection with the organism Giardia lamblia, which resides and multiplies in the duodenum (the upper small intestine). The parasite can be found either as the live protozoan stage or as the dormant cyst stage.

Severity of Problem: A very uncomfortable disease as the acute infection form, and the chronic diarrhea form (with malabsorption) leads to moderate to severe malnutrition, especially in children.

Contagious? Yes. Although most people get this infection from contaminated water, either from a city water supply or untreated water in recreation areas, it can be passed from person to person by direct contact. It passes through households and nursery schools quickly and has been transmitted by sexual contact (especially in male homosexuals). It is a particularly difficult problem for tourists. The organism is found in all areas of the world and in all climates.

Treatment: Once diagnosed, the infection can be treated with several possible medications. (All the medications have side effects that make them unpleasant to take, and they need to be taken under a doctor's supervision.)

Prevention: So far, it has not been possible to completely eradicate this organism from the water supply through usual methods. Treatment of all people who have the infection, whether they have symptoms or not, and treatment of household contacts helps control the spread from person to person.

Discussion: This is one of the most common of the intestinal parasites and is found in all areas of the world and among all types of people. Infants and children are particualrly susceptible. It can be very difficult to positively diagnose this parasite, even when it is suspected.

GINGIVITIS
Inflammation of the gums (gingivae).

Symptoms: Swelling and redness, tenderness of the gums at the base of the teeth. There may be bleeding with toothbrushing and later with chewing. Increasing swelling and inflammation lead to loosening of the teeth and full-blown periodontitis.

Cause: In most cases the gums are irritated by hard plaque (debris that forms at the base of the teeth, then hardens). Lack of good tooth cleaning (brushing, mouth rinsing, flossing) allows the problem to worsen. As inflammation and swelling increase, infection settles in. Some medications—phenytoin, used for seizures—make this problem particularly likely to occur.

Severity of Problem: Can be mild and uncomfortable or progress to serious periodontitis, which leads to tooth loss and chronic infection.

Treatment: Prompt care by a dentist to clean the plaque from the teeth. Afterward, vigorous toothbrushing, flossing and mouth rinsing, sometimes with water sprays, are important to keep the inflammation under control.

Prevention: Conscientious mouth care, including rinsing after eating, toothbrushing and flossing. Regular dental care. These measures are particularly important in people who must take Phenytoin.

Discussion: While poor dental hygiene is most often responsible for gingivitis and periodontal disease, some people develop it in spite of regular, conscientious care.

See also STOMATITIS—ACUTE;

GLAUCOMA—ACUTE
Sudden onset of increased pressure within the eye.

Symptoms: Sudden and severe pain in the eye, with blurred vision. The eye is intensely red and the pupil dilated. The cornea appears clouded.

Cause: Sudden blockage of the area at the side of the iris of the eye, which causes sudden, severe increase in the pressure inside the eye. This can result from sudden dilatation of the pupil, either because of drugs that dilate the pupil or for other reasons such as severe stress or a darkened room. In order for acute glaucoma to occur, the anterior chamber of the eye (the part between the iris—the colored part of the eye—and the cornea) must be more narrow than normal.

Severity of Problem: Leads to blindness if not corrected within several days.

Contagious? No.

Treatment: Requires immediate treatment by an ophthalmologist. Immediate reduction of the intraocular pressure (pressure within the eye) by using drugs that cause the eye pupil to get smaller and the pressure to go down. Surgery to remove part of the iris of the eye is done within a few days. If the pressure is reduced promptly, the risk for permanent visual damage is reduced.

Prevention: Avoid extreme dilatation of the pupils if a potential for this problem exists (if the anterior chamber of the eye—the part in front of the pupil and iris—is narrow). The potential for this problem can be detected through routine ophthalmological examination.

Discussion: Can be a complication of drugs used before anesthetic is given or to dilate the eyes. About 1 percent of people over 35 have a potential for this problem, although most of them never have an attack. Glaucoma can involve one or both eyes.

GLAUCOMA—CHRONIC

Consistent, chronic elevation of pressure inside the eyes, starting and developing gradually over a period of years.

Symptoms: Initially there are no symptoms. First symptom is gradual loss of ability to see to the sides and top, but with preservation of central vision. Gradually leads to tunnel vision. With very high pressures, people report seeing halos around lights.

Cause: The cause of the elevated pressure is not known, but the tendency to have glaucoma is inherited.

Severity of Problem: Leads to gradual loss of vision, which can progress to complete blindness over 10 to 30 years if not treated.

Contagious? No.

Treatment: Use of eye medications that keep the pupils of the eyes small, to increase the drainage of the fluid that is formed in the eye. Sometimes, other drugs that reduce the pressure are also needed. These must be used for life.

Prevention: There is no way to prevent the glaucoma itself, but early detection is critical to protection of vision. Periodic eye examination, which includes the measurement of intraocular pressure (pressure within the eye), measurement of vision and looking at the optic nerve through the ophthalmoscope, should take place every three to five years for all people over 20. People with a family history of glaucoma should have an examination every year.

Discussion: Glaucoma produces blindness because the elevated pressure within the eye presses on the arteries of the retina and the optic nerve, causing permanent damage. Unlike acute glaucoma, which can occur in one or both eyes, chronic glaucoma always involves both eyes. It has been estimated that there are about a million people with glaucoma, and one-fourth of these cases have not been detected.

GONORRHEA

A sexually transmitted disease and a serious public health problem. Approximately 720,000 cases reported yearly, but these do not in any way represent the total number of people infected each year (which is probably more like 2 million new cases).

Symptoms: Men experience burning with urination; irritation and pain; discharge from penis. Women usually have no symptoms or sign of infection. Unknowingly, then, they can have and transmit gonorrhea indefinitely. It is the required "reporting" system that may tell them they have the disease (for example, a male sees a doctor because he has symptoms and must report his sexual contacts).

Cause: Gonococcus bacteria that are transmitted by sexual contact.

Severity of Problem: Untreated gonorrhea may lead to further serious infection and to sterility in both men and women. Complications include arthritis, meningitis, septicemia and endocarditis—and women, besides the latter complications, may develop "pelvic inflammatory disease" (PID), a very serious infection. Gonorrhea can cause problems for the unborn child, so any pregnant woman who knows she has the disease or feels she may have contracted it should consult her physician immediately.

Contagious? Extremely.

Treatment: Once identified by a physician and verified by laboratory test, antibiotic therapy is 100 percent effective.

Prevention: Sexual contact (any type of genital contact) should be avoided with anyone who has the disease (even during the time of treatment). Routine use of a condom appears to be the best preventive measure for sexually active people.

Discussion: Honest and thorough "reporting" of all sexual partners is vital to alleviating the hideous complications that can occur as the disease festers.

Some professionals suggest periodic testing for gonorrhea in sexually active females, in particular, since symptoms do not occur. Once exposed to the infection, women have a much greater rate of getting the disease than men.

HEADACHE
Mild to severe and debilitating pain in the head.

Symptoms: The type of head pain experienced can often help in diagnosing the type of headache that is occurring. While many headaches are not particularly distinct, certain patterns are important. *Tension headaches* can be mild to painful and tend to feel like a constricting band has been wrapped in one or more directions about the head. *Migraine headaches* tend to feel throbbing or pulsating and can be quite debilitating when pain becomes severe. Often an "aura"—a set of symptoms that each person develops for seconds to minutes—occurs, along with one or more of the following: dizziness, nausea, vomiting and sensitivity to sound. *Cluster headaches* (also called histamine headaches) are usually one-sided and tend to occur when the person is relaxing (even asleep). These headaches tend to appear in clusters—a few times a day, often for many weeks (called a cluster period). There are then periods without any headaches (for days, weeks, months, years). While in a cluster period, the eating or drinking of anything with histamine in it will bring on a headache. *Other causes* of headache usually have distinct symptoms related to them, which can include blurring vision, other vision changes, nausea and vomiting, fever and nasal congestion.

Cause: There are many possible causes, including head injury or injury to the neck muscles and supporting structures (so-called whiplash); inflammation or infection of the structures of the head (sinusitis, meningitis, mastoiditis, tonsillitis); stress and anxiety (tension headache); changes in the size of the blood vessels (migraine headache, cluster headache); intoxicants, poisons; eye disorders; metabolic disturbances; and tumors or other causes of increased pressure inside the head. Persistent or severe headache requires a thorough medical evaluation in order to determine potentially serious causes of headache.

Severity of Problem: Pain can be nagging and mild, to very severe and incapacitating. Depends on cause, to a certain extent.

Contagious? No.

Treatment: Depends on cause, but general principles include rest, reduction of stress and stimulation, and use of pain relievers, varying in strength from aspirin or aspirin substitute to narcotics. Migraine headaches respond to certain medications (ergot preparations) that cause dilatation of the arteries. Migraine and cluster headaches can be prevented by taking a medication called methysergide. Indentification and treatment of the underlying cause of headaches is very important.

Prevention: Stress reduction is helpful for anyone with chronic headaches. Vascular headaches (migraine, cluster headaches) can be prevented by taking a drug, methysergide. Otherwise depends on cause.

Discussion: Headache is one of the most common symptoms and can be a response to almost any illness. Temporary, mild to moderate headaches probably should not cause undue alarm. However, particularly severe or recurrent headaches should always prompt a thorough medical investigation for a potentially serious, correctable cause.

HEART BLOCK

Block in the usual conduction pattern of heart impulses.

Symptoms: Can be none, or the patient may simply feel faint or actually faint.

Cause: The normal impulse conduction pattern is from the upper chambers (the atria) to the lower chambers (the ventricles) along specialized conducting tissue. The impulse conducted is basically electrical, thereafter causing contraction of the heart muscle and thereby pumping blood either to the next chamber or out of the heart to the body. A blockage in this conducting system can occur with age or infection or can result from drugs.

Severity of Problem: Can vary from no symptoms to long pauses without heartbeats and fainting or even death.

Contagious? No.

Treatment: Stop causative drug, if this is the problem. Application of appropriate medications or possible insertion of temporary or permanent pacemaker (an electrical source that makes the heart contract at a predetermined rate).

Prevention: None.

Discussion: A previously difficult problem in the aging population (particularly since medical therapy was ineffective). The advent of the pacemaker has now made therapy easy and effective.

HEART FAILURE (CONGESTIVE HEART FAILURE)

Ineffective pumping of the heart.

Symptoms: Shortness of breath at rest or with exertion; weakness; fatigue; ankle and abdominal swelling.

Cause: May be due to narrowing (stenosis) of valves, which doesn't allow the heart to completely empty (this results in backup in the lungs and elsewhere). The same results occur from failure of the cardiac muscle to contract forcefully enough. Heart failure may also be due to arrhythmias (see CARDIAC ARRHYTHMIA).

Severity of Problem: Requires medical evaluation and treatment. Can be a minor to quite serious problem.

Contagious? No.

Treatment: Medical treatment must be undertaken with diuretics and other medicines; valve abnormalities can be corrected surgically; heart muscle abnormalities are not amenable to surgical correction. Medical regularization of irregular beat or a pacemaker for slow beating may help the problem.

Prevention: Sodium (salt) intake restriction helps in controlling the problem.

HEAT EXHAUSTION

Excessive fluid and salt loss during particularly hot weather.

Symptoms: Occurs most often in hot weather. The set of symptoms include excessive sweating; cool, clammy skin; and sudden weakness and fatigue. Blurry vision, nausea, headache and dizziness may also be experienced. Extreme thirst and salt loss may occur. Exercise in hot weather makes one more susceptible to heat exhaustion.

Cause: Extreme heat coupled with excessive water and salt loss (through profuse sweating); eventual dehydration; inadequate fluid replacement; and inability to cool off.

Severity of Problem: If heat exhaustion gets out of control, heatstroke (a serious, life-threatening emergency) may occur. It is therefore imperative that steps be taken to avoid heat exhaustion and treat it immediately so a more serious problem does not arise.

Contagious? No.

Treatment: At the first signs of fatigue or weakness, immediate rest and replacement of fluids (in particular, water).

Prevention: Wear appropriate clothing to allow ventilation and evaporation for cooling purposes. Take special care to drink plenty of liquids (e.g., water) to maintain body fluids; assure adequate salt intake during hot weather; allow for frequent periods of rest and cooling down.

HEATSTROKE (HYPERPYREXIA, SUNSTROKE)

Serious, life-threatening emergency in which the body's temperature-regulation mechanism fails to work, most often during very hot weather.

Symptoms: Instead of sweating (releasing heat from the body) in hot weather, the person suddenly stops sweating, and the internal temperature rises to dangerous levels (well above 104° F). Skin becomes hot and dry. There is nausea; dizziness; headache; confusion; rapid heartbeat; breathing quickly; and sometimes listlessness; dehydration (depletion of body fluids); and drop in blood pressure. Eventually shock and collapse occur, and the brain and tissues essentially "cook" without prompt recognition and treatment.

Cause: Breakdown in the internal temperature-regulation mechanism and/ or excessive, unrelenting heat.

Severity of Problem: Life-threatening medical emergency. Death can occur suddenly if treatment is not prompt and aggressive.

Contagious? No.

Treatment: *At first signs of heatstroke*: The person must be immediately taken out of the heat (to a cool or shady area or an air-conditioned room); cool water should be poured over the person, and he or she must be encouraged to drink a substantial amount of water to replenish the body's fluids. *If symptoms persist*: Pack the person in ice or place loose ice over all areas of the body; immediately transport the person to an emergency facility either by paramedic, ambulance or private car (if necessary).

Prevention: Adequate water intake; periodic cooling-off periods in the shade or in an air-conditioned room; less activity or total inactivity (where indicated) on hot days with high humidity; cool and loose clothing should be worn; care should be taken to treat the first signs of a potential problem. Being overly cautious in this situation is prudent. Older people and young children are more at risk; they should be closely observed and care taken to prevent a potential problem.

HEMORRHOIDS (PILES)

Enlargement of the veins that are located just above and around the anal opening.

Symptoms: Initially, discomfort with bowel movement, protrusion of soft lumps around the anal opening and sometimes small amounts of bleeding with bowel movements. When severe, there can be chronic infection, itching, loss of control of bowel movement and chronic bleeding. The hemorrhoids may always be protruding outside the rectum, and the tissue may get caught there, causing sudden acute pain.

Cause: Enlargement of the veins of the rectum and anus is caused by many factors that are responsible for increased pressure inside the abdomen or on the rectum. These include pregnancy and delivery, prolonged constipation with straining to have a bowel movement, infection around the anal opening, liver disease and prolonged sitting.

Severity of Problem: Can be a very mild, intermittent problem or a serious one, with prolonged bleeding, discomfort and development of complications.

Contagious? No.

Treatment: For mild problems control of constipation and reducing friction against the hemorrhoids by softening stool is effective. This can be done by adding more liquid to the diet, reducing roughage in the diet and use of mineral oil or other laxatives, if recommended by a doctor. (Chronic use of laxatives is potentially harmful.) Soothing sitz baths, local ointments and careful cleansing without scrubbing and scratching are helpful. Try to avoid using hemorrhoid creams with anesthetics in them, because they can cause local skin irritation and allergy.

Severe hemorrhoids or those that bleed continuously or otherwise cause trouble should be surgically removed. There are many possible ways for this to be done, depending on the seriousness of the problem.

Prevention: If possible, avoid constipation by assuring regular bowel habits; avoid prolonged straining; take care to see a physician if symptoms are observed, so serious problems may be prevented by early management.

Discussion: A very common, bothersome condition that affects a large part of the population. Most of the time, the problem is nagging but mild. If bleeding is a symptom, however, always see a physician to be sure that hemorrhoids (and not another, more serious problem) are the cause.

HEPATITIS

Inflammation of the liver.

Symptoms: Severe loss of appetite, nausea and vomiting, fatigue. Abdominal discomfort or pain, jaundice (yellow skin color). Fever is common in the infectious forms, as is a particular aversion to cigarette smoking.

Cause: Several groups of causes, including viral infections, alcohol and other drugs, and toxic substances.

Severity of Problem: Hepatitis is usually a disease that lasts weeks to months. It may slowly disappear, leaving little permanent damage, or progress to cirrhosis and scarring. One form, called fulminant hepatitis, or acute yellow atrophy, leads to death rather quickly because of overwhelming liver failure.

Contagious? The infectious (viral) forms are.

Treatment: There is no specific treatment for any of the forms of hepatitis. Rest, avoidance of anything (especially alcohol) that will add further injury to the liver cells and a diet that is high in carbohydrates and contains adequate calories.

Prevention: Depends on the cause.

Discussion: While infection and alcohol are by far the most common causes of hepatitis, toxic hepatitis due to environmental toxins (like carbon tetrachloride, for example) and many drugs must be considered as possible causes whenever a person has symptoms that suggest hepatitis. Try to avoid unnecessary exposure to toxic drugs and chemicals.

HEPATITIS—ALCOHOLIC

Inflammation of the liver caused by the toxic effects of alcohol poisoning and abuse.

Symptoms: As with other forms of hepatitis, severe loss of appetite, nausea and vomiting, with onset of jaundice are the hallmarks of the disease. There is abdominal pain and tenderness in the upper right side. This group of symptoms often follows a bout of heavy drinking in a person who has been a chronic drinker.

Cause: Damage to the cells of the liver by alcohol, which is a poison. Certain people who drink heavily are more susceptible than others, especially women. While it usually occurs only after years of heavy drinking, alcoholic hepatitis can occasionally appear after only a year or two of alcohol abuse. Nutrition has been thought to play a part, but this is still unclear.

Severity of Problem: While alcoholic hepatitis can, in unusual situations, resolve without leaving significant liver damage, it most often progresses to scarring and cirrhosis of the liver. A severe case can lead to serious involvement of the brain and deterioration within days or weeks.

Contagious? No.

Treatment: General support, including providing adequate nutrition, either by mouth or by vein, is very important, as is complete avoidance of alcohol. Rest and prevention or prompt treatment of any stomach bleeding that might occur are also important.

Prevention: Avoidance of heavy alcohol use. Once alcoholic hepatitis has occurred, complete avoidance of alcohol is important if further damage is to be prevented.

HEPATITIS—VIRAL

Inflammation of the liver due to infection with one of a number of viruses known to cause this problem. There are several distinct types of viral hepatitis.

Symptoms: The early phases of hepatitis seem similar to any other viral illness, including "flu." There is fever, general aches and pains, nausea and vomiting, sometimes sore throat and headache. Loss of appetite is very severe, often way out of proportion to the amount of illness, and cigarettes taste especially bad. After about a week the fever falls, and jaundice appears, along with abdominal discomfort, especially in the right upper abdomen. The stools may appear light in color and the urine dark yellow or brown. There is profound fatigue and weakness, often accompanied by weight loss because of the loss of appetite and vomiting.

Cause: This type of hepatitis is caused by infection of the cells of the liver by certain viruses. There are several distinct types of hepatitis, based on both the course of the disease and the viruses that are found. *Hepatitis A*, previously called "infectious hepatitis," appears about two to six weeks after contact with someone who has it and lasts for several weeks to several months. *Hepatitis B*, previously called "serum hepatitis," appears six weeks to six months after contact and can last much longer, with a person carrying the virus for months to years. A recently recognized type of hepatitis, called *non-A, non-B hepatitis*, is known to be caused by a virus, but not by the previously indentified kinds. Hepatitis can also be caused by viruses that produce other diseases, such as infectious mononucleosis and cytomegalovirus disease.

Severity of Problem: Hepatitis is always a potentially serious disease that can progress to chronic hepatitis or permanent liver damage. It is also a public health hazard, because it is quite contagious and is often transmitted to others before a person knows he or she is ill.

Contagious? Yes, all forms of viral hepatitis are contagious. Hepatitis A virus is found in the stool and urine and is passed by contact with contaminated food. It is contagious for as long as two weeks before a person is ill and for several weeks after that. Hepatitis B is most often passed from one person to another through blood transfusions or shared drug paraphernalia but can also be transmitted through sexual contact and in saliva. (Hepatitis B is a particularly difficult disease among male homosexuals.) Hepatitis B is prevalent in certain groups of Orientals and can be passed from a carrier or infected mother to an unborn or newborn infant. Non-A, non-B hepatitis is transmitted through blood transfusions and is the most common cause of post-transfusion hepatitis.

Treatment: There is no specific treatment for viral hepatitis. Rest, avoidance of strenuous activity, a well-balanced, adequate diet and avoidance of substances that can further injure the liver (alcohol, certain drugs) are important.

Prevention: All forms of viral hepatitis are preventable by avoiding contact with persons who have the disease, especially by avoiding contact with their secretions. However, this is often not practical. While screening of donated blood will identify certain forms of hepatitis (hepatitis B), other forms cannot yet be identified. Injection of gamma globulin is helpful for people who have had known household exposure to someone with hepatitis A. There is a vaccine available (licensed in 1982) for use in people with particular risk for hepatitis B.

Discussion: Hepatitis in infants and children (especially hepatitis A) can be a "silent" illness—that is, the child may have what looks like intestinal flu (acute gastroenteritis) without ever becoming jaundiced. It is only when adults in the household become ill with jaundice that the real disease is identified. Hepatitis A is easily spread in group-care situations where babies are not yet toilet-trained.

HERNIA—HIATUS

Protrusion of abdominal contents, usually a portion of the stomach, through a gap in the diaphragm.

Symptoms: A sensation of fullness or pain behind the breastbone, especially after eating; heartburn and chest or upper abdominal pain are common. Symptoms commonly occur after a large meal or if there is pressure on the abdomen. Problem may be accentuated by lying down.

Cause: Protrusion of part of the stomach or abdominal contents through a gap in the diaphragm, often appearing in middle or old age. The potential gap may have always been present but did not cause symptoms. Anything that increases the pressure inside the abdomen will tend to push the abdominal contents into the chest.

Severity of Problem: Can lead to severe pain or discomfort, as well as to esophagitis if acid repeatedly spills up into the esophagus. Severe chest pain can cause justified worry about heart disease. Some people with this problem repeatedly regurgitate food and liquid, especially at night, and have chronic aspiration and pneumonia.

Contagious? No.

Treatment: Eating small, bland meals and staying upright after eating usually help prevent the pain of the hernia's becoming stuck. Avoiding caffeine, tobacco and alcohol tends to reduce the amount of acid produced and thereby reduces the discomfort if regurgitation is a problem. Surgery may be necessary in severe cases where food intake is not possible.

Prevention: None known.

HERNIA—INGUINAL

Protrusion of intestine or other abdominal contents through a gap in the muscles and tissues of the groin. The protruding mass can usually be felt in the groin or in the scrotum and may be large or small.

Symptoms: Swelling in the groin and/or scrotum, usually without discomfort if small. As the hernia becomes larger, it may cause a feeling of dragging in the groin or scrotum. Swelling may come and go, change in size.

Cause: Failure of the normal gap between tissues in the groin to close. The opening is normal in fetal life, especially in males, because the testicles needed to descend down through it. With increased pressure inside the abdomen, the intestine is pushed down through the gap, leading to swelling of the testicles. This may result from injury or straining.

Severity of Problem: A nagging problem that requires surgical correction. In infancy there is a significant risk for the hernia to incarcerate (get stuck in the gap), leading to probable damage to the bowel itself.

Treatment: Surgical repair is the only truly effective treatment and should be planned whenever an inguinal hernia is discovered in a young boy. Sometimes older men find the use of a trusslike device helpful.

Prevention: Probably no measures are effective.

Discussion: Inguinal hernias are more common in boys than in girls. They are also very common in babies who were premature and in families where hernias have occurred. Because of the tendency of hernias to incarcerate (get stuck), a lump or swelling in the groin should always prompt a thorough investigation.

HERPES SIMPLEX TYPE 1 (COLD SORE, FEVER BLISTER)

Acute, recurring viral infection in and around the mouth and face.

Symptoms: Painful blisters in or around the mouth, often on the lips. Cluster of small, water-filled blisters that can occur once or frequently. After several days, a crust forms and lasts for one to two weeks. Can involve other areas of the body, but usually occurs above the waist. Can cause inflammation and ulcers of the cornea of the eye (keratitis).

Cause: Infection with the virus Herpes simplex type 1. This virus lies dormant in the cells after the first infection and can reactivate to cause recurrent infections in the future.

Severity of Problem: A very painful, bothersome problem, usually with no serious consequences. Rarely causes brain inflammation (called encephalitis), especially in infants and children.

Contagious? Yes, through contact with the fluid from the blisters.

Treatment: No known cure. Some of the symptoms may be alleviated or lessened by use of a prescribed cream or ointment. Research continues to look for a cure, and there are frequent claims of success.

Prevention: Only by avoiding close contact (that is, kissing, sharing eating utensils, etc.) with people with active blisters. Some people seem more susceptible to this infection when exposed than others.

Discussion: The Herpes simplex 1 virus lives in the cells around the mouth after the first infection and is often dormant (inactive) for long periods of time. Such factors as fever, another type of infection, sun exposure, stress, tension and even menstrual periods have been associated with causing the virus to become active again (new blisters appear).

The first Herpes type 1 infection in young children is a very painful, serious disease. There is high fever for three to six days, with extensive, very painful ulcers in the entire mouth (called herpetic stomatitis). There is no cure, and treatment consists of pain relief and making sure the child drinks plenty of liquid. The major risk is of dehydration because of refusing to drink.

HERPES SIMPLEX TYPE 1—HERPETIC KERATITIS

Inflammation of the conjunctival membranes of the eye due to infection with herpes virus. Keratitis refers to inflammation of the cornea of the eye (the thin membrane over the pupil).

Symptoms: At the start, not very different from other forms of conjunctivitis: excessive tearing, redness, mucus in the eye, swelling of the lids, pain and irritation of the eye. Rapid development of the feeling of something in the eye and light sensitivity, then blurred vision. After a short time with corneal inflammation, the intense pain disappears, and the eye is not sensitive to pain.

Cause: Infection of the eye tissues, especially the cornea, with the Herpes simplex virus.

Severity of Problem: Inflammation of the conjunctiva alone is usually not serious and may be the first form of the disease. If not treated correctly, it can become a very serious disease that can lead to blindness. It, like other herpes infections, can cause further inflammation with later flare-ups and causes a particular type of ulcer (called dendritic ulcer).

Contagious? Yes, although not all people who get the virus from the infected person will get conjunctivitis or keratitis.

Treatment: *This disease must always be treated by a physician, usually an ophthalmologist.* Antiviral drugs (several available) can be used several times a day. If healing does not begin rapidly, surgery may be necessary to remove the debris from the mucous membranes.

Prevention: Avoid contact with people who have herpes virus flare-up (those with cold sores and fever blisters).

HERPES SIMPLEX TYPE 2 (GENITAL HERPES)

Painful, recurrent virus infection, with blisters or ulcers on or near the genital area. A sexually transmitted disease.

Symptoms: Water-filled blisters that may crust over or become ulcers, located on or near the genitals (penis in males and vulva or vagina in females). First infection is usually intensely painful and lasts one to three weeks. Recurrent episodes may not be as painful and may go unnoticed.

Cause: Infection with Herpes simplex type 2 virus. A sexually transmitted (venereal) disease except in newborn infants, who can contract the virus either while in the uterus or during vaginal delivery.

Severity of Problem: Intensely painful, but usually not otherwise a problem in the adult. However, can be insidious and life-threatening for the unborn or newborn baby if contracted from the mother near or during delivery.

Contagious? Yes. Extremely contagious when disease is active (blisters present). Transmitted by contact with blister fluid.

Treatment: No known cure or effective treatment. Pain relief is sometimes necessary (physician prescription), and sitz baths may be helpful. Encouraging research developments are on the scene for effective treatment. Antiviral drug treatment is available and is partially successful for generalized herpes infection in the infant.

Prevention: Avoid sexual contact with a person who has active herpes (lesions present). Use of condom protection even when the virus is inactive is highly recommended to prevent transmission to either partner. (Often the active virus is in an unseen area, so protection is advisable even without symptoms.)

Discussion: Genital herpes is the most common sexually transmitted disease today. It is at an epidemic level. The virus usually resides in the tissues of the genital tract and can live dormant (inactive) for long periods of time. Most commonly, lesions are located on the genitals, but can occur on the skin below the waist.

Since the unborn/newborn is at great risk for problems, the pregnant woman with genital herpes must be followed closely. It is imperative that her personal physician be aware that she has genital herpes or has any reason to believe that she may have come into contact with someone who does have the virus.

HERPES ZOSTER (SHINGLES)

Painful eruption of blisters that are caused by the same virus that causes chicken pox.

Symptoms: Chills, fever and general bodily weakness are present several days before the watery blisters appear. Blisters are located on one area of the skin and are sometimes in a line.

Cause: The varicella-zoster virus. Shingles are the reactivation of chickenpox virus that has been inactive but is still present in certain nerve cells.

Severity of Problem: Shingles last from 10 days to 5 weeks and can be very painful. The disease usually lasts longer in adults (especially the elderly) than in children. If all of the blisters appear within 24 hours, the length of the disease is shortened.

Contagious? Yes. Requires direct contact with blisters. Shingles can cause chickenpox in persons who have never had it.

Treatment: Pain medication prescribed by a doctor is usually needed. Try to make the person as comfortable as possible and keep rash clean and dry to prevent additional infection.

Prevention: None.

HICCUPS

Rhythmic contraction of the diaphragm (the muscle between the abdomen and the chest), causing sudden, noisy escapes of air.

Symptoms: Sudden onset of forceful hiccups, lasting for short or long periods of time. When hiccups persist for hours to days, they can cause exhaustion and soreness of the muscles of the abdomen.

Cause: Rhythmic reflex contraction of the diaphragm, caused most often by irritation of the nerve that controls it. This irritation can result from many possible factors, such as eating too rapidly; eating spicy or irritating foods; swallowing air, causing over-expansion of the stomach; peptic esophagitis; ulcer; anxiety; and many other generalized problems (nervous system problems, liver disease, kidney failure, certain infections).

Severity of Problem: Most incidents of hiccups occur in healthy people, last for only a few minutes and are embarrassing and a nuisance but not a serious problem. In a few unfortunate people, they can persist for hours, days, weeks, months or years. In these people a careful search for unusual causes is needed. They are extremely common in young infants and should not cause worry.

Contagious? No.

Treatment: Many things have been tried with varying success: breath-holding, distraction, sudden scares, drinking water. Most often the hiccups go away in a short time, regardless of what is done. For severe, long-lasting hiccups, medical evaluation and treatment (for the underlying problem as well as for the hiccups) is needed. Sedative drugs, antacids, and medications that reduce intestinal movement are most often tried. On rare occasions surgery to cut the nerve that supplies the diaphragm is needed.

HYDROCELE

Fluid-filled cyst in the scrotum.

Symptoms: Painless enlargement of the scrotum, on one or both sides. The scrotum is filled with fluid, and the testicles are surrounded by this fluid collection.

Cause: Often present in newborn babies, because of persistence of a space through which the testicle descended into the scrotum. Later in life, it may result from overproduction of fluid because of inflammation of the testicle or after injury to the scrotum. (Blood in the scrotum can also result from injury.)

Severity of Problem: Swelling is usually small and does not produce difficulty. Hydrocele may be associated with a hernia.

Contagious? No.

Treatment: Many hydroceles, especially in young infants, disappear with time. Large collections of fluid may need to be removed by surgery. Hydroceles that are found along with hernias need to be repaired. Surgery may be recommended if there is any question about whether the swelling is a tumor or a fluid collection.

Prevention: Usually none.

HYPERLIPIDEMIA

Elevated blood levels of fats (lipids), of which cholesterol is one.

Symptoms: None due to the elevated fat levels alone.

Cause: May be related to dietary intake of fats or to a family tendency to high blood lipids.

Severity of Problem: Controversial. A risk factor in coronary artery disease.

Contagious? No.

Treatment: May benefit from limitation of foods containing high levels of saturated fats. Certain drugs may be helpful in lowering blood lipids.

Prevention: Limitation of amount of saturated fats in the diet.

HYPERTENSION

High blood pressure.

Symptoms: May have no symptoms, or there may be headache and fatigue.

Cause: Can be seen with kidney disease or rarely with correctable deformities or hormone-secreting tumors. Most commonly, the cause is unknown—"essential hypertension." The heart must contract very forcefully to pump blood against very high resistance in the blood vessels. Runs in families.

Severity of Problem: Can be mild with few long-term effects or with secondary damage to organs.

Contagious? No.

Treatment: Other than the rare curable types of hypertension, high blood pressure usually requires both treatment with drugs and restriction of sodium (salt) in the diet.

Prevention: Reduced salt intake is thought to reduce the likelihood of developing high blood pressure.

Discussion: High blood pressure is a very common medical problem associated with long-term harm to various organs (the brain, kidneys and heart). People with poor blood pressure control have increased incidence of stroke, heart attack and kidney failure. If blood pressure can be brought under effective control with medication and diet, there is good reason to continue that regimen.

HYPERTHYROIDISM (THYROTOXICOSIS)

Overactivity of the thyroid gland, with overproduction of thyroid hormone.

Symptoms: Weakness, tremors, sweating, weight loss in spite of a ravenous appetite, and nervousness. Heat intolerance can be profound. Rapid and irregular heartbeat, diarrhea and warm, moist skin all are indicators that the body metabolism has speeded up. The eyes may protrude (exophthalmos), and the person may tend to stare. There may be blurred or double vision. The thyroid gland is usually enlarged (goiter).

Cause: Most often the cause is unknown and associated with the enlargement of the thyroid gland and exophthalmos (a disease called Grave's disease). Other causes include tumors that secrete thyroid hormone, tumors of other endocrine glands and inflammation of the thyroid gland.

Severity of Problem: The eye complications are potentially serious if the disease is not controlled, and heart problems can be persistent and severe. Complications of treatment are also possible and depend on what type of treatment is used. Certain people with thyrotoxicosis go on to have other endocrine difficulties.

Contagious? No.

Treatment: The goal of treatment is to reduce the amount of thyroid hormone that is being produced. This can be done with medications that suppress or destroy the thyroid gland, irradiation (in the form of radioactive iodine) or surgery to remove the overactive gland. Often a combination of these is used. Treatment is very complicated and depends on the individual.

Prevention: Probably none.

Discussion: Hyperthyroidism most often appears in women between 20 and 40 years of age. Grave's disease progresses in some people, even if the thyroid overactivity has been controlled. Hypothyroidism (underactivity of the thyroid gland) is a common result of treatment.

HYPOGLYCEMIA
Abnormally low blood sugar.

Symptoms: Tremulousness, sweating, irritability and restlessness; feeling of extreme hunger; headache and nausea; chronic fatigue and weakness. With severe hypoglycemia the person may lose consciousness.

Cause: There are many possible causes. Hypoglycemia that occurs after the person has been *fasting* for several hours may be related to having too much insulin, either because the pancreas is secreting too much or because there is a tumor that is secreting insulin; certain liver diseases; and certain endocrine conditions. Low blood sugar that occurs *after meals* can have multiple causes: That which happens within two or three hours (called *reactive hypoglycemia*) results from rapid passage of carbohydrates from the stomach into the intestine and may follow surgery on the intestine. It can also occur in certain people without apparent cause. So-called *late hypoglycemia* (four to six hours after ingestion of a high-carbohydrate meal) is considered evidence of a prediabetic condition. Another form of hypoglycemia occurs in people who have had a large amount of *alcohol* to drink, either without eating or along with very high quantities of sugar-containing mixes.

Severity of Problem: Potentially life-threatening if severe drop in the blood sugar occurs, because of loss of consciousness. Lack of sugar supplied to the brain over long periods of time can lead to brain damage.

Contagious? No.

Treatment: Depends on the cause, but almost all types respond to a balanced diet that is relatively low in carbohydrates and high in protein, eaten in small, frequent meals.

Prevention: Depends on cause.

Discussion: There are certain people who seem to have symptoms that are similar to those seen in hypoglycemia but have normal tests of glucose metabolism. These people tend to be anxious and may or may not respond to dietary changes.

HYPOTHERMIA

Serious decrease in the body temperature that can be life-threatening.

Symptoms: Initial symptoms: Weakness, slurred speech, confusion, shivering and clumsiness. Progressive symptoms: Weakness is replaced by stiff muscles; the person feels unable to move; drowsiness and sleepiness occur.

Cause: The body is no longer able to conserve heat, and the body temperature falls rapidly. High risk: Swimming or other water activities (where water is below 50° F); mountain climbing; skiing; other activities that couple cold, wetness and wind with exertion and sweating; being out in the cold weather without proper protective clothing (must provide both warmth and protection from wetness). The very young and the elderly must take careful precautions. Also, drunkenness, exhaustion, hunger, disease and illness are things that make people at greater risk for hypothermia.

Severity of Problem: Severe hypothermia is a major medical emergency and requires prompt action. Death can occur rapidly if steps are not taken to reverse the process.

Contagious? No.

Treatment: It is critical to stop the process immediately: Remove all wet clothing (it retains the cold and wetness); if possible, rewarm the body with whatever is available (dry clothing, towels, blankets, jackets, sweaters, even paper); use the warmth (body heat) of others; and a warm (not hot) bath is helpful. The person should be seen by a doctor as soon as possible.

Prevention: Wear proper clothing (both warm and waterproof) when going out into cold or wet weather. Be extra cautious when this involves exercise that causes sweating or over-exertion. A hat is always a good idea, since a great deal of heat loss is by means of the exposed head. At the first signs of hypothermia, take steps to reverse the process.

HYPOTHYROIDISM

Underactivity of the thyroid gland, with deficiency of thyroid hormone.

Symptoms: Symptoms depend on the time of onset. In *infants and chil-*

dren: Failure to gain weight; failure to grow in height; hoarse cry; poor appetite; sluggishness; pot belly; dry, coarse skin; constipation; and mental retardation. In *older children*: Failure in school, sluggishness and anemia may be seen. In *adults*: Sluggishness, cold intolerance, weakness, fatigue, hoarseness and disturbances of menstruation, usually excessive menstrual bleeding. In the later stages of the disease: heart failure, extreme puffiness; dry, pale or yellow skin; weight gain; and constipation. Enlargement of the thyroid gland—called a goiter—may or may not be present in any age group.

Cause: In infants failure of the thyroid gland to develop or its destruction or failure to produce thyroid hormone due to a variety of causes. In adults the gland has either been destroyed or is deteriorating for any number of reasons.

Severity of Problem: In infants and children, can lead to permanent mental retardation and growth failure if not recognized and treated promptly. In adults the primary complication of non-treatment is heart failure, which can lead to early death. A rare complication called myxedema coma is life-threatening.

Contagious? No.

Treatment: For all types treatment with thyroid hormone in the amounts that would usually be produced by the body is basic. With the correct amount of hormone, the hypothyroid person will return to normal in activity and appearance very quickly. Most people with hypothyroidism require medication with thyroid hormone for the rest of their lives.

Prevention: Avoidance of thyroid-suppressing medications during pregnancy (to prevent congenital hypothyroidism, called cretinism); otherwise, probably none.

Discussion: There are many people who are treated with thyroid hormone for somewhat shaky reasons. If there is no hypothyroidism, the body will slow down or stop producing thyroid hormone when thyroid medication is administered. Not only is this not necessary, but it may be harmful because of the potential for complete suppression of thyroid production. Newborn screening procedures are now used to try to detect congenital hypothyroidism, so infants can be treated quickly and mental retardation can be prevented.

IMMUNIZATION (VACCINATION)

Way of preventing disease by giving a person a small dose of a material derived from a bacterium or virus that causes a particular disease, so the body can make immunity against it.

Common Vaccines: There are vaccines available that prevent many of the more common so-called childhood diseases. These vaccines are usually given to infants and children at recommended times, when their bodies are able to make immunity against the particular diseases. Some of the vaccines produce what seems to be long-term immunity, while others need "booster" doses to keep up the immunity. While each of the usual vaccines has known risks and complications, the overwhelming recommendation of the American Academy of Pediatrics and the Center for Disease Control of the U.S. Department of Health is that children should be routinely immunized. The following are the commonly used vaccines in childhood, with recommendations for when they are given and their usual side effects.

Diphtheria, tetanus and pertussis (whooping cough) (DTP) is a vaccine that must be injected into the muscle. The first dose is usually given at 2 months of age, and repeat doses are administered at 4 months, 6 months, 18 months and 5 years of age. The injection is avoided if a baby is ill with fever or if there is suspicion of a serious nervous system problem. Reactions to the vaccine include a sore injection spot, irritability or sleepiness, fever and general crankiness for 24 to 48 hours. More severe reactions, with high fever (over 103°F) or convulsions, are usually the result of a reaction to the "P" (pertussis) portion, which is then left out of the subsequent immunizations.

Polio vaccine is usually given as trivalent oral vaccine (Sabin) in the United States, but the killed virus vaccine (Salk) is used frequently in other parts of the world. The oral vaccine is a living but modified virus and actually sets up a mild case of polio in order to stimulate the body's immunity. There are no known immediate reactions, but a very rare (less than one case in 3 million doses of vaccine) case of vaccine-associated polio occurs. Oral polio vaccine is given twice in the first year of life, usually at 2 and 4 months, with a booster at 18 months and again at 5 years. Injections of killed Salk vaccine have no significant side effects and are given as injections at the same time as the DTP (2, 4, 6 and 18 months of age, with boosters needed every few years). This vaccine can be used for adults, while the oral vaccine is usually not recommended for adults.

Vaccines against measles, mumps and rubella are usually given as a single combined injection at 15 months of age or afterward. Only one injection is required, based on studies so far. Vaccines against each of these diseases can be given separately if needed. The vaccines contain living, modified viruses, which set up a minor case of the disease. Side effects from the mumps portion are not known. The measles portion can cause a mild illness with fever and rash about a week after the vaccine was given. The rubella portion can cause mild aches and pains, with joint pains and swelling several weeks after the immunization. (This is the same reaction that can be seen with the disease rubella, especially in adult women.) Rubella vaccine is recommended for all women of childbearing age who are not immune to rubella, as long as pregnancy can be prevented for several months after it has been given. Mumps vaccine can be given to adults, usually males, who have not had the disease.

Specialized Vaccines: Certain vaccines are available or being tested for special situations in which certain groups of people are at particular risk for a given disease. Some of these include the following: *pneumococcal vaccine*, which protects against a particular type of bacteria, the pneumococcus. This vaccine is of use in people with sickle-cell disease and those without a spleen. *Meningococcal vaccine*, which is used in the military to protect against a particularly deadly bacteria that causes epidemic meningitis. *Hepatitis B vaccine*, which has recently become available to protect people who are at particular risk from hepatitis B virus. *Influenza ("flu") vaccine*, which can be given to prevent or modify influenza, and is usually administered only to those at risk for complications of influenza.

Immunizations for Travel: There are a multitude of vaccines available for use by people who will travel to areas where certain contagious diseases are found frequently. Each area of the world differs in the risks to its travelers, and recommendations change often. Therefore, check with your local health department for the latest recommendations for the area to which you will be traveling, and find out where you can obtain necessary shots. You should be aware, however, that smallpox vaccine, which previously was not only required for travel but also given routinely, is no longer recommended for use for travel anywhere, since the disease is considered to have been eradicated. The vaccine itself is quite dangerous and should therefore not be used for other reasons either.

Discussion: Immunization against diseases has been a very effective means of preventing some of them. In particular, there is no reason that children should ever get certain diseases that in the past were a hazard of childhood. Be sure your child is adequately immunized. If you're not certain about his or her status, call your doctor or health department.

IMPETIGO

Skin infection common in children. There are two forms.

Symptoms: First form is bullous impetigo: small, pus-filled blisters that quickly break, leaving a red, circular area with broken skin attached. Starts on diaper region of small infants (first few weeks of life). Other form (impetigo contagiosa) occurs in older children: Small blisters quickly form yellow crusts, usually on face around nose and mouth or on lower legs.

Cause: Skin infection. Bullous impetigo is caused by staphylococcus bacteria. Impetigo in older children is caused by streptococcus, with or without staphylococcus as well; this form may follow insect bites, scabies or skin injuries that are scratched.

Severity of Problem: Bullous impetigo of newborns occasionally leads to generalized septicemia in small infants. Impetigo caused by streptococci can lead to kidney inflammation (glomerulonephritis) and, rarely, rheumatic fever if not treated.

Contagious? Yes, very much. By contact with blisters or crusts.

Treatment: Wash infected areas well several times a day; soak off any crusts with soap and water. If *one* small sore only in older children, antibiotic ointment may be used on it. If more than one crust or if the bullous form, see a doctor for antibiotic treatment, which is given by mouth or injection.

Prevention: Avoid contact with people with skin infections. Wash insect bites and cuts and scrapes well, especially if children scratch them.

Discussion: Recurring infection in older children may mean that someone in the house carries the bacteria that is causing it. Consult a doctor. Bullous impetigo in the newborn can be a one-time problem with no apparent cause or can occur in outbreaks related to infection from a single hospital source.

IMPOTENCE

Inability of the male to have or maintain an erection.

Symptoms: Failure of the penis to become erect or maintain an erection, resulting in the male's inability to have sexual intercourse.

Cause: Ninety percent of the time impotence is a psychosomatic disorder (no physical basis for the problem, but a psychological one). *Some psychological causes include* stress, anxiety, tension; fatigue, exhaustion or a feeling of overall physical weakness; end product of a poor self-image, lack of confidence or fear of rejection; attitude that sexual activity is "performance" and therefore fear of performing poorly; fear of not satisfying sexual partner; end product of constant criticism from a sexual partner; guilt due to moral or religious convictions; and ill feelings, dislike or conflict with sexual partner. *Physically based causes include* prostate failure; some serious chronic diseases (including diabetes); anemia; leukemia; exposure to excessive amounts of radiation; use of certain drugs (tranquilizers, alcohol, antidepressants and others); and some vitamin deficiencies.

Severity of Problem: Can be devastating psychologically if not put into perspective and the "cause(s)" identified and resolved. The fear of continued impotence usually adds more stress, anxiety, tension and frustration to an often already difficult and painful situation for the man. Occasional failure to have or maintain an erection is common and does not indicate a serious psychological or physical problem.

Contagious? No.

Treatment: Depends upon the basis for the condition. A physician should be consulted if impotency persists, to determine if any underlying physical problems exist. If there is no physical basis for impotency, then a psychologist or counselor may be recommended.

Prevention: Attention to overall general health: stress reduction and control; good nutritional habits; exercise; adequate rest and relaxation; a positive self-image; excellent communications between sexual partners; and seeking professional consultation before a situation becomes extremely difficult or painful.

INDIGESTION (DYSPEPSIA)

Essentially a set of symptoms that together define a nonspecific condition called indigestion or "upset stomach."

Symptoms: Bloated or full feeling; heartburn, nausea or vomiting; belching or regurgitation; gas or "upset stomach"; less often may include abdominal and intestinal cramping, constipation or diarrhea; and lack of appetite.

Cause: Many possible causes: spicy or rich foods; overeating; eating too fast; excessive stomach acid; inadequate digestive function; stress, anxiety and tension; excessive use of alcoholic beverages or other liquids (such as coffee, soft drinks, etc.); insufficient bile secretion to aid in digestion; underlying liver disease.

Severity of Problem: May be mild to severe, chronic to infrequent. Most often a temporary problem where someone "overdid it" at dinner by overeating spicy foods and indulging in alcoholic beverages. However, it may be a warning signal for another underlying problem or for developing peptic ulcer.

Contagious? No.

Treatment: Sometimes antacids are recommended. Also important to reduce stress; change diet to less spicy foods; reduce or stop consumption of alcohol and other acidic liquids; and eat smaller amounts of food. If condition persists or becomes problematic, a physician should be consulted to determine if any underlying problem (liver disease, bile production, etc.) is to blame and can be treated.

Prevention: Proper diet; stress control; moderate intake of alcohol, coffee and other acidic beverages. If due to other underlying cause, preventive steps may or may not be possible.

INFERTILITY, MALE AND FEMALE

Inability to produce offspring. May be due to problem in either partner.

Symptoms: Lack of conception in a couple.

Cause: Variety of possible causes. In the female, ranges from congenital abnormalities to psychological and emotional disturbances. Among the more common specific causes are blockage of the Fallopian tubes because of scarring; polyps blocking the cervical canal; failure of the ovary to release eggs; vaginal and uterine inflammation; unusual composition of vaginal secretions that is damaging to sperm; and problems of the uterus that prevent implantation of a fertilized egg. Male infertility problems can result from congenital factors such as abnormal development of the testes or cryptorchidism; damage to testicle by infection; or any factors that lead to impotence or loss of sexual desire. Sperm production may be absent or reduced, or the sperm may not be as movable or hardy as normal. Sometimes a result of the anxiety of "trying too hard."

Severity of Problem: From a health standpoint, the damage is primarily psychological.

Contagious? No.

Treatment: Depends upon the identification and correction of causes of the condition, if possible.

Prevention: Depends on cause.

Discussion: Infertility is a very complex problem that requires thorough evaluation of both partners without making assumptions about cause or which person is responsible. Problem is often solved with relief of anxiety and stress of "trying too hard" to conceive. Many couples who appear to be infertile during the first year or two of a relationship will conceive within three to four years.

INFLUENZA

Virus infection that primarily involves the respiratory tract.

Symptoms: Sudden appearance of high fever, chills, headache, aches and pains, congestion and cough. There might be mild intestinal symptoms of nausea, loss of appetite, vomiting and diarrhea, but the symptoms of congestion and cough are most prominent. The fever lasts for three to four days, with the cough going from dry and hacking to loose and mucousy.

Cause: Infection with one of many influenza viruses. The influenza virus tends to infect people in epidemic proportions during the winter months, and as people start to become immune, the virus changes itself so it can continue to exist. This accounts for the large epidemics that occur every five to seven years.

Severity of Problem: Usually an uncomfortable disease but one that disappears within a week for people who are usually healthy. In elderly people, or those with chronic heart or lung problems, it tends to be a more severe disease with many complications, some leading to death.

Contagious? Yes, by contact with respiratory secretions carried in the air.

Treatment: There is no specific treatment. Rest, treatment of the cough if it is severe and preventing sleep, and treatment of complications if they arise are all that can be done. Elderly people or those with chronic disease should be evaluated by a physician if there are anything but very minor symptoms.

Prevention: Influenza virus vaccine is available each year and is given in two injections about two weeks apart. It is especially recommended for those people who are at risk for complications but can be taken by anyone. Its effects last no more than a year, and the vaccine is changed every year in anticipation of what viruses will be a problem.

Discussion: Antibiotic therapy is not effective for influenza that is not complicated by a bacterial infection. Bacterial pneumonia is the most common complication of influenza.

KIDNEY STONES

Stones (can be hard, soft, sharp or smooth) present in one or both kidneys. These vary in size from tiny particles to masses one inch or more in diameter. May require immediate medical intervention.

Symptoms: Sudden, severe and unexpected low back pain that can radiate to the abdomen and groin; pain can be excruciating in some cases; nausea, vomiting, chills, sweating and even shock may also occur; tenderness and inflammation of the kidneys; abdominal distention; blood in the urine; frequency of urination if a stone is trying to pass down the ureter; and difficulty of urination if a stone has obstructed the ureter.

Cause: No structural or other abnormality is found to account for kidney stones in at least 50 percent of people afflicted. Some associated or possible causes for stones forming seem to be inadequate calcium metabolism; problems in uric acid metabolism; parathyroid malfunction; consumption of large quantities of vitamin D; and excessive consumption of dairy products (in particular, milk and cream). Kidney stones are principally composed of oxalates, phosphates and carbonates.

Severity of Problem: If a stone obstructs the ureter as it attempts to leave the body and urine backs up, this can result in serious infection or uremia (poisoning of the body). These can ultimately lead to death without prompt medical intervention. Severe pain can also result in shock (which is always potentially life-threatening). Since there is almost always more than one stone involved, even if you feel you have already passed a stone, call your doctor for consultation. At the first signs of possible kidney stones, a doctor should be consulted. If pain is severe, immediate medical care at an emergency facility is vital.

Contagious? No.

Treatment: Hospitalization is most often required; large amounts of fluids are given to help the stone pass; pain medication is administered, as is antispasmodic medication; and the person is watched carefully. If the stones are too large to pass, the aforementioned method is not effective, complications have occurred or complete obstruction has taken place, surgery is necessary to remove the stones.

Prevention: Usually the problem must occur first, then prevention of further stone formation depends on whether or not a cause has been identified. If diet is responsible, changes are made; other causes would require further investigation to determine if preventive measures could be taken.

LARYNGITIS

Change in the voice that makes it more harsh, or coarse.

Symptoms: Change in tone or quality of voice to a coarse, harsher sound; need to clear the throat; sometimes fever, swallowing difficulty and throat pain or discomfort, depending on cause.

Cause: The voice box (larynx) becomes inflamed as a result of inhaling smoke, chemical fumes, gases, vapors or dust; overuse or abuse of voice; excessive use of alcohol; diseases such as sinusitis, tonsillitis, bronchitis, flu, the common cold, pneumonia and pharyngitis; polyps in the throat; cancer; and others.

Severity of Problem: Is most often a temporary, minor problem. However, chronic or persistent hoarseness may signal a minor to serious underlying problem. If hoarseness continues for two weeks, it is best to have the problem evaluated.

Contagious? No, except for infectious causes.

Treatment: Depends on basis for problem. However, initial treatment usually includes "not talking" in order to rest the larynx; no smoking or drinking; an increase in fluids; and medication if deemed necessary. Further treatment would depend on the cause of the hoarseness.

Prevention: Avoid abuse of larynx: Do not smoke; drink moderately; avoid chemical and other fumes that can cause problems; and seek medical consultation where indicated.

LEPROSY

Chronic infection that involves the skin, its adjacent structures and the nerves that supply it.

Symptoms: Gradual development of flat skin sores, which may eventually thicken and form ulcers. The sores may be numb or have unusual sensations in them. Small tumors under the skin may occur, and the infection progresses gradually, destroying skin, underlying tissue and even the ends of fingers and toes.

Cause: Infection with the bacteria Mycobacterium leprae, a relative of the tuberculosis bacteria. It is believed that the infection is usually caught during childhood.

Severity of Problem: Advances slowly, progressively destroying tissue. Can lead to severe deformity and disfigurement over time. The more serious form results in death in 10 to 20 years without treatment, while the less severe skin form may suddenly stop advancing after 3 to 5 years. Some people with the more serious form are at more than the usual risk for tuberculosis.

Contagious? Yes, but not as much as people have thought through the ages. Probably caught during childhood by prolonged contact with the bacteria. There is no need to isolate people who are under treatment.

Treatment: Drug treatment is possible and effective, but treatment takes years in order to be effective. Deformities will persist after treatment. Care of the sores and nodules as well as surgical treatment of ulcers are important.

Prevention: Avoiding prolonged contact during childhood is probably effective, but not very practical in areas where leprosy is found. There has been some success with immunizing children with BCG, the vaccine used against tuberculosis.

Discussion: Leprosy is found in tropical and subtropical climates, such as the southern United States, Central and South America, tropical portions of Asia, Africa and the Pacific Islands.

LEUKOPLAKIA

Development of white patches inside the mouth.

Symptoms: Roughening of the lining of the mouth, then development of painless white patches inside the mouth. There may be one or more patches.

Cause: Usually, irritation of the mucous membranes of the mouth. Common substances that can cause it are tobacco smoke, poorly fitting dentures and broken teeth. It can be a sign of cancer in the mouth.

Severity of Problem: Can be a small patch or extensive involvement of the entire mouth lining. If cancer, the problem is serious. Leukoplakia is thought to be a premalignant change in the tissue.

Contagious? No.

Treatment: Biopsy with removal of patches is important in finding out whether they are malignant. Removing all irritants is the basis for treatment. This involves quitting smoking, repairing or replacing dentures, and avoiding trauma to the inside of the mouth.

Prevention: Avoid repeated irritation of the mouth lining.

Discussion: Treatments other than surgical removal (when possible) have not been very successful. After leukoplakia is first discovered, it is important that periodic evaluation occur, so any change in the patches can be monitored.

LICE (PEDICULOSIS)

Infestation with lice, small parasites that live on the skin.

Symptoms: Usually, itching is the most prominent symptom and involves the area where the lice are living (this may be the head, the skin of the midsection of the body or the pubic area). Rash, infection of the skin where it has been scratched are common.

Cause: Contamination and infestation with small insects called lice. There are three types of louse that infest humans: Pediculus capitis (head louse), Pediculus corporis (body louse) and Pthirus pubis (pubic louse or crab louse). These are spread by contact with someone who has them or with articles of clothing that are contaminated. Usually a disease of poor hygiene and crowding.

Severity of Problem: Very itchy problem. May lead to skin infections when scratched. Lice can also carry other infections, such as relapsing fever.

Contagious? Yes, by contact with a person who has them or sharing of clothing.

Treatment: Application of lotions or creams that destroy the parasites. Gamma benzene hexachloride (by prescription only) or pyrethrins (over-the-counter) are effective. Clothing and bedclothing must also be disinfected and all infested people who are in contact must be treated at the same time.

Prevention: Good personal hygiene, avoidance of close contact with people who have lice.

LICE (PEDICULOSIS)—BODY LICE

Infestation of the body with the body louse, Pediculus corporis.

Symptoms: Intense itching, usually of the body around the chest and abdomen. Often worst at the waistline. Scratched skin may become infected, with pus-containing sores. If clothing is inspected, tiny brown bugs may be seen in the seam lines.

Cause: Infestation with the body louse, Pediculus corporis, by coming into close contact with someone who has it or by sharing clothing that is contaminated (often underclothing). Most common in people who have poor personal hygiene and live under very crowded conditions.

Severity of Problem: A nuisance, uncomfortable. Possibility of infection of scratched skin. Lice can also carry certain diseases, such as relapsing fever.

Contagious? Yes, by direct close contact with someone who has lice or by sharing clothing and bedclothing.

Treatment: Application of anti-louse preparations to the entire body below the neck. Gamma benzene hexachloride (prescription only) or pyrethrins (nonprescription) are both effective. Disinfect clothing, bedding at the same time and treat all who are infected.

Prevention: Avoid contact with people who have lice; practice good personal hygiene. Avoid sharing clothing or bedclothes with those who might be infested.

LICE (PEDICULOSIS)—CRAB LICE (PUBIC LICE)

Infestation of the pubic area with the crab louse, Pthirus pubis.

Symptoms: Itching, rash in the pubic area. Occasionally, there are blue spots seen on the insides of the thighs or lower part of the abdomen. Lice that are slightly larger than body lice may be seen crawling in the pubic hair, and the little white pearly nits can be seen attached to the very base of the hair shafts. Enlargement of the lymph nodes in the groin is common.

Cause: Infestation with the pubic louse through contact with an infected person.

Severity of Problem: Very bothersome. The louse can occasionally carry other diseases, such as relapsing fever.

Contagious? Yes, by contact with someone who has crab lice. These lice are easily passed on to others, by personal contact (sexual contact), sharing of contaminated clothing or even sitting on a contaminated toilet seat. Lice are often found where personal hygiene is poor.

Treatment: Application to the skin of lotion or cream that will kill the lice. Gamma benzene hexachloride (prescription) or pyrethrins (nonprescription) are both effective. Clothing must be disinfected, and all sexual partners must be treated at the same time.

Prevention: Avoid contact, especially sexual, with infested persons. Practice good personal hygiene.

LICE (PEDICULOSIS)—HEAD LICE

Infestation of the scalp with the head louse, Pediculus capitis.

Symptoms: Itching of the scalp. Often, the lice, which are small, shiny insects about 1/8 inch long, can be seen crawling in the scalp. The nits, which are the eggs of the lice, are usually found as tiny, pearly gray particles firmly attached to the hairs near the scalp. Nits are usually easiest to find near the nape of the neck and around the ears. The lymph nodes at the base of the skull are often enlarged because of the irritation and inflammation the lice cause.

Cause: Infestation with the head louse, Pediculus capitis, which lives in the scalp and feeds by biting the scalp.

Severity of Problem: Very bothersome and itchy. Can be extremely widespread, especially among children. Can spread to involve the eyelashes, causing reddened, sore eyelid margins.

Contagious? Yes, by contact with a person who has lice. Very easily passed from one person to another and can be spread by using the same comb or wearing the same hats. Often travels through schools in epidemic proportions and can be difficult to get rid of because of re-exposure.

Treatment: Shampooing with gamma benzene hexachloride (prescription) and removing the nits from the hair shafts with a very fine comb are usually successful. Several treatments are generally needed, because the nits that have been missed will hatch in a week or so. If the lice have infested the eyelashes, petroleum jelly can be rubbed onto the eyelids.

Prevention: Avoid contact with persons with lice. Teach children not to share hats and combs with other children.

LYMPH NODES—ENLARGED

Swelling of the lymph nodes, which are small, firm lumps located in many parts of the body. Lymph nodes are part of the body's immune system.

Symptoms: Swelling, usually painless, of one or more lymph nodes. This is discovered by feeling lumps that were not there before. They may vary anywhere from pea-sized to golf ball-sized and may seem either separated or matted together. The node(s) may become tender if felt often. Depending on cause, there may or may not be other symptoms.

Cause: The basic cause of lymph node enlargement is as the body's defense against a threat—which may be infection, inflammation or tumor. Which lymph nodes enlarge depends on where the "threat" is—because certain lymph nodes guard certain areas. So the location of the enlargement gives a clue as to where to look for the underlying problem. For example, with a sore throat the lymph nodes right under the jaw near the ear (one on each side) enlarge; with an infection on the knee the swollen node is in the groin; and with severe conjunctivitis a node right in front of the ear may swell.

Severity of Problem: Usually a mild problem in itself and just an indicator of a mild to more severe problem elsewhere. Sometimes the node itself might form an abscess. Enlarged lymph nodes, while usually a "healthy" response to infection, should be evaluated if they persist, since this may be one of the early signs of cancer (especially leukemia and lymphoma).

Contagious? Not as such. Underlying infection may be contagious.

Treatment: Usually the treatment for the underlying cause.

Prevention: Only possible if the underlying problem is preventable.

Discussion: Lymph node enlargement is especially common in some children, who have generalized lymph node swelling with common, minor infections. This causes worry for their parents but is part of normal development. (Enlarged tonsils—very similar in structure to lymph nodes—are seen at the same age, for the same reasons.) The lymph nodes shrink after puberty unless there is a continued or new infection.

MACULAR DEGENERATION

Deterioration of the macula, which is the part of the retina that allows us to see clearest in the middle area of our vision.

Symptoms: Gradual blurriness and dimness of vision, especially at the most central area of vision.

Cause: Thought to be a result of damage to the retina's circulation as part of the aging process for some people.

Severity of Problem: Can vary but usually does not lead to complete blindness.

Contagious? No.

Treatment: Nothing is available to slow or stop the process of deterioration of the macula. However, there are many low-vision aids to help people with this problem cope with normal day-to-day activities.

Prevention: None known.

Discussion: One of the most common causes of decreasing vision among the elderly, it rarely leads to complete blindness but can limit function.

MALOCCLUSION

Condition in which the upper and lower teeth are malaligned, so they don't meet each other in the proper way.

Symptoms: Crooked teeth, irregular appearance to the teeth. Pain or discomfort in chewing is occasionally a problem, as is aching or discomfort in the jaw area.

Cause: There are many causes, including teeth that are too large or crowded in the mouth; missing teeth that have allowed the remaining teeth to shift into bad position; congenital deformities of the jaw (such as cleft palate, some disorders in which there are extra or missing teeth); and some habits (thumb sucking, finger sucking or habitual pressure from the tongue on the teeth).

Severity of Problem: Can vary from mild and cosmetic to severe enough to interfere with chewing.

Contagious? No.

Treatment: Depends on the cause, but the earlier the condition is corrected by orthodontic procedures, the easier the correction and the better the results. Orthodontic work usually involves devices that apply pressure to the teeth gradually, so they shift in the jaw. Sometimes it also involves removing extra teeth or putting in spacers or bridges.

Prevention: Depends on cause. Prevention of periodontitis and dental decay, which lead to loss of teeth, is important, since these are among the most common causes of malocclusion. Interruption of habits like thumb sucking may be helpful, if they persist after 3 or 4 years of age.

MEASLES (RUBEOLA, "RED MEASLES")

Very contagious, serious viral infection identified by its characteristic symptoms and rash. This disease (MEASLES [RUBEOLA] "RED MEASLES,) is often confused with German measles, also called "three-day measles" (and known as rubella). However, they are two very different diseases. For information on German measles ("three-day measles"), see RUBELLA (GERMAN MEASLES, "THREE-DAY MEASLES").

Symptoms: High fever (104° F +), runny nose and cough for three to four days before rash. Red, painful eyes that are sensitive to light. Cough becomes harsh, hollow-sounding and severe. On the fourth day a red, flat rash begins on neck and around ears and spreads to rest of body quickly. Koplik's spots, which are diagnostic of measles, appear the day before the rash and may be seen on the day of the rash. They are tiny white sandlike spots in the mouth stuck to the inside of the cheeks near the top molar teeth.

Cause: Infection with measles virus.

Severity of Problem: Moderate to severe illness, with several possible complications: otitis media; pneumonia; encephalitis; appendicitis. Death can occur, although rarely. Very rarely the virus can cause a very severe encephalitis that gradually worsens over time.

Contagious? Yes, very much, by contact with secretions and by airborne spread.

Prevention: Can be completely prevented by immunization of infants and children. Measles vaccine is recommended at or after 15 months of age. During epidemics, vaccine is given to adults and children who are not immune. Gamma globulin given to exposed people can lessen the severity of the illness.

Treatment: No cure. Symptoms are treated with aspirin or aspirin substitute for fever and discomfort; rest and fluids are recommended. Antibiotics are used for ear infections or pneumonia, if they occur.

Discussion: Disease previously occurred most in young children. Now seen in unvaccinated teen-agers and young adults as well.

MENIERE'S DISEASE OR SYNDROME

Very uncomfortable chronic condition in which there are episodes of severe dizziness and loss of balance.

Symptoms: Sudden onset of incapacitating dizziness or spinning sensation, with loss of balance. There is usually severe nausea and vomiting as well. Almost all people with Meniere's syndrome eventually have some loss of hearing as well. There might be ringing in the ears or a feeling of fullness in the ears at the start of an attack. The episodes of dizziness may happen frequently or only every few years. They may be as short as a few minutes or as long as several days.

Cause: A variety of possible causes, including acute or chronic ear infection, tumor, allergy, medications, stress, many systemic diseases and unknown factors. Attacks may be precipitated by acute ear inflammation or stress.

Severity of Problem: Attacks are always incapacitating for as long as they last. Depending on the frequency and the length of time attacks last, the person may be miserable and unable to function or may have very few attacks and do well.

Contagious? No.

Treatment: Many have been tried, with varying success. Medications that are effective against motion sickness, antihistamines and those that cause fluid loss are often successful. Reduction of salt in the diet may help certain people. In very severe cases surgery to remove the structures of the inner ear may offer the only possible relief. However, this surgery leads to complete loss of hearing in that ear and is therefore a drastic step. Newer treatments such as ultrasound may provide promise for this difficult problem.

Prevention: None known.

MENINGITIS

Inflammation and infection of the meninges, the membranes that cover the brain and spinal cord.

Symptoms: Gradual or sudden onset of illness, with fever, headache that is usually severe, nausea and vomiting, generalized aches and pains, and stiff neck. With worsening infection, increasing lethargy and sleepiness, irritability, progressing to coma if not treated.

Cause: Infection with several possible germs, either bacterial or viral. Infection may spread from the respiratory tract or be carried to the meninges through the blood.

Severity of Problem: Depends on type of meningitis (see separate entries for the bacterial and viral forms). Bacterial forms are life-threatening if not treated and may leave permanent damage, mild to severe. Viral forms are usually mild.

Contagious? Yes, although the amount of threat to others varies with the type of meningitis. Certain forms potentially cause epidemics (meningococcus, sometimes Hemophilus influenzae).

Treatment: Immediate medical care to determine type and cause if symptoms are suggestive of meningitis. For the bacterial form hospitalization with intravenous antibiotics given for several weeks is needed. May require intensive medical support. Viral meningitis may require hospitalization for observation, but there is no treatment except for relief of fever and headache.

Prevention: Avoid contact with persons who have the germs that cause meningitis. Treatment of close family contacts (or those spending much of day together, for example, in day-care centers) with preventive antibacterial medicine for certain kinds of infections.

Discussion: Diagnosis requires immediate lumbar puncture (spinal tap) to determine what type of meningitis is present, so effective treatment can be begun as soon as possible. A very frightening disease for most people. Antibiotics available today make most forms of meningitis potentially very treatable. Death rate decreases each year, and with early treatment residual damage is less.

MENINGITIS—BACTERIAL

Severe infection of the membranes covering the brain and spinal cord with one of several bacteria.

Symptoms: Rapid onset of fever, increasing headache, lethargy and irritability. Stiff neck, vomiting and progressive loss of consciousness occur over hours. Infants and young children usually refuse to feed and appear very ill. Signs of shock may be present. A rapidly developing skin rash with bleeding spots may occur and indicates a very serious infection.

Cause: Infection with one of several types of bacteria. These include meningococcus and pneumococcus (in adults); Hemophilus influenzae and pneumococcus (in infants and children); and various other more rare types in newborn infants, people with poor immunity and the chronically ill.

Severity of Problem: Potentially life-threatening. Prompt treatment with the correct antibiotic can reduce this risk, but there is a significant problem with long-term effects, from mild to severe brain damage.

Contagious? Most forms are contagious, but degree depends on the bacteria. Two types, meningococcus (the form of meningitis people usually associate with epidemics) and Hemophilus influenzae (which affects primarily infants and young children), are definitely contagious. Other forms are less so.

Treatment: Immediate medical evaluation in an emergency facility if there are signs of meningitis. Treatment with intravenous antibiotic(s), intensive support and observation, and treatment of complications.

Prevention: Isolation of people with the contagious forms of meningitis for 24 hours after the start of treatment. Treatment of close family contacts for meningococcus and Hemophilus influenzae forms.

Discussion: One of the most severe and life-threatening of infections. Diagnosis requires lumbar puncture (spinal tap) quickly, in order to determine which type of meningitis is present. Complications include fluid collection inside the head, seizures, infections and abscesses in other parts of the body, deafness, blindness, mental retardation or various forms of nervous system damage.

MENINGITIS—VIRAL (ASEPTIC MENINGITIS)

Inflammation and infection of the meninges with one of several possible viruses.

Symptoms: Gradual development of fever, headache and sensitivity of the eyes to light. Nausea and vomiting, stiff neck. General aches and pains, listlessness and irritability. Increased sleep. Occasionally a mild, fine red rash.

Cause: Infection with one of several types of viruses that can invade the central nervous system. These viruses include the group known as enteroviruses, which are most commonly seen in the late summer and early fall. Mumps and measles infections can also produce a meningitis.

Severity of Problem: Uncomfortable, but mild and resolving without treatment. Almost never leaves any serious aftereffects. Partial deafness may be seen after mumps and measles.

Contagious? Yes, but not all people who get the virus will contract meningitis.

Treatment: Relief of headache, intravenous fluids if vomiting is severe. May require hospitalization for observation. Antibiotic treatment is not effective.

Prevention: Only possible if infection with viruses can be avoided.

Discussion: The most important thing about aseptic meningitis is being sure that the infection is not caused by bacteria. This requires a lumbar puncture (spinal tap) with examination of the spinal fluid. Occasionally the diagnosis is not clear, and hospital observation with antibiotic treatment and repeated lumbar puncture will be needed.

MENOPAUSE

Phase in a woman's life when her menstrual periods cease. It may be natural, premature or artificial. It may occur between the ages of 39 and 59, but the average age seems to be around 47.

Symptoms: Cessation of menstrual periods and symptoms may take place over a one- to five-year period of time. Some women experience no symptoms other than lessening of menstrual period flow and days; greater length of time between periods; then total cessation of menstrual periods. Others may experience occasional hot flashes (flushing or redness and hot feeling on face and neck) and sweating; sometimes a feeling of being cold follows a hot flash. Other possible symptoms include nervousness; menstrual disturbances; fatigability; lassitude; depression; irritability; insomnia; palpitation of the heart; numbness and tingling in limbs; urinary frequency; and varied gastrointestinal disturbances (gas, constipation or diarrhea).

Cause: The ovaries shrink and cease to function (do not ovulate) because of a decrease in estrogen production. Surgical removal of the ovaries will also cause what is called artificial or premature menopause, unless estrogen is replaced (by pills or injections).

Severity of Problem: Menopause is a natural aspect of a woman's life, but uncomfortable symptoms depend on each individual woman. Those who are experiencing severely uncomfortable problems should see a physician for evaluation.

Contagious? No.

Treatment: Estrogen therapy prescribed by a doctor if symptoms are severe. The risks and benefits of taking estrogen should be explained fully so each woman can determine what is best for her.

Prevention: None. It is a natural phase in a female's life.

Discussion: There have been a lot of myths about menopause over the years, and they have led to many misgivings, undue stress and fear. Sexual function is not compromised, nor is femininity. Some women feel better than ever, and because pregnancy cannot occur, feel more at ease sexually. Others require or prefer the support of estrogen therapy. But in no way should menstrual cessation (menopause) cause fears or concern about one's femininity or sexuality.

MENORRHAGIA

Excessive vaginal bleeding during menstrual cycles. Sometimes the length of the cycles also changes.

Symptoms: Excessive menstrual blood flow, sometimes with clot formation and "gushing." There may be fever, abdominal pain or uterine cramps as well, depending on the cause.

Cause: This type of bleeding usually results from problems in the uterus itself, including endometriosis, polyps (growths) and pelvic infections, especially pelvic inflammatory disease (PID). It occasionally results from hypothyroidism.

Severity of Problem: Repeated episodes of excessive bleeding can cause anemia. If bleeding is severe, it can lead to a rapid fall in blood pressure and shock, although this is unusual.

Contagious? No, unless the underlying cause is pelvic inflammatory disease due to untreated gonorrhea (which is contagious).

Treatment: Depends on the cause, which must be looked for promptly. For a severe episode of bleeding, the usual treatment is the administration of hormones for several days to stop the menstrual flow, then treatment depending on the specific cause. Dilatation and curettage (scraping of the lining of the uterus) may be needed in some situations and can help with making the diagnosis.

Prevention: Depends on cause. However, most causes cannot be prevented.

Discussion: Sometimes no specific cause for the bleeding can be found, but the problem persists. In this case the doctor will often recommend use of hormone therapy—combined estrogen and progesterone in the form of so-called birth control pills—for several months to attempt to regulate the menstrual flow.

METRORRHAGIA

Uterine bleeding, regardless of amount, that occurs between regular menstrual periods.

Symptoms: Uterine bleeding between menstrual periods, with or without other symptoms. This term is usually used for women who are still having normal periods but occasionally is also used for those past the menopause who again have vaginal bleeding.

Cause: This is the most common symptom of malignant tumors of the reproductive organs, especially of the uterus (endometrium). This is especially true of women past menopause. Other causes include cervicitis, ovulation, withdrawal of hormones (forgetting to take birth control pills, for example), pregnancy, hypothyroidism and a few other rare endocrine disorders.

Severity of Problem: The bleeding itself can range from a trickle or spotting to severe hemorrhage. The underlying cause can also vary in severity.

Contagious? No.

Treatment: Depends on determining and treating the underlying cause. Bleeding between periods or after menopause should *always* prompt a medical evaluation. If no specific underlying cause is found, treatment often involves use of hormones to stop the bleeding and establish normal menstrual cycles without metrorrhagia.

Prevention: Depends on cause.

MONONUCLEOSIS INFECTIOUS, (GLANDULAR FEVER)

Acute infectious disease that primarily affects the lymph nodes and causes overall weakness and fatigue.

Symptoms: Enlarged, often painful swelling of the lymph nodes (in particular, those under the jaw, under the arm and in the groin); enlarged spleen; high fever; fatigue; headache; sore throat; cough; general weakness; a general rash sometimes occurs; and some people become jaundiced. Most people have no appetite and feel poorly overall.

Cause: Epstein-Barr (EB) virus, which is a herpes virus. Similar symptoms and findings can result from another related virus, cytomegalovirus (CMV).

Severity of Problem: Mild to severe. The spleen is extremely vulnerable to rupture with this disease, and great care must be taken to avoid a blow to the spleen (including no strenuous exercise, contact sports or risk-taking that could possibly result in trauma to the spleen). The fatigue and weakness can continue for weeks and even months. Although usually not life-threatening, it can be a miserable, debilitating disease until recovery is reached. Sometimes complications are seen, such as hepatitis, neuritis, encephalitis and myocarditis.

Contagious? Yes. However, studies have shown that the disease is not as easily transmitted as once was thought. Usually spread through close contact (and that's why it has been called the "kissing disease"). More frequent in the 10 to 35 age group; it is seen infrequently after the age of 35. Can be seen in young children but is harder to recognize.

Treatment: Bed rest is imperative during the period of fever and weakness. Exercise or any strenuous activity must be avoided as long as the spleen is enlarged. A doctor should first approve any kind of physical activity to avoid trauma to the spleen. A well-balanced, nourishing diet is important to maintain.

Prevention: None. However, as with all diseases, fatigue and exhaustion seem to make people more susceptible to mononucleosis.

MOTION SICKNESS

Nausea and queasiness, often with vomiting, resulting from sensitivity to motion.

Symptoms: Feeling of light-headedness, nausea and sleepiness, often with vomiting, as a result of motion. There may be headache, tendency to yawn and swallow air, and paleness as well. These symptoms usually come and go during the exposure to motion.

Cause: Repetitive motion, especially to-and-fro or rocking, causes increased stimulation of the balancing portion of the inner ear. This produces a sensation of dizziness, and the nausea and vomiting follow.

Severity of Problem: Many people are sensitive to excessive motion, as is felt in sailing or boating, flying or on amusement rides. Others have difficulties with riding in cars. Symptoms can vary from mild to severe, from temporary to prolonged. Most people, when exposed to motion for a long period of time, adjust to it and do not feel ill any longer.

Contagious? No.

Treatment: Simple measures, such as reducing the amount of motion that is perceived by sitting in areas of a vehicle that have the least motion or by looking at objects far in the distance so little motion is seen are helpful for most people. Sucking or chewing on hard candy or sipping a cold drink helps nausea for some. Nonprescription drugs for motion sickness (such as Dramamine®, Marezine® or Bonine®) can be quite effective if taken regularly by people who are susceptible to the problem.

Prevention: Use of all the treatment measures before the start of dizziness and nausea. Medications should be taken 30 to 60 minutes before exposure to motion. Currently there is a drug available by prescription that can be applied to the skin behind the ear, where it releases medication that is absorbed through the skin to combat sickness.

Discussion: Most people are at least somewhat sensitive to the effects of motion, especially when the motion is violent or severe.

MULTIPLE SCLEROSIS

Chronic, progressive disease of the nervous system that affects scattered parts of the brain and therefore produces symptoms in scattered parts of the body.

Symptoms: The earliest symptoms are often unrecognized because they are so subtle. Some of the early symptoms include temporary weakness of an arm or leg, changes in sensation (numbness, tingling); sudden loss of vision in one eye, double vision or blurriness; slurred speech; loss of bladder control. Later, weakness tends to remain. Late in the disease, there are mood alterations, especially inappropriate cheeriness and euphoria, lack of awareness of the severity of the disease.

Cause: Degeneration of the coverings of the nerves scattered throughout the nervous system. The cause is unknown. Many theories have been tested, including viral infection, drug or toxin exposure, stress and various dietary deficiencies. None of these explain the disease.

Severity of Problem: The disease progresses over time, with people often living 10 to 30 years after its detection. During bouts of active disease, the disability is great. Bouts of the disease have a tendency to come and go.

Contagious? No.

Treatment: There is no curative treatment, although many drugs have been tried. Plenty of rest, avoidance of stress and a nutritious diet are all important, both during and between episodes of worsening. Sometimes cold temperatures help people with this disease, while excessive heat makes the symptoms worse. Physical and occupational therapy are very important to help people recover as much function as possible after an acute episode and to help them learn to live with residual weakness and disability.

Prevention: No known prevention for the disease.

Discussion: Multiple sclerosis usually begins in early adulthood, in the 20s or 30s, but may not be recognized until several years later. It is marked by episodes of worsening and improving nervous system function and symptoms that strike different parts of the body randomly. Most people with the disease gradually worsen over years but live 20 to 30 years after the disease has appeared.

MUMPS (EPIDEMIC PAROTITIS)

Viral infection of salivary glands and sometimes of other organs.

Symptoms: Mild fever, with swelling of the parotid glands, which are located in the cheeks, just in front of the ears and extending around the bottom of the ears. Pain on eating sour substances and generalized discomfort are common. There may also be symptoms of inflammation of other organs: abdominal pain, nausea and vomiting if there is pancreatitis; headache, stiff neck and lethargy if meningitis is present; swollen, painful testicle(s) if orchitis is present.

Cause: Infection with the mumps virus.

Severity of Problem: Usually a mild disease that is uncomfortable but leaves very few aftereffects. In fact, many infections are not recognized, and many people who don't think they have ever had the disease have immunity. Complications of aseptic meningitis, pancreatitis and orchitis are common.

Contagious? Yes, by contact with infected person. Contagious for about one day before the start of illness and then until the signs of illness have disappeared. Lag time between exposure and illness is two to three weeks.

Treatment: No specific treatment. Relief of discomfort with mild pain relievers and heat or cold applied to the areas of swelling are important.

Prevention: Immunization of infants and children against the disease is successful and is recommended at or after 15 months of age.

Discussion: Mumps is often confused with infection or enlargement of the lymph nodes of the neck, where the swelling is below the jaw, not in front of the ear. Mumps aseptic meningitis is very common and usually has no long-term complications except for occasional mild hearing loss. Mumps orchitis (inflammation of the testicle) occurs in about 25 percent of adult men who get this disease and is very uncomfortable. However, sterility due to this infection, often feared, is very rare. About 75 percent of people with mumps have both parotid glands affected, but permanent immunity is obtained even if only one side is involved. (You don't need to get mumps on both sides, as is commonly believed.)

MUMPS (EPIDEMIC PAROTITIS)—
MUMPS ORCHITIS

Inflammation of one or both testicles as a complication of mumps.

Symptoms: Swelling and pain in the scrotum during the course of mumps. There is usually fever, generalized weakness and tenderness of the testicles.

Cause: Involvement of the testicles in the infection by the mumps virus.

Severity of Problem: Very painful problem. Sterility, even after inflammation and infection of both testicles, is rare.

Contagious? Yes, by contact with saliva of a person with mumps.

Treatment: Rest in bed, elevation and support of the swollen scrotum.

Cold packs are helpful in relieving pain, and aspirin or aspirin substitute (sometimes a stronger pain reliever) is important.

Prevention: Prevention of mumps by immunizing infants and susceptible children against the disease. Adult men who are not immune to mumps can also receive this vaccine. If not immune, men should avoid contact with people who have mumps.

Discussion: This complication of mumps if often blamed for sterility in men. In fact, sterility from this cause is rare, even if both testicles have been involved with orchitis.

MUSCULAR DYSTROPHY

Progressive muscle disease in which there is gradual weakening and wasting of the muscles.

Symptoms: Gradual weakness of the muscles, with enlargement of the muscles because of accumulation of fat and scar tissue in them. The most common form (called Duchenne's type) causes weakness of the hips and upper legs, with inability to walk. Weakness of the shoulders and upper arms, as well as of the back and trunk muscles, follows. Other less common forms involve the muscles of the face, the shoulders and upper arms, and then the rest of the body.

Cause: Gradual deterioration of the muscles, with resulting weakness. The various forms of muscular dystrophy are inherited. The most common form (Duchenne's muscular dystrophy), which affects young boys, is inherited as a sex-linked recessive—it is passed on the X-chromosome from the mother, who does not have the disease. Other inheritance patterns exist for the other forms.

Severity of Problem: Muscular dystrophy is slowly progressive and leads eventually to profound weakness and inability to move. Death usually results from pneumonia becasue of inability to cough, but heart failure because of involvement of the heart muscle is also common. Most boys with muscular dystrophy are completely unable to walk within ten years of the onset of the disease but can live into their thirties with good, supportive care.

Contagious? No.

Treatment: There is no cure. Any treatment is aimed at physical and occupational therapy to help a person adapt to the weakness and to prevent complications of pneumonia and deformities of the spine (curvatures) and legs (tightness of joints because of inability to move).

Prevention: None known.

Discussion: The various forms of muscular dystrophy are slowly progressive over time and can continue to advance over 20 to 30 years. Genetic counseling is important for families with a history of these diseases.

NEARSIGHTEDNESS (MYOPIA)

Eye condition in which a person can see close objects but is unable to focus on objects farther away.

Symptoms: Objects more than a few feet away are "fuzzy" or blurry, and person is unable to correctly focus. People often blink, rub eyes or crane neck. Headaches at times occur. Children or young people may do poorly in school (because they can't see the blackboard). Others sit close to televisions or squint while driving an automobile.

Cause: Nearsightedness results when the eyeball is too long to enable correct focusing on the retina or the refractive power of the eye is too strong.

Severity of Problem: Ranges from mild to severe but requires evaluation and correction.

Contagious? No.

Treatment: Corrective lenses can be prescribed by an ophthalmologist or an optometrist.

Prevention: None. Myopia is due to the shape of the eye, and this cannot be changed.

Discussion: Nearsightedness is found in people of all ages. Prompt attention in children will help to ensure the attainment of educational goals and avoid frustration and feelings of inadequacy.

NEPHRITIS—ACUTE

Inflammation of the glomeruli of the kidneys (the structures which filter the blood of waste products to make urine).

Symptoms: Smoky, dark or bloody urine; decrease in the amount of urine; mild puffiness or swelling, usually of the face, hands and feet; sometimes headache, loss of appetite and fever. Occasionally mild disease produces no symptoms, and severe disease leads to severe headache (because of hypertension), difficulty with vision and marked edema. There is often a history of a respiratory infection or sore throat about two weeks before the start of the urine changes.

Cause: The underlying cause for many cases of acute glomerulonephritis, especially in children, is previous streptococcal infection (either strep throat or impetigo). Other causes include so-called immune diseases, of which there are several. All these diseases cause the production of antibodies against the glomeruli, which deposit along the membranes of the glomeruli in the kidneys. These membranes interfere with the function of the kidneys and lead to bleeding from the kidneys.

Severity of Problem: Can vary from producing no symptoms, to severe disease with progressive renal failure (uremia). One of the most serious immediate dangers is hypertension, which needs to be detected and treated when severe. Heart failure because of excessive accumulation of fluid is a possible complication.

Contagious? No. The glomerulonephritis that follows streptococcal infection is due to the body's making antibodies against the strep germ, not a direct infection of the kidneys.

Treatment: Depends on the severity of the disease, but mild restriction of salt in the diet, and occasionally limitation of liquid intake to minimum amounts might be recommended. Bed rest is usually recommended during the very early stages. Treatment of hypertension, medications to cause urine production might be tried.

Prevention: For most causes, there is no specific prevention. For post-streptococcal acute glomerulonephritis, elimination of strep from the community is a goal, to reduce the number of individuals who are at risk for this complication.

Discussion: Most people with acute glomerulonephritis slowly recover over one to two years. However, as many as 20 percent will have chronic glomerulonephritis, with repeated flareups in the acute disease. Some of these will have progressive kidney failure.

NEPHRITIS—CHRONIC

Chronic inflammation of the glomeruli, the kidney structures that filter the blood of waste products.

Symptoms: Usually there are no specific symptoms, although there has been a past episode of acute glomerulonephritis. The abnormalities are found in the urine, and consist of abnormal substances being "leaked" into the urine. Repeated flareups of acute inflammation can be seen after infection or injury or excessive fatigue.

Cause: Failure to heal the glomeruli after an episode of acute glomerulonephritis. A person is said to have chronic glomerulonephritis if there are abnormalities of the urine and kidney function (as measured by certain blood values and urine tests) after two years following a bout of acute nephritis. Many causes of chronic glomerulonephritis are due to obscure diseases.

Severity of Problem: Chronic nephritis invariably leads to progressive deterioration in kidney function, but this can occur very gradually over many years (20 to 30 years) or over just a short time.

Contagious? No.

Treatment: Depends entirely on whether the person has severe disease, with hypertension and severe lack of renal function or not.

Prevention: A few cases might be preventable by vigilant care of acute nephritis, but most cases are probably not preventable.

Discussion: A certain number of people with chronic nephritis ultimately need dialysis ("artificial kidney") treatment and a kidney transplant.

NEPHROTIC SYNDROME (NEPHROSIS)

A condition in which the kidney membranes are "leaky" and lose a large amount of protein into the urine.

Symptoms: Moderate to large degree of water retention and swelling of the body—usually the legs and feet first, then of the face, hands and abdomen. There is usually loss of appetite and shortness of breath because of accumulation of fluid in the abdomen. There may be weakness and a very pale color.

Cause: Nephrotic syndrome can be caused by a number of kidney diseases, with glomerulonephritis among the most common. Damage to the kidney membranes causes them to become leaky, allowing protein to escape. Loss of protein leads to the puffiness and swelling in the tissues. One form of this problem occurs in young children (about two to five years old) and has no specific cause, but usually goes away with treatment after several years.

Severity of Problem: Can be variable, depending on the cause. In children, about half do very well, with return of normal kidney function after several years. Adults often go on to develop kidney failure and have persistent hypertension.

Contagious? No.

Treatment: When fluid accumulation is great, restriction of salt and water intake, high protein diet, and intravenous diuretics (drugs that stimulate urine production), with or without added protein are usually needed. If infection has occurred (a risk in nephrotic syndrome), vigorous treatment is usually carried out. Sometimes steroid hormones (cortisone relatives) or other strong drugs are used, depending on the cause of the nephrosis.

Prevention: Probably not possible.

NOSEBLEED (EPISTAXIS)

Bleeding, whether minor or major, from the nose, for a variety of reasons.

Symptoms: Onset of bleeding, usually from the front of the nose. This may be minor and resolved without specific treatment, or profuse, requiring medical intervention. There may be associated stuffiness of the nose. If the blood has drained down the throat, vomiting of blood may be the first symptom.

Cause: The most common cause is irritation of the nose from picking and trauma, infection of the nose, injury from the outside or dryness. Serious underlying diseases, such as hypertension, bleeding disorders, infections like measles and rheumatic fever, leukemia and tumors might be responsible, but are much less common.

Severity of Problem: Usually a minor problem, without serious consequences. Occasionally, bleeding is profuse, especially when the bleeding starts in the back of the nose rather than the front. Severe blood loss may lead to shock and anemia.

Contagious? No.

Treatment: Have the person rest and apply pressure over the side of the nose, holding steady pressure for 10 minutes, without releasing to check whether there is still bleeding. After 10 minutes, check for further bleeding. If bleeding starts again, repeat the pressure for another 10 minutes. If there is still bleeding, contact your doctor or go to an emergency facility. Do not blow the nose or pick at it after bleeding has stopped, in order not to disrupt the clot that has formed.

Prevention: Try to keep the nose lining moist and do not pick at it. Use a soothing gel on the inside of the nose if dryness or cracking is a problem.

Discussion: Nosebleeds are a very common cause of concern among parents of small children with colds or an allergy involving the nose. These nosebleeds are almost always due to nose-picking and dryness or cracking of the nose because of constant irritation. Adults with persistent nosebleeds are more likely to have hypertension or a more serious underlying disease.

OSTEOMYELITIS

Infection of the bone.

Symptoms: Pain in the affected bone, fever. There may be swelling, warmth, redness and tenderness over the bone and often in a nearby joint.

Cause: Infection in a bone with bacteria (often Staphylococcus, sometimes Hemophilus influenzae, beta streptococcus, tuberculosis or Salmonella). Bacteria may spread from a nearby sore or wound or an infected joint, or may spread from a distant place via the bloodstream.

Severity of Problem: Needs prompt medical care. May require long-term antibiotic therapy to eradicate. Can potentially progress to bone destruction and deformity if not treated promptly.

Contagious? No.

Treatment: Antibiotic treatment for several weeks to months, depending on severity and type of infection. Initial treatment is given intravenously (for several weeks), with later treatment sometimes possible by mouth. Protection of the infected bone from injury is important (because there is a potential for further infection and fracture). Rest, fever control, elevation of the infected bone, heat to the bone and pain control are important. Sometimes surgery to remove pus and debris from the bone is necessary.

Prevention: Treatment of local infection with antibiotics before the spread to bone occurs may prevent some cases.

Discussion: The incidence of osteomyelitis has decreased since the advent of antibiotics, and the infection is usually successfully treated without long-term aftereffects.

OSTEOPOROSIS

Loss of the calcium (mineral) portion of the bones, especially of the spine and hips.

Symptoms: There may be no symptoms, or there may be severe pain, especially backache, which signals that a fracture has occurred. This disease accounts for the prevalence of fractures of the vertebrae, hips and arms in older people, particularly older women.

Cause: The most common cause is the loss of minerals (especially calcium) from the bones as a result of aging. In women who have passed the menopause, there is an association between lack of the hormone estrogen and osteoporosis. This can also result from poor diet, inadequate calcium and protein intake, prolonged inactivity or immobilization, and certain drugs and hormones (especially cortisone and its relatives).

Severity of Problem: Can be a relatively minor problem without consequences or can lead to multiple fractures, particularly of the back, hip and arms. These fractures can occur with recognized injury, or they can happen spontaneously with minimal if any trauma.

Contagious? No.

Treatment: Good, nutritious, balanced diet that contains adequate protein, calcium, phosphorus and vitamin D. Women who are past the menopause may benefit from hormone therapy, and research is being done on the use of fluoride for this condition.

Prevention: Hormone therapy after menopause often prevents osteoporosis or reduces its severity. A balanced diet is also beneficial.

OTITIS, EXTERNAL (SWIMMER'S EAR)

Infection of the skin of the ear canal. Most common in the summer months in swimmers, therefore the name *swimmer's ear*.

Symptoms: Itching, pain and burning of the ears. Swelling and redness of the skin in the ear, discharge of debris and pus, sometimes small amounts of blood. The outside part of the ear is tender when touched or moved because of the severe skin inflammation.

Cause: Infection of the skin of the ear canal with bacteria and sometimes fungi. Most likely to happen when the skin is kept wet and when there is injury to the skin (for example, from use of cotton swabs). Irritation from chemicals in the ears can also be a problem.

Severity of Problem: Very bothersome and painful, but does not cause serious long-term problems if treated.

Contagious? Probably not.

Treatment: Have problem evaluated by a doctor, to be sure there is no otitis media (middle-ear infection) associated. Antibiotic ear drops are usually prescribed to treat the infection.

Prevention: Keep the ears dry, especially after swimming and if there is irritation of the skin. Avoid picking and poking in the ears with cotton swabs and other objects. Rubbing alcohol or diluted vinegar may be used in the ears after swimming if there is a tendency to get swimmer's ear often.

OTITIS MEDIA (MIDDLE-EAR INFECTION)—ACUTE

Most common in younger children (aged 3 months to 3 years), acute otitis media is a middle-ear infection that can be caused by bacteria or viruses.

Symptoms: Severe earache; often high fever, vomiting, diarrhea and irritability; the eardrum sometimes ruptures, with some bleeding and drainage from the ear; temporary hearing loss may occur.

Cause: Infection of the middle ear (behind the eardrum) with bacteria or virus. Often follows a cold or congested nose from other causes.

Severity of Problem: Serious complications can occur without prompt identification and treatment. Some serious complications include chronic otitis media, hearing loss, meningitis, brain abscess and facial paralysis.

Contagious? Not in the usual sense, but the organisms that cause it are carried in the nose and can be passed on to others.

Treatment: Requires doctor's evaluation and treatment. Antibiotics are usually used.

Prevention: Sometimes possible in people who know they are at risk. (See "Discussion.")

Discussion: Prompt treatment reduces the risk of serious complications. It is important that follow-up evaluation be performed to assure that the infection has cleared up. Allergies, certain abnormalities (such as cleft palate, Down's syndrome) and possibly abnormal functioning of the Eustachian tube (the opening that equalizes pressure between the middle ear and the outside— the cause of your ears popping) increase the risk for acute ear infection.

OTITIS MEDIA, ACUTE—WITH PERFORATION

Untreated acute otitis media may progress to chronic collection of pus in the middle ear. This usually leads to rupture of the eardrum and a chronic hole in the eardrum.

Cause: Continued infection and pus in the middle ear after an acute infection. Can also result from mechanical injury to the eardrum, as can be seen with blast injuries and diving, especially scuba.

Severity of Problem: Most serious problem is the tendency to have infection continue and spread to other areas (see OTITIS MEDIA [MIDDLE-EAR INFECTION]—ACUTE). Chronic hearing loss is common. May result in development of a growth called a cholesteatoma in the middle ear.

Contagious? No.

Treatment: Requires medical treatment, usually with antibiotics to control infection. Important to keep an ear with a perforated eardrum dry. Surgery is sometimes needed to close a hole in the eardrum.

Prevention: Be sure that acute ear infections are treated promptly.

Discussion: Can be a serious problem with long-term consequences. Often easier avoided than treated.

OTITIS MEDIA (MIDDLE-EAR INFECTION)— CHRONIC SECRETORY ("GLUE EAR")

Chronic condition involving thick fluid in the middle ear, with resulting hearing loss that can be permanent if the "glue" is not removed.

Symptoms: Hearing loss; sensation of fullness or fluid in the ears; rarely intermittent mild earache.

Cause: Continued fluid in the middle ear. Can result from an acute infection or from anything that keeps the Eustachian tube blocked (such as allergic rhinitis, cleft palate, Down's syndrome, abnormal functioning of the Eustachian tube).

Severity of Problem: Can lead to chronic hearing loss, occasionally to repeated acute infections.

Contagious? No.

Treatment: Removal of fluid. Sometimes medications that "dry up" the nose are tried. Usually requires surgery to place small plastic tubes through the eardrum to drain the fluid and prevent it from collecting again.

Prevention: Get medical attention for any earache or suspected ear infection. Be sure to have the infected ear looked at again at the end of treatment to be sure the infection has cleared up.

Discussion: This is a preventable cause of hearing loss and a very common problem. No earache should be taken lightly.

OTOSCLEROSIS

Most common cause of conductive hearing loss in adults who have a normal tympanic membrane (eardrum).

Symptoms: Most noticeable initial symptom is difficulty understanding voices at a distance or when others are whispering. Other symptoms include: Own voice seems so very loud (because of bone conduction) that person tends to speak very softly; sounds of chewing food are exaggerated so much that person tends not to hear dinner discussions and no longer takes part in conversations; person becomes frustrated at having to constantly ask others to repeat what was said; and often withdrawal and seclusion become the person's only defense against progressive hearing loss.

Cause: A malformation or overgrowth of spongy bone in parts of the middle ear. This bone surrounds and immobilizes the stirrup-shaped "stapes" that deliver the vibrations to the inner ear. If the stapes cannot vibrate, sound cannot be transmitted to the auditory nerves, which send the signals to the brain.

Severity of Problem: Can be mild hearing loss (muffling of sounds) to severe hearing loss (no sounds at all). Medical evaluation should be sought at the onset of any symptoms.

Contagious? No.

Treatment: Because otosclerosis is a conductive type of hearing loss, it can often be improved with the use of a hearing aid. Surgery is sometimes recommended in very severe cases. Careful evaluation and selection of surgical candidates is important. The objective is to restore free vibration of the stapes so that sound can be properly received. Several surgical options are usually considered, including removal of the stapes and replacement with a plastic device or a vein graft. The hope of surgery is to substantially improve hearing or return it to normal.

Prevention: None.

Discussion: Otosclerosis usually causes progressive hearing loss, and the problem appears to be hereditary. It most commonly affects those between the ages of 15 and 40 and is experienced more by women than by men. Those with known otosclerosis in their families should advise their physician of this family history so careful ear examinations and hearing tests can be performed routinely.

PANCREATITIS—ACUTE

Inflammation of the pancreas (which produces both hormones and digestive juices).

Symptoms: Severe and often progressive abdominal pain (can be in upper area of abdomen or generalized, and may radiate through abdomen to the back). Severe attacks may include fever, shock, vomiting, reduced blood pressure, elevated pulse rate and clammy skin.

Cause: In one-half of people biliary tract disease is the cause. In one-third cause cannot be identified. Passage of gallstones into duodenum is related to acute pancreatitis attacks. Other causes include infectious diseases (such as mumps, infectious mononucleosis, meningitis); hyperparathyroidism; some drugs; heavy alcohol use; trauma; and hyperlipidemia. Surgery on the biliary tract and stomach may also cause an acute attack.

Severity of Problem: Can be life-threatening. Very painful problem that requires immediate medical intervention.

Contagious: Pancreatitis is not contagious. If the cause is mumps or infectious mononucleosis, these are contagious.

Treatment: Requires prompt, intense medical intervention in a hospital. Eat or drink nothing until physician has evaluated the basis for severe abdominal pain and discounted pancreatitis. Continual pain relief with strong drugs may lead to addiction.

Prevention: Avoid alcohol consumption, overeating and obesity; small, low-fat, frequent meals help minimize chance of recurrence.

PARKINSON'S DISEASE

Chronic, progressive nervous disease, generally developing in later life, marked by tremors and weakness of resting muscles.

Symptoms: Weakness of facial muscles; lack of facial expression; hand tremors while at rest; shuffling gait; infrequent blinking; tendency to have vacant stare and open mouth; drooling.

Cause: Unknown. May be a late effect of a virus infection in some situations (especially influenza). Some tremors cause same kinds of symptoms.

Severity of Problem: May suffer mild impairment of mental faculties; may eventually become totally unable to function physically or mentally because of slowness and tremor.

Contagious? No.

Treatment: While not curable, Parkinson's can be treated by drug therapy. In some cases, surgery may be helpful in alleviating tremor. Requires close medical supervision.

Prevention: None known.

Discussion: Parkinson's disease occurs during middle-age and later years. Affects men far more often than women and is slowly progressive. May not be incapacitating for several years.

PARONYCHIA (INGROWN NAIL)

Inflammation of the tissue surrounding the nail (finger or toe).

Symptoms: Local pain, tenderness, redness, swelling. In chronic cases the nail can become distorted.

Cause: Infectious organisms enter the skin surrounding a nail through a crack or break caused by injury, hangnail or persistent irritation. Inflammation and infection follow.

Severity of Problem: Ranges from minor soreness to extreme inflammation and infection. If left to fester, systemic infection may occur.

Contagious? No.

Treatment: With acute infection: hot compresses; soaking in warm-to-hot water; antibiotics are prescribed when infection occurs; drainage is often necessary to release accumulated debris and relieve pain. With chronic infections vigorous treatment and management by a physician are necessary. More extensive infections require prompt surgical incision and drainage.

Prevention: Any cuts or hangnails should be kept sterile (clean with soap and warm water), and any signs of infection should signal the need for consultation with a doctor before the infection worsens.

PELVIC INFLAMMATORY DISEASE (PID)

Inflammation and infection of the Fallopian tubes, sometimes extending into nearby pelvic organs.

Symptoms: High fever and chills; progressively severe pain in the lower abdomen and pelvis; tenderness of the abdomen, especially the cervix and nearby structures (during examination). Symptoms often start during a menstrual period.

Cause: Infection, most often bacterial. Can follow or complicate gonorrhea. Increased risk with intrauterine device (IUD) in place or after an abortion. Sometimes a complication of delivery.

Severity of Problem: Can be a very serious disease when acute. Can lead to generalized infection (sepsis); abscess of the Fallopian tubes and ovaries; peritonitis. A late complication is sterility because of blockage and scarring of the Fallopian tubes.

Contagious? PID is not *itself* contagious; however, if gonorrhea was the original cause and has not been treated, this may be transmitted by sexual contact.

Treatment: Requires immediate medical care in a hospital. Intravenous antibiotics are essential. Surgery may be needed to drain abscess if present or to treat infection not responding to antibiotics. If IUD is present, it must be removed.

Prevention: Since PID is a complication of gonorrhea in women, avoiding sexually transmitted diseases is the best means of prevention. If a sexually transmitted disease is contracted, prompt medical treatment is imperative.

Discussion: A disease of the sexually active woman. Very rare before puberty and after menopause. Goal of treatment is controlling infection in order to prevent tube obstruction and infertility.

PERICARDITIS

Inflammation of sac that surrounds the heart (peri = around; cardium = heart).

Symptoms: Severe chest pain, sometimes worse with inspiration (breathing in) and improved with position change. Not associated with exercise, nausea, vomiting or sweating. Constant.

Cause: Can be secondary to viral infection, bacterial infection or inflammation without infection. Can occur after heart attack or after heart surgery. Occurs commonly in end-stage kidney disease.

Treatment: Medical care should be sought. Bacterial infection is very serious and must be carefully treated and eradicated. Inflammatory pericarditis needs to be treated with medicine against inflammation until symptoms resolve (as long as large accumulation of fluid does not occur). If so, it may require drainage.

Severity of Problem: Can be quite serious. Requires prompt medical evaluation and treatment.

Contagious? Viral infection is thought to be contagious.

Prevention: None.

Discussion: Pericarditis can be confused with other sources of chest pain. It is therefore imperative that chest pain be evaluated immediately to determine its cause.

PERIPHERAL VASCULAR DISEASE

Disease of the minor arteries of the legs and arms.

Symptoms: Cramping in the buttocks, calf or thighs with exercise. Cramping is relieved by rest.

Cause: Blocking of blood flow because of plaque formation (see CORONARY ARTERY DISEASE).

Severity of Problem: May be minor to more serious. Requires medical evaluation.

Contagious? No.

Treatment: Strong improvement when cigarette smoking ceases and prescribed, strenuous exercise program is undertaken. If conservative treatment is unsuccessful, the condition can be surgically repaired.

Prevention: No definite preventive measures. However, avoiding cigarette smoking and following a diet low in fats, sugars and, in particular, cholesterol may have some potential preventive effect.

PERITONITIS

Chemical irritation and/or bacterial infection of the lining of the abdominal cavity.

Symptoms: Severe localized or diffuse abdominal pain with fever, cramping, tenderness and muscle spasm. Area very tender when palpated (examined by feel).

Cause: Usually seen in the presence of perforation or rupture of the bowel or pelvic inflammatory disease. May also occur as a complication of kidney or liver failure. Due to bacterial infection and/or to exposure of the peritoneum to chemicals.

Severity of Problem: Usually severe. The cause and the condition need early medical attention.

Contagious? No.

Treatment: Antibiotics administered in a hospital and drainage of stomach juices and air by tube through the nose. If there is a large amount of pus, surgical drainage may be necessary.

Prevention: None.

PHARYNGITIS—ACUTE

Inflammation of the throat.

Symptoms: Constant dull soreness of the throat and a sharper pain on swallowing. Fever usually present.

Cause: Infection, usually with a virus. May be bacterial, caused by Group A beta hemolytic streptococcus ("strep throat").

Severity of Problem: Strep throat may lead to rheumatic fever or kidney inflammation.

Contagious? Yes, whether viral or strep.

Treatment: If strep throat is diagnosed, antibiotic therapy is advised. Otherwise, treatment will include rest, aspirin, warm salt water gargles and plenty of fluids. Antibiotics are not effective against viral sore throat.

Prevention: Avoid contact with people known to have sore throats, and during winter months it may be prudent to avoid large crowds when possible.

Discussion: While strep throat is always feared, viral sore throats are more common. It is almost impossible to tell the difference between them by symptoms and examination—a throat culture to grow the strep bacteria in the laboratory is needed. People with high fever and sore throat, especially children, should be seen by a doctor.

PINWORM (ENTEROBIASIS)

Infestation of the intestines by small parasitic worms, most frequently seen in small children.

Symptoms: Itching of the anus and surrounding area.

Cause: The eggs of the pinworm enter the body via hand-to-mouth contact. After they hatch in the intestines, a parasitic relationship is established with the new "host." Adult female pinworms leave the intestine at night while the host (person) is asleep and lay eggs on the skin around the anus. Reinfection occurs from scratching the anal area and unknowingly depositing the eggs in the mouth (thereby maintaining the parasitic cycle). Others become infected by the eggs through contact with the infected person or objects he or she has touched.

Severity of Problem: Seldom harmful; minor irritation may result from anal scratching; occasionally worms will also infest the vulva, causing inflammation. Although rare, the worms may cause an obstruction of the appendiceal lumen, and this may result in appendicitis.

Contagious? Yes. Contact with an infected person or egg-infested objects (for example, food, clothing, bedding) may result in transmission of the parasite.

Treatment: Pinworms are difficult to eradicate totally, since their eggs can remain viable for up to three weeks. The entire household must be treated. An extended vacation with daily changes of location may be necessary to break the reinfesting cycle. A doctor-prescribed medicine may be necessary to aid in the destruction of the parasite.

Prevention: Avoidance of contact with infected person and egg-infected objects.

Discussion: Pinworm (Enterobiasis) is the most common parasite found in warm climates. Children comprise the primary population for this condition (with one in five being infested). Often, infestation ceases without formal treatment.

PLACENTAL ABRUPTION

Premature separation of the placenta that occurs late in pregnancy, mostly among older women and those who have had more than one child.

Symptoms: Characterized by painful bleeding associated with either uterine contractions or cramping; or just constant, very severe pain in the uterus.

Cause: Women who are older, those with chronic hypertension and those who have had many other children are at greater risk for premature separation of the placenta than other expectant mothers. Trauma to the mother's abdomen may also cause placental abruption, although this is uncommon.

Severity of Problem: Blood loss is usually from the mother's side of the placenta, so she can develop shock, which also decreases the oxygen supply to the baby. With massive abruption, fetal death can occur rapidly, even with prompt intervention. It is very important to remember that if bleeding occurs during pregnancy, the doctor should be called immediately for consultation; if bleeding is severe, a trip to the nearest emergency room is in order.

Contagious? No.

Treatment: When a significant placental abruption occurs (unless it happens very early in pregnancy), the recommended treatment is most often prompt delivery, before the fetus dies and the mother experiences a serious loss of blood. Rapid vaginal delivery or emergency cesarean delivery is performed, and blood transfusion is often necessary to manage shock from blood loss.

Discussion: It is very important, if bleeding occurs, for the woman to call her doctor immediately. Significant bleeding and pain require immediate evaluation at an emergency room. If the problem is placental abruption and the placenta has only partially separated, immediate delivery of the baby may save his or her life. Therefore, a very rapid response to bleeding on the woman's part is paramount.

PLACENTA PREVIA

Most often, painless bleeding experienced during the last three months of pregnancy due to a portion or all of the placenta's lying in the lower part of the uterus near or directly over the cervix.

Symptoms: Placenta previa is most often recognized when it causes painless bleeding. (Although a small number of women experience minor cramping or contractions with bleeding from placenta previa, this problem is painless in most cases.)

Cause: A portion or all of the placenta is lying in the lower part of the uterus near or directly over the cervix. The reason this occurs is unknown.

Severity of Problem: Any bleeding during pregnancy should signal the need to call the doctor for consultation. Most bleeding from placenta previa is not massive. However, if severe, uncontrollable bleeding occurs, shock can result, and immediate cesarean delivery is necessary.

Contagious? No.

Treatment: Complete bed rest is recommended, most often in the hospital, until delivery. The goal in managing placenta previa is to stop the bleeding, carefully monitor the mother and baby (as necessary), and keep both in good condition until approximately the 37th week of pregnancy. At this time fetal lung maturity is determined, and if the fetus is mature, cesarean birth is performed.

Prevention: Nothing specific known.

Discussion: At times blood loss from the mother may be serious enough that she will need one or more blood transfusions. Placenta previa increases the risk for prematurity and its many associated problems, as well as perinatal death. With today's technology and knowledge, however, the outlook is vastly improved for the baby, and maternal death due to placenta previa has become increasingly rare.

PLAGUE (BUBONIC, PNEUMONIC)

Very severe infection that causes massive enlargement of lymph nodes and sometimes pneumonia.

Symptoms: Sudden development of fever, severe aches and pains, and sometimes delirium. There may be a sore at the site of a flea bite, with enlarging of a lymph node nearby. Breathing difficulties and severe cough may develop.

Cause: Infection with the Yersinia pestis bacteria, which is transmitted by the bite of an infected flea. The flea acquires the infection from rodents, which are the natural host for these bacteria.

Severity of Problem: The recovery rate is good if the disease is confined to the lymph nodes and is treated promptly. If pneumonia occurs, the death rate can be as high as 60 percent (although it is usually around 20 percent with treatment).

Contagious? Usually not from human to human, unless a flea bites the infected person, then a healthy person. Disease is passed from animals to humans via the flea.

Treatment: Rapid treatment with antibiotics is effective. Other support measures are also important and are based on how extensive the problem is.

Prevention: Best preventive measures are those that are aimed at controlling rodent populations (rat control, in particular) and fleas. Vaccines are available but are not very effective.

Discussion: Plague is characterized as "bubonic" or "pneumonic," depending on the major symptoms and signs. Bubonic plague refers to the more common form, which involves a sore and severe enlargement and inflammation of one or more lymph nodes (these masses are called buboes). When pneumonia occurs, either along with or instead of buboes, the plague is called pneumonic, by far the more serious form.

While this infection is very serious and still occurs, the fear people have of it is often out of proportion. Plague is most often seen in crowded city areas with poor rat control, and in rural and mountainous areas of the Southwest, where rodents may be uncontrolled at times.

PLEURISY

Inflammation of the lining surrounding and covering the lungs.

Symptoms: Sudden, intense stabbing pain in the side or shoulder, aggravated by deep breathing, coughing, sneezing or moving. Breathing is usually rapid and not very deep.

Cause: May result from injury or irritation of the underlying lung; entry of an irritating substance into the pleural space; entry of infection either from the lung or through the bloodstream; or leakage of tumor cells into the pleural space.

Severity of Problem: Not serious of itself if treated properly. Depends on underlying cause.

Contagious? No.

Treatment: Depends on treating underlying cause. Heat applied to chest, and pain relievers help with symptoms. Antibiotics are used if infection suspected or proved.

Prevention: No specific measures known.

Discussion: Inflammation of the pleura, the membranes lining the chest and covering the lungs, causes pain when the lung moves back and forth over the inflamed area. Sometimes, friction is irritating enough that fluid gathers in the chest between the ribs and lungs (called pleural effusion). This kind of fluid collection, if present, can be drained by needle or tube and the fluid studied for infection and abnormal (cancer) cells. Depending on cause, pleurisy can occur one time only or be a recurring problem.

PNEUMOCONIOSIS
Group of lung diseases due to occupational exposure to small particles that are inhaled over a long period of time. These include meat packer's lung, asbestosis, black lung, farmer's lung, silicosis, coal miner's lung and others.

Symptoms: Chronic cough, particularly on re-exposure to offending particles; progressive shortness of breath; fatigue after slight exertion; cyanosis; changes of the fingers and toes called clubbing.

Cause: Chronic inhalation of irritating particles causes a slow inflammatory process in the fibrous tissues of the lung. This inflammation increases over time and compromises the air-exchanging ability of the lungs. It also reduces the lungs' expandability. Some of the offending particles may become deposited in the lung tissue itself.

Contagious? No.

Treatment: After the disease is established, no specific treatment other than avoidance of infection, if possible. Use of oxygen and other breathing supports may be necessary.

Prevention: Avoidance of exposure to dust and other irritating airborne substances. Use of masks when exposure cannot be avoided may be helpful. If disease is known to be present, its progression may be stopped if further exposure is avoided. This may require changing jobs.

Discussion: A major health issue today, occupational lung disease has only recently become understood and to some degree preventable.

PNEUMONIA
Inflammation of the lung, with or without infection. Is also called pneumonitis.

Symptoms: Varying degrees of fever, cough and difficulty breathing. Sometimes there is also pleurisy (chest pain made worse by deep breathing and cough).

Cause: There are many possible causes of lung inflammation, including infection (bacterial, viral, mycoplasma, fungal); hypersensitivity to inhaled substances; and aspiration (inhalation) of stomach contents or foreign material.

These various factors can lead to two different patterns of pneumonia: *interstitial* pneumonia, which is inflammation involving the tissues between the air sacs, and usually involving a good portion of one or both lungs; and *lobar* pneumonia, which is inflammation of the air sacs and connective tissues of a localized segment of the lung. The pattern of the pneumonia can help the doctor determine its possible causes.

Severity of Problem: Varies with the cause and extent of the inflammation. Some pneumonias are life-threatening, while others are comparatively mild illnesses. Also depends on the general health and immunity of the person.

Contagious? Very few of the pneumonias are truly contagious, in the sense of passing from one person to another. The organisms that cause most are already present in the environment and in other people.

Treatment: Depends on the cause. General measures include rest; support of breathing, if needed; drinking of much liquid; medications to fight infection, stop cough and open up airways, as needed.

Prevention: Depends on cause. Many pneumonias that are infectious occur for no apparent reason in a person who has often been exposed to the same organism. Temporary stress, weakness or other change in resistance (which usually cannot be detected) influences the person's getting pneumonia.

Discussion: Many people panic when they hear the word *pneumonia,* because in past decades it was indeed a disease to be feared. While certain forms of pneumonia are still devastating, many can now be easily and successfully treated (even without hospitalization).

PNEUMONIA—ASPIRATION

Inflammation, usually accompanied by resulting infection, of the lungs following the aspiration (inhalation) of irritating substances, especially stomach contents.

Symptoms: Respiratory difficulty starting after a choking or vomiting episode in a person who has difficulty with swallowing, is not fully conscious (ill, recovering from anesthetic, a drug abuser, mentally deficient, neurologically handicapped) or has a problem with regurgitation of food and liquid because of an intestinal problem. There is usually mild fever as well.

Cause: Irritation and damage of the lining of the airways and the lungs because of the aspirated material. Stomach acid is particularly damaging to the lungs. Bacteria may invade and cause infection of the damaged lungs, although this does not always occur.

Severity of Problem: A very serious problem, especially if it occurs repeatedly. A single episode can cause enough damage to lead to death, and repeated episodes usually result in chronic lung damage. This is often what leads to death in chronically ill, debilitated persons.

Contagious? No.

Treatment: Oxygen, breathing support with a machine (respirator), if needed. Suctioning the lungs with a tube inserted through the windpipe may help to remove some of the irritating material if done shortly after the choking or aspiration episode. Sometimes antibiotics and steroids (cortisone-related drugs) will be used, although their use is controversial among doctors.

Prevention: Treatment or control of any underlying problems that make a person susceptible to aspiration.

PNEUMONIA—BACTERIAL

Lung infection caused by any of a variety of bacteria.

Symptoms: With most bacterial forms of pneumonia, there is sudden onset of high fever, chills and cough, followed by varying degrees of difficulty breathing. There may be production and coughing up of sputum, which is sometimes rust-colored. There is often chest pain located over the inflamed area of the lung. This may follow mild respiratory symptoms (stuffy nose, mild cough) by several days. Sometimes infection is generalized in the blood, which makes the person appear very ill.

Cause: Infection of the lung with any of a variety of bacteria. Most common in those people who are otherwise healthy is pneumococcus infection. In those who are chronically ill, malnourished, alcoholic, very young or very old, or have underlying lung disease, the pneumonia may be caused by very unusual bacteria, which can be difficult to treat. The bacteria may enter the lungs from the respiratory tract (by inhaling them) or, rarely, by spread from another part of the body through the blood.

Severity of Problem: Depends on the bacteria involved and the general state of health of the person. Pneumococcal pneumonia in a healthy person is easily treated, with only a few side effects. Pneumonia caused by more unusual bacteria in people with poor resistance is often associated with severe problems, even death.

Contagious? Not as such, for the most part. Bacteria responsible for pneumonia are everywhere in the environment and cause disease only in people who are particularly susceptible or as an unexplained event.

Treatment: The mainstay of treatment is antibiotics, with the specific drug used depending on the type of pneumonia present. Often this requires hospitalization for intravenous therapy, but occasionally treatment can be done at home with mild disease. Rest, fever and cough control (when needed), as well as high liquid intake are all important. Some people need intensive care with support of breathing (with a respirator) and other treatments.

Prevention: Only as far as can be done to control any underlying disease that makes a person susceptible to pneumonia. Asthma and chronic lung disease of other kinds need to be under as good control as possible.

Discussion: The pneumonias caused by bacteria tend to be lobar pneumonia—localized areas of intense infection, sometimes with formation of pleural effusion or pus. These were the pneumonias most often associated with death in the past and are still serious problems.

PNEUMONIA—VIRAL

Lung infection caused by a virus.

Symptoms: Fever, usually less than 103° F, cough and chest discomfort. Usually there is less chest pain than with bacterial pneumonia, and the person does not feel or look as sick. General weakness, loss of appetite and aches and pains are common. There have usually been symptoms of a cold for a few days before the coughing becomes severe. Most people with viral pneumonia, while feeling ill, can continue many of their usual activities.

Cause: Infection of the lungs with a virus. There are many types of viruses that can cause pneumonia.

Severity of Problem: Viral pneumonia is usually a mild to moderately severe disease, which goes away on its own in time. There are very few complications. Exceptions to this occur in small infants, in people with underlying lung disease and in those people with abnormal immunity, where viral pneumonia can be a serious disease. Pneumonia due to the chickenpox virus and the measles virus tends to be more severe, especially in adults.

Contagious? Yes, by contact with the virus spread through the air. However, not all people who are exposed to a particular virus will get pneumonia from it.

Treatment: Rest, fluids, control of fever and cough. Sometimes oxygen and other support measures for breathing will be needed. Most people with viral pneumonia can be treated at home and do not need hospitalization. Antibiotics do not help viral pneumonia, although many doctors prescribe them.

Prevention: None, other than avoidance of the viruses that might cause it.

Discussion: Viral pneumonia is usually an infection that involves the connecting tissue in the lungs (interstitial pneumonia). It is viral pneumonia that people most often refer to as "walking pneumonia," because they did not feel bad enough to stay in bed and continued to walk around.

PNEUMOTHORAX

Collection of air in the chest cavity preventing expansion of the adjacent lung.

Symptoms: Sudden onset of severe stabbing pain in the chest associated with shortness of breath.

Cause: Air can enter the chest cavity through a traumatic perforation of the chest wall (e.g., crushed chest or broken rib), or this may occur spontaneously when a small pocket in the lung leaks into the adjacent cavity.

Severity of Problem: Variable; needs medical attention.

Contagious? No.

Treatment: Small air pockets will usually reabsorb spontaneously. Larger ones, particularly those that compromise respiratory capacity, are treated by insertion of a chest tube, which drains the air.

Prevention: None.

POLIOMYELITIS (POLIO)

Acute infection that can cause paralysis.

Symptoms: At the start of the disease, polio is very similar to other flulike illnesses, with fever, nausea and vomiting, diarrhea or constipation, headache and sore throat. Severe muscle pains with spasms of the muscles, weakness and stiff neck, followed by paralysis of various muscles may follow.

Cause: Infection by one of three types of polio viruses.

Severity of Problem: Can be a very mild disease, but more often severe, with small or large areas of muscle being permanently paralyzed. Most serious type of polio is bulbar type, with paralysis of breathing. This can be temporary or permanent. Death can happen during the acute phase of the disease or later because of complications of bacterial infection.

Contagious? Yes, by contact with respiratory secretions. The virus can either be inhaled or swallowed.

Treatment: Initially and in mild disease, general measures to make the person comfortable: aspirin or aspirin substitute for pain, fluids, fever control. If there are severe muscle pains and spasms, hot packs and changing positions with movement of the painful parts are helpful. Careful observation for weakness of breathing or swallowing muscles is important, with suctioning and breathing support by machine if needed. As the disease improves, physical therapy to help with recovery from weakness and muscle spasms begins.

Prevention: The disease can be completely prevented by immunizing people against it. Infants and children, as well as adults who are not immune and are exposed to a person with the disease, should be immunized with live virus vaccine (Sabin). Adults who travel to areas of the world in which polio is still common should also be immunized. People with immune problems can be immunized with killed vaccine (Salk).

Discussion: Polio is most commonly seen in the summer and late fall and is still common in many areas of the world. The virus can cause a mild illness that resembles other flulike illnesses; a mild aseptic meningitis; paralytic polio, with permanent paralysis of muscles of the trunk and extremities; and bulbar polio, with paralysis of muscles that control breathing, swallowing, gagging, eye movement, talking and facial expression. The mild, flulike form cannot be told apart from other illnesses with similar symptoms.

POLYPS—COLON AND RECTAL

Small growths that arise from the lining of the colon (large bowel) or rectum. May be flat or on a stalk, large or small, single or multiple.

Symptoms: The most common symptom of a polyp is rectal bleeding. The blood is usually bright red and may coat the surface of the stool or be mixed in with it to a certain extent. Polyps are painless.

Cause: Usually a benign (noncancerous) growth that develops at any age. Certain disorders that occur in families are marked by multiple polyps in the colon and sometimes by associated problems as well. These are usually genetically inherited diseases.

Severity of Problem: Most polyps are benign and cause no problems other than bleeding. Occasionally, a flat polyp is actually a cancer that has metastasized (spread) from somewhere else. People with multiple polyps are bothered by many problems, and their disease may make them at risk for developing cancer.

Contagious? No.

Treatment: Most simple polyps can be removed easily using an instrument called a sigmoidoscope or colonoscope, which is used to look inside the rectum and colon. People with multiple polyps may require abdominal surgery to remove the polyps or even the entire colon.

Prevention: None known.

Discussion: Polyps can occur at any age but are increasingly common with advancing age. The vast majority cause no symptoms at all and are not detected until autopsy. (As many as 10 percent of people have a polyp found at the time of autopsy.)

POLYPS—NASAL

Growth with stemlike protrusion found in the mucous membrane of the nose and/or sinuses.

Symptoms: Breathing obstruction; possible bleeding; profuse nasal discharge; sometimes swelling of the face; headaches are possible; some loss of smell; teardrop-shaped growth(s) may be visible in the nose.

Cause: May occur as a result of acute or chronic infections of the mucous membranes of the nose or sinuses.

Severity of Problem: Secondary infection may occur, with possible pressure damage to surrounding facial areas. Difficulty in breathing may result from nasal obstruction.

Contagious? No.

Treatment: Surgical removal is the most reliable treatment. The use of corticosteroids is sometimes effective in reducing the size of the polyp(s).

Prevention: None.

POLYPS—VOCAL CORD

Stemlike growth(s) on the vocal cord(s).

Symptoms: Hoarseness; raspy voice; other changes in voice.

Cause: Can develop from voice abuse or overuse; inhalation of irritating material in the atmosphere; smoking; or from chronic allergic reactions of the larynx.

Severity of Problem: Can be extremely uncomfortable; may affect ability to speak normally.

Contagious? No.

Treatment: Surgical removal may be needed to restore the voice to normal. Treatment should be aimed at the cause to minimize or prevent recurrence.

Prevention: Care should be taken not to overuse or abuse the voice. Sometimes training with a voice therapist is helpful. Smoking and other irritants should be avoided. However, in some cases there are no possible preventive steps.

POSTNASAL DRIP

Dripping of secretions from the nose down the back of the throat.

Symptoms: Sensation of dripping in the back of throat; scratchy throat or sore throat, especially in the morning; frequent throat clearing; hacking cough, especially in the morning; bad breath; usually nasal stuffiness or congestion.

Cause: Most often caused by allergic rhinitis or chronic sinusitis.

Severity of Problem: A nuisance but usually not a serious problem. Rarely, a person with this kind of congestion may also have chronic bronchitis.

Contagious? No.

Treatment: Treatment of the underlying cause is the key to success. Avoiding substances or situations that lead to allergic symptoms or use of antihistamines for allergic rhinitis; treatment of sinusitis with antibiotics and/ or decongestant medications; drinking liquids and use of numbing gargles or sprays for discomfort.

Prevention: Depends on the underlying cause. Can often be controlled, but if due to an allergy, cannot be cured.

See also ALLERGIC REACTIONS AND DISORDERS (ATOPY)—ALLERGIC RHINITIS; SINUSITIS, ACUTE AND CHRONIC.

PREGNANCY—ECTOPIC

Pregnancy in which the embryo implants (attaches) outside the uterus. This may occur in the Fallopian tube (most common) or rarely in the cervix, on the ovary or in the abdominal or pelvic cavity.

Symptoms: Symptoms of early pregnancy, then intermittent vaginal spotty bleeding and crampy abdominal pain soon after the first menstrual period is missed. Increased pain and sometimes weakness over the next two to four weeks. If not treated, sudden abdominal pain with collapse occurs around six to eight weeks after conception. (This usually means rupture of the tube with shock and severe hemorrhage.)

Cause: In about half of ectopic pregnancies, the embryo implants in the tube because of scarring from previous tubal infection. Otherwise, cause usually unknown for tubal and for other more rare forms of ectopic pregnancy.

Severity of Problem: Potentially life-threatening. If not treated early, rupture of the tube can lead to shock and death from hemorrhage.

Contagious? No.

Treatment: Surgery to remove the ectopic embryo and products of conception as soon as diagnosis is made. If tubal rupture has occurred, general intensive support, blood transfusion and immediate surgery.

Prevention: None specific. Treatment of pelvic infections when they occur may prevent tubal scarring and potential risk of future ectopic pregnancy.

Discussion: Surgery for tubal pregnancy almost always involves removal of the Fallopian tube on that side. The ovary frequently must be removed also. This potentially affects subsequent pregnancy by limiting ovum release to one ovary (that is, ability to conceive is probably reduced).

PREGNANCY—MINOR DISORDERS

Fatigue, muscle cramps, sore breasts, swelling and puffiness, irritability and dizziness are all minor problems experienced during pregnancy. The following is a description and discussion of each of these minor disorders. Morning sickness is discussed separately (see PREGNANCY—MORNING SICKNESS).

Fatigue: Tiredness is a very common affliction of the pregnant woman, and interestingly, for many it seems to be more acute during the first three months than later in pregnancy. Some women report a loss of energy and a desire to sleep a lot. A change in hormones may play a role in these feelings of fatigue. Planning to rest every day could be of benefit, although this does not work for all women.

Muscle Cramps: Leg cramps are very common during pregnancy, and often calcium supplementation, whether through diet or through calcium tablets, may be helpful. Never add calcium to your diet without a doctor's recommending it, though. When cramps occur (most often at night), they can be relieved by stretching the cramping muscle. Usually this can be accomplished by extending your leg or foot and then pushing your foot against resistance.

Sore Breasts: Breast enlargement and tenderness is a normal part of pregnancy and takes place in preparation for milk production. Although it can be very disturbing if you bump into something, there is really nothing you can do to prevent the everyday, normal discomfort and tenderness. Wearing a support bra will usually help during pregnancy and while nursing.

Swelling and Puffiness: The discomforts of swelling and puffiness in pregnancy are related to an increase in body fluid. Some swelling, especially late in pregnancy, is expected, because the size of the uterus prevents the blood from draining from the tissues as efficiently as before pregnancy. On the other hand, serious swelling is not normal and may signal a problem, especially during the last three months. Report this to your doctor.

Irritability: Most women experience times of irritability off and on throughout a pregnancy. Irritability is partly due to changes in hormones and is sometimes the result of the minor aches and discomforts associated with a pregnancy. As women get closer to term, irritability is often due to the desire to "get this show on the road." Too, some women cannot continue to be as active as they were before pregnancy and sometimes do not have the energy they used to have and respond by off-and-on irritability. It helps most women to have someone listen to what is bothering them and be understanding.

Dizziness: Some women feel faint (off and on) during their pregnancies, and others actually faint or lose consciousness temporarily. Light-headed feelings and faintness may result from poor diet, low blood sugar or anemia. In some cases, especially late in pregnancy, these feelings may occur when a woman is lying on her back. This is caused by the pressure of the uterus on the large blood vessels that return blood to the heart and brain. In all cases, when you feel dizzy or faint, immediately lie down on your side, and keep your head at the same level as your heart. If you have not eaten recently, get something to eat or drink, as well. Notify a doctor immediately if you ever lose consciousness.

PREGNANCY—MORNING SICKNESS

Nausea and vomiting usually restricted to the first three months of pregnancy.

Symptoms: In some cases the "off-and-on" sensation of having a touch of the flu, not feeling well or bouts of dizziness arrive even before the first period is missed and pregnancy is confirmed.

Cause: Morning sickness got its name because so many women experience problems in the morning (probably due to lack of food intake for so many hours). Lengthy periods of time without food seem to be one of its causes, as may also be the many hormonal changes that take place during pregnancy. There is no basis for the claim that morning sickness is an overt sign that a woman does not want a pregnancy. Many myths have developed about morning sickness, and this is one of them.

Severity of Problem: Morning sickness isn't pleasant and can be downright miserable. The best part of the condition is that it is almost always self-limited. The bouts of vomiting and nausea usually stop after the first three months of pregnancy. It seems that a woman's body has by then adjusted to the pregnancy and its hormonal changes. If, however, the nausea or vomiting become excessive and food and liquids cannot be kept down, then the doctor should be consulted. If it continues beyond the third month of pregnancy, it is best to discuss the problem with the doctor.

Contagious? No.

Treatment: Sometimes drinking small volumes of liquid frequently and eating a few crackers now and then helps control the problem. It is best, however, to have a physician recommend the steps to take, since these may depend on special dietary restrictions for certain women. If the problem is out of control and the mother's and baby's health are potentially jeopardized by lack of adequate food and liquid intake, a drug may be prescribed to control the morning sickness. The pros and cons should be discussed with a woman's personal physician. Also, one of the best treatments for temporary and uncomfortable morning sickness is understanding and support from those close to the woman.

Prevention: None.

PREMENSTRUAL SYNDROME

Group of symptoms that occur in certain women several days to two weeks before the onset of menstrual periods.

Symptoms: Irritability, changes in mood, anxiety, inability to sleep, inability to concentrate, and depression or aggression. Nausea, vomiting, breast soreness and swelling of breasts and ankles, with weight gain of as much as 10 pounds in some women.

Cause: Exact cause is unknown, although wide changes in hormone levels with retention of fluid is probably responsible, at least in part.

Severity of Symptoms: Can be mild and intermittent for some women or very severe and interfere with the lives and relationships of others.

Contagious? No.

Treatment: No treatment is completely effective, although there have been trials of a certain diuretic, spironolactone, which has shown some promise. Restriction of dietary salt helps with keeping the weight gain down. Some women do well with birth control pills, which prevent ovulation and the resultant wide hormone changes. It is important for those close to the woman to understand that her behavior is based in physical problems.

Prevention: Probably no effective prevention for those who are destined to have this, other than salt restriction, suppression of ovulation.

Discussion: Almost all women have some of the features of this syndrome at least occasionally during their menstrual years. However, it can be a particularly severe problem for some, especially those in their thirties who have never been pregnant.

PRESBYOPIA

Loss of near vision as part of the natural aging process.

Symptoms: Blurriness is the major symptom. Headaches, redness, tearing and other eyestrain symptoms may also be experienced.

Cause: The lens of the eye loses its ability to change shape, which decreases one's ability to focus on near objects. When this occurs, the eye muscles must do more work to help the eye focus clearly. This causes eyestrain. Occurs after the age of 45.

Severity of Problem: Unfortunately, loss of near vision is part of the natural aging process. Glasses most often correct this problem. Presbyopia itself does not result in total blindness. If other problems (for example, cataract, retinal degeneration) are present, then these must be evaluated and corrected, where possible.

Contagious? No.

Treatment: See an ophthalmologist or optometrist for evaluation and corrective glasses. Bifocal lenses are often necessary, while others need "reading glasses" for close-up work.

Prevention: None.

PROLAPSED UTERUS

Condition in which the uterus drops or slips down and may even protrude into and out through the vagina.

Symptoms: *Early symptoms*: a feeling of dragging in the lower abdomen; backache while standing or during exertion or exercise; frequency of urination; and a feeling of a large internal weight between the vulva and anus. *Later symptoms*: swelling of the vulva; uncomfortable to painful sexual intercourse; vaginal pain and sometimes discharge; at times abdominal cramping may be experienced.

Cause: Weakness and/or stretching of the pelvic ligaments and muscles due to childbearing (usually many pregnancies) or as a result of the aging process; may also be a result of an inherent weakness of the pelvic structures present at birth (congenital); although less frequently, this can be due to injury (such as lifting heavy objects incorrectly, chronic straining to move the bowels and overstress of the pelvic structures).

Severity of Problem: If the prolapse affects the uterine blood circulation or supply, then abnormal bleeding can occur. Severe bleeding can be life-threatening if not controlled. Pain and discomfort can become chronic and severe in some cases.

Contagious? No.

Treatment: For those who could not tolerate surgery, have high surgical risks, or those where temporary treatment is warranted, a pessary (a device inserted into the vagina) is used to support the pelvic structures. Most often surgical removal of the uterus and repair of other pelvic structures (where indicated) are recommended. If the prolapse is more minor and the woman is still within childbearing age, surgical repair without removing the uterus may be possible.

Prevention: Muscle-strengthening exercises may be helpful after childbirth, especially if they are continued and become part of one's life-style. In some situations prevention is not possible.

See also CYSTOCELE:

PROSTATISM

Enlargement of the prostate gland in men, causing difficulty with urination.

Symptoms: Usually occurs in older men. Increasing difficulty starting a urinary stream, dribbling of urine, urination during the night, urinary frequency are experienced. If severe, may cause urinary retention, infection and uremia (poisoning by release of toxins in the blood).

Cause: Blockage formed by progressive enlargement of the prostate as a normal process due to aging; or it may be due to cancer of the prostate.

Severity of Problem: Depends on basis for enlargement. Should be evaluated by a physician.

Contagious? No.

Treatment: Medications and, where necessary, surgery.

Prevention: None.

Discussion: Enlargement of the prostate gland is a normal part of aging in men. When the gland becomes obstructive to urination, serious problems can arise, and medical care should be sought.

PROSTATITIS—ACUTE

Inflammation of the prostate gland.

Symptoms: High fever and chills, general weakness and malaise. Pain or burning on urination. Difficulty in starting to urinate; frequency of urination; feeling of needing to urinate constantly or without delay. Pain in the low back, in the pelvis and in the genitals behind the scrotum. Pain with bowel movement.

Cause: Bacterial infection from organisms that reach the prostate through the urethra (penile opening) or bloodstream. May be a complication of a lower urinary tract infection.

Severity of Problem: Very uncomfortable. Can lead to chronic prostatitis if not treated promptly.

Contagious? No.

Treatment: Antibiotics, rest and plenty of liquids. Pain relievers, stool softeners and sitz baths help with discomfort. Intercourse should be avoided for several weeks.

Prevention: None.

Discussion: Prompt treatment of acute prostatitis may reduce risk of chronic, or recurring, prostatitis.

PSORIASIS

Chronic skin disease characterized by red patches covered with dry, white or gray scales.

Symptoms: Characteristically involves the scalp, extremities (elbows and knees), back and buttocks. Fingernails and eyebrows may also be infected. Lesions are highly visible, although non-itching, showing as rough, red skin covered with overlapping silver-white skin scales of a hard, dry nature.

Cause: Psoriasis commonly runs in families and can be triggered by local trauma, severe sunburn, reaction to certain chemical compounds and general irritation to the skin.

Severity of Problem: Except for any psychological damage (being self-conscious, embarrassed, etc.) caused by the unsightliness of the exposed skin, general health is not affected. A physician consultation may be helpful in severe cases.

Contagious? No.

Treatment: Since the number of truly effective remedies is limited, the traditional treatments such as lubricants, topical corticosteroids and keratolytics should be tried first. Extensive cases should be seen by a dermatologist. A new treatment called "PUVA" (medication plus ultraviolet light) shows promise.

Prevention: While acute outbreaks can usually be expected to subside, complete and permanent disappearance of the disease is rare. Chemical compounds and environmental conditions suspected or known to be factors should be avoided. Lesions should be treated as soon as possible.

Discussion: Generally starts during preteen years, and it comes and goes over a period of many years. It rarely starts after middle age.

PTERYGIUM

Small, triangular growth on the eyeball.

Symptoms: Appearance and enlargement of a soft, triangular-shaped growth on the conjunctiva of the eye, located at the inside of the iris (colored portion). As it grows, it may begin to cover the cornea, causing a defect in vision at the nasal side of vision.

Cause: Frequent irritation of the conjunctiva, usually seen with constant exposure to sun, wind and sand.

Severity of Problem: Not a problem unless it grows to cover the cornea and interferes with vision.

Contagious? No.

Treatment: None is necessary unless pterygium extends onto the cornea. If it does, surgical removal is required so vision can be preserved.

Prevention: Avoidance of exposure to wind and sand, when possible. Eye protection may be helpful.

Discussion: This small growth can occur on one or both eyes and has a tendency to return if surgery is performed, unless the irritating wind and sand exposure are avoided.

RAYNAUD'S DISEASE (PHENOMENON, SYNDROME)

Condition in which there is episodic pallor or cyanosis of the fingers (and sometimes toes) because of arterial spasm.

Symptoms: Sudden onset of intense pallor and/or cyanosis of the tips of the fingers following exposure to cold or, occasionally, emotional upset. The fingers are usually uncomfortable, with burning pain, tingling or numbness. When this kind of attack, which can recur frequently, ends, the skin turns bright red, and there may be slight swelling, throbbing and pain.

Cause: Arterial spasm from a variety of causes leads to *Raynaud's phenomenon* or *Raynard's syndrome,* which is this symptom complex found in association with other diseases such as scleroderma, carpal tunnel syndrome, peripheral artery disease and systemic lupus erythematosis. *Raynaud's disease* is a similar problem but without underlying cause. An abnormality of the sympathetic nervous system is probably involved.

Severity of Problem: Episodes can occur only occasionally, or frequently, and can lead to chronic ulcers and deterioration of the fat at the tips of the fingers. Raynaud's disease tends to be less severe and disabling than Raynaud's phenomenon.

Contagious? No.

Treatment: Rewarming of the hands and body by returning to a warm environment or putting the hands in warm water. Any skin irritation or dryness should be relieved using hand lotion or cream. Drugs that dilate the peripheral arteries can be helpful. Sometimes surgery to sever the lumbar sympathetic nerves is suggested for intractable arterial spasm. It is important that a doctor watch anyone with Raynaud's phenomenon closely for signs of other underlying diseases.

Prevention: Individual attacks can be prevented by using very warm clothing and mittens or gloves when going outside. Care needs to be taken to protect the hands from injury, because sores on the hands heal slowly when the arterial blood supply is questionable.

Discussion: Raynaud's disease, which has no known specific cause, usually affects women between 15 and 40 years old and is a relatively minor problem. Raynaud's phenomenon or syndrome, on the other hand, can occur in both men and women and may lead to scarring and deformity.

RENAL FAILURE—ACUTE

Sudden failure of the kidneys to perform their normal blood-cleaning function.

Symptoms: Cessation of urinary output, edema and water retention. Loss of appetite, nausea and vomiting, lethargy, elevation of blood pressure. There may be many other symptoms, depending on underlying cause of kidney failure.

Cause: Causes are varied, including massive or crushing injuries, blood loss, dehydration and surgical shock; poisoning from chemicals, natural substances (such as wild mushrooms) and certain antibiotics; tissue destruction from burns; incompatible blood transfusions; infectious disease; complications of pregnancy; water and electrolyte depletion; and bone marrow tumors.

Severity of Problem: Extremely critical. Certain untreated causes could result in death.

Contagious? No.

Treatment: Hospitalization and close medical supervision are required, as are immediate identification and treatment of causes. Normal body fluid composition is the goal of treatment. The person is protected from new infections when possible. Special diet, salt and water restriction are usually required. Appropriate antibiotics are given if infection is present. (Poisonous waste products may need to be removed from the body by a special technique called dialysis).

Prevention: Prevention of causes is required.

Discussion: Shock from any cause is the most common reason for acute renal failure. At other times the problem progresses to chronic kidney failure.

RETINA, DETACHED

Separation of the retina (the back part of the eye on which images are focused in order to see) from the structures that lie under it. This results in tearing of the tiny nerve endings and blood vessels.

Symptoms: Sudden partial or complete loss of sight in one eye. May start like a "curtain" that blocks sight in just one part of the area of vision. There is no pain and no redness of the eye.

Cause: Most often retinal tears occur without warning and without apparent cause. Injury to the eye, severe nearsightedness and absence of the lens (as a result of cataract surgery) may lead to retinal detachment.

Severity of Problem: Can lead to permanent loss of vision, although most often treatment is effective if done quickly after the retina has detached.

Contagious? No.

Treatment: Requires immediate evaluation and treatment by an ophthalmologist. May involve use of ultrasound or laser treatment to reattach the retina by causing inflammation and development of tiny amounts of scar tissue. Cryosurgery (treatment with cold) and conventional surgery are also possible forms of treatment.

Prevention: None in most cases.

Discussion: When a small part of the retinal membrane tears and separates from the structures behind it, fluid forms in the space and causes further separation of the retina. The last area to separate is the macula, the area that is involved with central vision. Without treatment, retinal detachment will become complete in several months, with total blindness. More than three-fourths of victims will have a successful recovery with surgery.

RETINOPATHY

Damage to the retina of the eye (the back portion on which the image of what we see is projected).

Symptoms: Blurriness, then progressive loss of vision. The visual loss may be generalized over the eye or may be worse in some parts than in others.

Cause: Damage to the retina is usually caused by damage to the blood vessels of the eye, with narrowing and loss of blood supply, congestion of veins with formation of aneurysms, and rupture of blood vessels, leading to blockage of vision by blood in front of the retina. There are many possible causes for these changes, including hypertension (both chronic and temporary, such as pre-eclampsia of pregnancy), diabetes mellitus and generalized arteriosclerosis.

Severity of Problem: Can be mild to severe, but in most cases the damage from generalized disease is gradual and progressive. Can lead to blindness unless the underlying disease is controlled.

Contagious? No.

Treatment: Consists of all measures needed to control the underlying problem.

Discussion: People with arteriosclerosis, diabetes and hypertension should have regular eye examinations to determine whether there is eye damage related to their underlying problem. Hypertension of pregnancy (pre-eclampsia and eclampsia) can cause retinae changes that usually revert to normal after the pregnancy has ended and the blood pressure has returned to normal.

RHEUMATIC FEVER

Group of symptoms that occur several weeks after and as result of streptococcal throat infection.

Symptoms: Usually in childhood several weeks after streptococcal sore throat: primarily fever, migratory joint pains; leaking of heart valves; skin nodules; rash; uncontrolled movements of the extremities (St. Vitus' dance).

Cause: Thought to be due to the body's immune response to the streptococcal infection.

Severity of Problem: Variable. Can be mild, with little or no long-term damage, or severe.

Contagious? Yes. Streptococcus sore throat is contagious. Both carriers and those exposed should be treated with penicillin.

Treatment: During acute episode, patient is treated with anti-inflammatory agents and whatever medical therapy is required for the acute heart problem. Over time, the acute problems subside. Thereafter, the patient should take daily oral or monthly intramuscular penicillin until the mid-twenties to prevent repeated streptococcal infection.

Prevention: Preventing the spread of streptococcal sore throat in the community with penicillin.

Discussion: The acute episodes of rheumatic fever usually resolve, leaving no symptoms until the eventual further problems with the valves that were damaged originally. How serious the rheumatic heart disease is afterward depends in part on how many additional bouts of rheumatic fever occurred and the person's socioeconomic level. The lower the socioeconomic level, the faster the rate of progression. Since the advent of penicillin, there has been a steady drop in the incidence of rheumatic fever in this country.

RHEUMATIC HEART DISEASE

Disease of heart muscle and heart valves resulting from acute rheumatic fever.

Symptoms: Symptoms vary, depending on which valve is affected. There may be shortness of breath, heart failure (see HEART FAILURE, dizziness, blackouts.

Cause: A consequence of heart inflammation due to rheumatic fever. Rheumatic fever is caused by the body's immune response to a streptococcal infection.

Severity of Problem: Variable. Valve and muscle damage can be major or less severe.

Contagious? No.

Treatment: Depends on which valve is affected and if it is narrowed (stenosis) or leaking (insufficient, regurgitant). Initially, medical treatment with control of heart failure, if present. With severe forms, valve-replacement surgery may be needed.

Prevention: None. Detection and treatment of strep infections have an indirect effect by preventing some cases of rheumatic fever.

Discussion: Other than valves that are abnormal at birth, the most frequent cause of valvular heart disease in this country is rheumatic fever. With the advent of penicillin therapy for prevention and surgical therapy for the eventual valve problems, the picture for rheumatic fever is improving. The valves usually affected are on the arterial (left) side of the heart (namely, the aortic and mitral). The condition is seen in adults, sometimes with no sure history of past acute rheumatic fever.

ROCKY MOUNTAIN SPOTTED FEVER

Acute infection with high fever and rash.

Symptoms: Abrupt development of chills, weakness, muscular aches and pains, and intense headaches. Within two days, fever marked by temperature of 103° F or 104° F. Fever lingers for two to three weeks, with rash extending over entire body, including soles of feet.

Cause: A virus carried by hard-shelled ticks. Virus attacks blood cells and skin. In some cases the heart, liver and lungs may be affected.

Severity of Problem: Rash can develop into large ulcers and gangrenous areas. Extended periods of high fever can result in insomnia, delirium and coma. In extreme cases pneumonia, circulatory failure, and brain and heart damage are possible.

Contagious? No. Passed on by the bite of a tick.

Treatment: Prompt diagnosis and antibiotic treatment, usually with tetracyline or chloramphenicol.

Prevention: Tick repellants (e.g., dimethyl phthalate) for individuals entering tick-infested areas. While a vaccine is available, its use is recommended only for those with frequent exposure to ticks.

Discussion: Rocky Mountain spotted fever is limited to the Western Hemisphere, in a broad area ranging from the Atlantic Coast to the Southwest.

ROSEOLA

An illness of infants and young children, thought to be a virus infection.

Symptoms: Sudden onset of very high fever (103° F to 105° F), which lasts for three days. Often the disease starts with a short convulsion due to the fever. Infants do not appear as ill as the fever might indicate and have no other symptoms of illness for the first three days. As the fever falls abruptly, a fine, red rash may be seen over the face, neck and chest. Rash lasts for only a short time and may be missed. There may be slightly enlarged lymph nodes at the base of the skull and the back of the neck.

Cause: Presumed to be a virus disease, although this has not been proved by identifying a specific virus.

Severity of Problem: Actually a mild disease without serious complications other than the possibility of febrile seizure because of the height of the fever.

Contagious? Probably mildly contagious to infants who have not had it.

Treatment: Control of fever with medication (usually aspirin substitute with or without aspirin also), light dressing and sponge baths with lukewarm water when needed. If convulsion occurs, drug treatment may be needed for that (but this is controversial).

Prevention: Possibly by avoiding contact with an infant who may have this disease.

Discussion: While this disease can be very frightening to parents because of the height of the fever, it is a mild problem, with no serious complications and no deaths. Many children who have convulsions with it do not have any with other febrile illnesses. Disease most often occurs in infants between 6 months and 2 years of age.

RUBELLA (GERMAN MEASLES, "THREE-DAY MEASLES")

Virus disease with fever and rash, usually mild for children and adults but potentially devastating for fetuses of pregnant women.

Symptoms: Mild fever, generalized fatigue and weakness, mild nasal congestion. A fine, pink to red, slightly bumpy rash appears on the face, neck, chest, back and upper arms and legs, worsening over several hours, and may itch mildly. There may be joint pains and mild swelling in adults. Rash and symptoms usually last for three days, although joint pains may last for several weeks. There are usually several lymph nodes at the base of the skull and back of the neck that are slightly enlarged and tender.

Cause: Infection with rubella virus.

Severity of Problem: A very mild disease for children and adults. Occasionally adults, particularly women, are bothered by joint pains for days to weeks after infection. Most serious complication is infection of a pregnant woman's fetus, especially during the first three months.

Contagious? Yes, by contact with respiratory secretions of a person with the disease. It is contagious for about a week before the rash appears or for many months in the case of congenital rubella.

Treatment: No specific treatment. Symptomatic treatment of fever, aches and pains. Rash requires no treatment.

Prevention: Can be completely prevented by immunizing susceptible children and adults with live modified rubella virus vaccine. Immunization is recommended for infants 15 months of age and older. It is especially important that girls be immunized before puberty. Adult women should know whether or not they are immune to this disease (by blood test) and be immunized if they are not. If vaccine is given to an adult woman, pregnancy must be prevented for three months.

Discussion: Rubella is a very mild disease that cannot easily be distinguished from other viral diseases that cause rash and fever, except in epidemics. Epidemics still occur and are particularly risky for young women who are not immune and may be pregnant but not yet aware of it.

SALMONELLA GASTROENTERITIS

Infection of the intestinal tract with Salmonella bacteria.

Symptoms: Sudden high fever and chills; vomiting; profuse liquid diarrhea, usually bloody or streaked with blood and mucus; crampy abdominal pain. May lead to severe weakness and delirium, as well as dehydration.

Cause: Acquired by eating food or liquid contaminated with infected human waste; disease usually starts within 12 to 48 hours after eating the tainted substance. Can be carried in pet turtles (a possible source of infection for children).

Severity of Problem: Very serious disease, especially in very young infants and children or severely ill or malnourished adults. Infection can enter blood and travel to other parts of the body. People with sickle-cell anemia are prone to bone infection from salmonella.

Contagious? Yes, as mentioned. Also, people who do not have symptoms but carry the germ can pass it on to others through food that has been handled.

Treatment: Rest; intravenous fluids if needed; fever control with medications. Antibiotic treatment only for very critically ill people; very young infants; or malnourished, chronically ill adults.

Discussion: The acute infection usually lasts three to five days and goes away by itself. Antibiotic treatment may prolong the carrying of the bacteria in the intestine. This is a common cause of "food poisoning" and should be thought of if a large group of people become ill after a common meal. May be carried in uncooked or improperly cooked poultry.

SALMONELLOSIS—TYPHOID FEVER

Generalized, serious infection caused by the bacteria Salmonella typhi. Disease lasts three to four weeks if untreated and can occur in epidemics.

Symptoms: (1) During the first week: gradual weakness and listlessness; headache; sore throat; cough; gradually rising fever, with daily increase in the height of fever (can go to 105° F+ at its worst). (2) During second week: abdominal pain, swelling and development of either constipation or liquid green diarrhea; there is decreased awareness and stupor; an unusual rash may also be seen on the abdomen. (3) During the third week: Complications of intestinal bleeding or intestinal rupture may occur. (4) During the later part of the disease: Fever slowly returns to normal, and symptoms gradually disappear.

Cause: Infection with Salmonella typhi bacteria. The origin is contaminated food or water due to poor sanitation or food handling by carriers of the bacteria. Bacteria invade the blood through the bowel and spread to other parts of the body.

Severity of Problem: Very serious disease, with high rate of complications (¼ to ⅓ of victims). Death may occur without treatment. Complications include intestinal bleeding, perforation, pneumonia, gallbladder infection, meningitis, inflammation of heart muscle, phlebitis and bone infection.

Contagious? Yes, through food and drink contaminated with infected human waste.

Treatment: Treatment of symptoms, usually in a hospital. Isolation to prevent spread by contaminated waste. Antibiotic treatment for severe infection *only,* not for carrier state.

Prevention: Avoid contaminated or questionable food and water, especially when traveling in areas with poor sanitation. Asymptomatic carriers (see "Discussion") should not handle food. Immunization is available for those traveling to or living in high-risk areas.

Discussion: A person may carry the bacteria for months or years after the acute infection without knowing it. The germ is usually found in the gallbladder or intestine. This asymptomatic carrier state is risky to others who can get the disease from food or drink contaminated by the carrier. Removal of the gallbladder may eliminate this problem. Treatment with antibiotics does not cure this carrier state and may prolong it.

SCABIES (MITES)

Contagious skin disease, with oozing crust.

Symptoms: Intensely itching, bumpy red rash found on finger webs; wrists; elbows; buttocks; around the nipples in females and on genitals in males.

Cause: Scabies is caused by the female itch mite, which tunnels into the layers of the skin and deposits her eggs. The larvae hatch within days and cluster around the hair follicles. The mites are irritating and lead to the skin inflammation and rash.

Severity of Problem: Continuous scratching can lead to secondary rash and skin infections.

Contagious? Yes. The disease is easily transmitted by skin-to-skin contact with an infected person.

Treatment: Recommended treatments include complete body cleansing, followed by applications of 25 percent benzyl benzoate, 1 percent gamma henzene hexachloride or 10 percent crotamiton (this must be obtained by doctor's prescription) over the entire body surface overnight. Clothes and bedding should be disinfected.

Prevention: Improved sanitary conditions; avoidance of suspected "carriers."

SCARLET FEVER (SCARLETINA)

Contagious disease that is really strep throat with a characteristic rash.

Symptoms: Sudden onset of fever, sore throat, headache, generalized aching, abdominal pain and fatigue. Rash begins to appear during the first day of the illness as a red, fine, rough (sandpaper-feeling) rash starting on face, neck, armpits and groin. It rapidly spreads to the rest of the body, and the spots run together. Swollen tonsils with pus; strawberry tongue. Rash peels at the end of the disease (about 10 to 14 days later).

Cause: Infection with group A beta hemolytic streptococcus bacteria. Certain groups of this bacteria produce a toxic substance that causes the scarlet fever rash.

Severity of Problem: A serious disease, but one that can be successfully treated with antibiotics. Complications include glomerulonephritis, an acute inflammation of the kidney. Rheumatic fever happens only rarely after this strep infection.

Contagious? Yes, by contact with infected person's secretions.

Treatment: Must be treated by a doctor. Antibiotic treatment (usually penicillin by mouth or injection) is very effective.

Prevention: Avoid contact with people with strep infections.

Discussion: Before penicillin was available, scarlet fever was a much more serious disease. It can follow infection in a cut or surgical wound.

SEBORRHEA

Inflammation of the scalp, with crusting and scaling.

Symptoms: Reddish or yellow scaly patches on the scalp, which may be dry or greasy. In advanced cases scaling can appear along the hairline, behind or in the ears, on the eyebrows, on the nose and on the forehead. Itching common. Can also be accompanied by acne.

Cause: Seborrhea can be caused by both genetic and climatic factors. Exposure to certain chemical compounds and low humidity can affect the incidence and severity of the disease.

Severity of Problem: Seborrhea is not a physically threatening disease, but it can be one of extreme discomfort. A rash called seborrheic dermatitis can complicate this problem.

Contagious? No.

Treatment: Depending on the severity of the resulting seborrheic dermatitis or its location, sulphur and salicylic acid ointment or selenium sulfide shampoo should be used. A shampoo schedule of every other day is recommended until the scaling is controlled, then once or twice a week. Facial areas below the hairline can be treated with a steroid cream until improvement occurs.

SEIZURE (CONVULSION, FIT, EPILEPSY)

Sudden, abnormal brain electrical activity that is associated with involuntary movements or jerks and usually loss of consciousness.

Symptoms: One or more episodes with loss of consciousness followed by stiffness, then rhythmic jerking of the body parts (either as a whole or limited to one area); may urinate and have bowel movement; breathing is stopped or labored; may turn blue; teeth are clenched. Afterward, person is temporarily not able to be awakened and does not remember the seizure. Other forms of seizures are described in the "Discussion" section.

Cause: Rapid, abnormal electrical discharge in the brain from a number of causes: brain injury (severe or minor, before or after birth); fever (see SEIZURE—FEBRILE); infections, such as meningitis, encephalitis, shigellosis; chemical disturbance, such as low blood sugar, low body sodium, very low blood calcium, uremia; tumors; withdrawal from drugs or alcohol. Sometimes a cause is never found, as in so-called idiopathic epilepsy. In some seizure disorders certain lights, sounds or temperatures may set off a seizure. May run in families.

Severity of Problem: Seizures can happen only once or be a chronic, recurring problem. Mild lack of oxygen may occur with severe, prolonged convulsion. Injuries may occur as a result of loss of consciousness (falls, fractures). Emotional problems may be seen in response to having a seizure disorder. *Most seizure disorders can be well controlled with appropriate medication.*

Contagious? No.

Treatment: During a seizure, lay the person down on his or her side or face down in a safe place (to prevent injury and to allow secretions to drain out of mouth). *Do not* try to put something between the teeth or open the mouth; it is not necessary. If seizure lasts longer than several minutes or blueness is severe, call paramedics. Get medical evaluation and treatment, even if convulsion stopped by itself. Treatment consists of taking medication every day for years or sometimes for life. Type of medicine is determined by kind and frequency of convulsions. Some people require the use of more than one drug.

Prevention: In a person with a known seizure disorder, taking medication as prescribed usually prevents seizures. The most common cause of repeated seizure in someone already on seizure medicine is failure to take the medicine. Otherwise, no prevention is known.

Discussion: Seizures are among the most misunderstood of medical problems. They do not mean a person is crazy, and they are not contagious. Most people who have them are otherwise *completely* normal.

There are several kinds of seizures, each with its own type of treatment:

1. *Grand mal (generalized seizure)*—involves shaking of whole body and loss of consciousness. Person may know it is coming on but can't stop it. Most common type.

2. *Petit mal (absence seizure)*—occurs mostly in children and consists of blank stares, momentary lapses of consciousness. These have a very specific brain wave pattern. Person often has grand mal seizures, too.

3. *Jacksonian (focal or partial seizure)*—involves jerking starting in one part of the body (twitching of mouth, jerking of one arm) and may move to involve other parts of the body or become a grand mal seizure.

4. *Psychomotor seizure*—is a very complex and variable form. May include patterned behavior, lip smacking, outbursts of activity, head turning and others. Among the most difficult to recognize and control.

People with uncontrolled seizure disorders must avoid activities and occupations (for example, driving, skydiving, flying aircraft, swimming alone) in which they or others might be injured.

SEIZURE—FEBRILE

Loss of consciousness with jerking movements of arms and legs lasting seconds to minutes and associated with high fever in children under the age of six years.

Symptoms: Loss of consciousness with jerking movements of the arms and legs. Eyes roll back; skin color is often blue. Fever is high, usually over 103° F. After the jerking has stopped, the child is sleepy and unresponsive for several minutes. Usually urinates and may have a bowel movement during the seizure.

Cause: Basically unknown. There is some tendency for febrile convulsions to occur in certain families more than in others.

Severity of Problem: Not severe. Seizures themselves are usually short, and the tendency to have them disappears as the child grows. Very frightening for parent.

Contagious? No.

Treatment: During convulsion, turn child on his or her side or face down, in a place where he or she cannot injure self. *Do not* try to put something between the teeth or jaws. If the child is very blue or seizure does not stop in five minutes, call paramedics for help. Begin CPR (cardio-pulmonary resuscitation) if both breathing and heartbeat stop. (This is *very* rare.)

As soon as the seizure has stopped, measure the temperature and begin to lower it if it is over 103° F. Use cool, wet towels over the child, or put him or her in a lukewarm tub for about 30 minutes. Contact physician immediately.

Prevention: Possible by control of fever.

Discussion: Most commonly seen in infants and children between 6 months and 6 years of age. Most children have only one febrile convulsion, while others have them with each fever. Most children with simple febrile convulsions are otherwise totally normal and do not go on to have other types of convulsions or epilepsy.

SEPTICEMIA (BLOOD POISONING, SEPSIS, BACTEREMIA)

Profound bacterial infection spreading through the bloodstream to the entire body.

Symptoms: High fever, chills and skin eruptions initially. Eventually associated with profound shock, low blood pressure, kidney failure, death.

Cause: May be seen wherever bacteria can spread via the bloodstream from infected source, including during procedure where a diagnostic instrument is inserted into an area of infection (e.g., insertion of a urinary catheter into a bladder full of infected urine).

Severity of Problem: Septicemia is very severe and should be treated by immediate administration of appropriate antibiotics and support measures in a hospital setting.

Contagious? No.

Treatment: Needs hospitalization, positive identification of the source and type of infection, administration of antibiotics and support measures.

Prevention: Prevention or early treatment of infection.

SINUSITIS—ACUTE AND CHRONIC

Inflammation and usually infection of one of the sinuses of the face and head.

Symptoms: Pain, swelling and tenderness over the involved sinus. Pain may be mild or severe. Can be located over the forehead, cheekbones, behind the eyes or in the back of the head, or can feel like a toothache of the upper jaw. Congestion of the nose is common. There may be fever, chills and a generally poor feeling.

Cause: Acute sinusitis is usually caused by a bacterial infection that complicates a common cold. Chronic sinusitis is a smoldering inflammation and infection that has not been treated effectively. Chronic nasal congestion caused by allergic rhinitis or deviated nasal septum may also lead to sinusitis.

Severity of Problem: Mild to moderate, although can lead to generalized infection (sepsis) occasionally.

Contagious? The initial viruses are.

Treatment: Requires medical diagnosis and treatment. Antibiotics are usually prescribed for 10 to 14 days and perhaps longer. Nasal drops or spray may be suggested to open the passages to the sinuses and drain the pus and mucus. Rest and pain relief with aspirin, aspirin substitute or stronger drugs will help.

Prevention: Treatment and relief of nasal congestion due to allergies or common cold if possible. Recognition of early symptoms and early treatment of acute symptoms and infection.

SLEEP DISORDERS—INSOMNIA

Inability to fall asleep, sleep soundly or get enough sleep.

Symptoms: Person simply can't sleep; lies awake in bed for long periods of time; tosses and turns; seemingly awakens at every noise; wakes frequently throughout the night; or feels tired a great deal because of inability to sleep well.

Cause: Generally due to stress and anxiety; emotional problems; medical conditions that involve pain or physical discomfort; and/or an interruption or change in normal routine or habits. Sometimes stimulants such as coffee, cola, tea (with caffeine), cigarettes or other tobacco products (nicotine), and others cause sleeplessness.

Severity of Problem: Insomnia *itself* is not a significant health problem, since exhaustion will bring on sleep (although this is not a healthy way to approach sleep). What may be a problem is "the cause(s)" for the insomnia. Also, sleep deprivation, anxiety and stress make people more susceptible to illness and/or injury. Temporary or infrequent sleep disturbances are usually normal.

Contagious? No.

Treatment: Professional consultation (physician, psychiatrist or psychologist) should be sought for chronic problems. Treatment is specific to the underlying cause(s). Sometimes exercise, proper diet, stress control, behavior modification and an emphasis on overall mental health may also be recommended as part of treatment. If the use of stimulants (coffee, cigarettes, etc.) is the problem, then they should be avoided in the evening hours.

Prevention: Overall emphasis on good health habits, wellness and stress control.

SLEEP DISORDERS—NARCOLEPSY

Condition in which short, involuntary periods of sleep occur repeatedly during the day.

Symptoms: Continually falling asleep under conditions not normally associated with sleep: at work; while driving; at public events; while shopping; or even in the morning after a complete night's sleep.

Cause: Unknown.

Severity of Problem: Potential injury and extreme harm to the person with narcolepsy and others, since falling asleep under certain conditions (e.g., while driving) can be very dangerous.

Contagious? No.

Treatment: Stimulant medications are sometimes prescribed by a physician.

Discussion: Symptoms usually begin in adolescence with no previous history of a problem. No pathologic changes can be detected in the brain. Symptoms usually persist throughout life, but sleep durations do not change. Although narcolepsy is rare, four times as many men as women are affected.

SLEEP DISORDERS—NIGHTMARES

Occurrence of terrifying or unpleasant dreams during sleep.

Symptoms: Dreams of terror, fear, apprehension or general unpleasantness during sleep. Particularly traumatic nightmares will interrupt sleep; some people may awake startled, anxious, breathing rapidly, heart beating rapidly, agitated and sweating.

Cause: Subconscious factors, fears, pressures and/or emotional disturbances may cause nightmares.

Severity of Problem: Constant nightmares may signal anxiety, stress, fear of something, undue pressure or even deep-seated emotional disturbances that may indicate the need for a professional evaluation (by a psychiatrist or psychologist).

Contagious? No.

Treatment: The underlying cause must first be identified and then treated.

Prevention: Control of stress; proper diet; routine exercise program; emphasis on overall wellness; prompt recognition that a problem may exist and the seeking of professional help before a situation worsens or becomes problematic.

SLEEP DISORDERS—SLEEP APNEA (ADULT)

Episodes of stopping breathing during sleep.

Symptoms: Very loud snoring, occasional snorting and startling during sleep, often unknown to the sufferer. Daytime sleepiness, need to nap, irritability, some memory disturbance related to lack of sleep.

Cause: This recently recognized problem is commonly caused by obstruction of the upper airway during sleep. Usually results from relaxation of the muscles and structures of the mouth and airway, with the tissues falling back into the throat. May be worsened by being overweight. In this form there may be much movement and apparent struggling to breathe, with no air being moved.

A second form of sleep apnea occurs because of a central nervous system abnormality in which the mechanism that controls breathing is abnormal. With this form breathing efforts stop momentarily, and there are no respiratory movements of the chest.

Severity of Problem: Causes severe sleep disturbance and disruption of function because of lack of sleep. Also can cause difficulties because of chronic lack of oxygen during these episodes of apnea, depending on how often they occur.

Contagious? No.

Treatment: Obstructive apnea is treated by removing any blockages in the upper airway if possible. When not possible, tracheostomy (a surgical operation in which a breathing opening is made in the windpipe in the neck) is performed to bypass any upper airway blockage.

Central apnea may be treated with medication that alters the sleep pattern and stimulates the brain center that controls breathing.

Prevention: Potentially, avoidance of blockage of the upper airway or recognition and treatment when it occurs. No prevention for central apnea.

Discussion: Sleep apnea has recently been recognized as one of the more serious of the sleep disturbances and insomnia. There is a tendency for this type of condition to run in families. It is a difficult problem that requires medical evaluation and treatment, usually in a large center, because of the need to do very sophisticated tests to determine if it is present.

SLEEP DISORDERS—SNORING

Often loud, hoarse-sounding breathing during sleep (caused by vibration of the soft palate).

Symptoms: Most often people are told they snore, or someone complains about their snoring; some people complain that they have a sore throat in the morning or that their mouth feels dry or dusty because they are breathing through their mouth instead of their nose.

Cause: Possible causes include anything that causes a "stuffy" nose; hay fever; common cold; nasal polyps; small nasal passages; structural defect of the inside of the nasal passages or septum; sinusitis; allergic rhinitis; pharyngitis; swollen or enlarged tonsils and adenoids; or a growth in the nasal passages. Most often people snore while sleeping on their back or sitting up with their head extended backward. This naturally allows the jaw to drop or fall open.

Severity of Problem: Snoring itself is more often a problem or irritant to those around the snorer than to the person who snores. However, the underlying cause for the snoring may need to be evaluated if it is causing discomfort or if persistent sore throats occur due to constant snoring.

Contagious? No.

Treatment: For the snoring itself, there is no treatment, but some underlying causes may merit treatment if they result in breathing difficulties.

Prevention: None. Attempting *not* to sleep on one's back may alleviate the problem to a point.

SPERMATOCELE

Mass in the scrotum caused by a cyst on the spermatic cord.

Symptoms: A painless enlargement of the scrotum, usually in adolescent or adult males. The swelling may be high, above or at the top of one testicle.

Cause: The formation of a cyst (fluid-filled pocket) in or near the spermatic cord, which carries sperm from the epididymis to the prostate gland. There may have been mild injury that led to the cyst formation. The cyst usually contains sperm.

Severity of Problem: Swelling generally causes worry. May become large enough to be uncomfortable.

Contagious? No.

Treatment: None is required unless the cyst is very large or causes discomfort. Surgery to remove the cyst is the treatment and may be needed if there is any question about whether the lump is a tumor or a cyst.

Prevention: None.

SPONDYLOSIS

Degenerative changes in the discs, the small pads that cushion the space between vertebrae in the back and neck.

Symptoms: Pain and stiffness in the back or neck, especially in the morning or after prolonged inactivity. Activity improves the pain. There is no fever and no apparent deformity. Tends to occur in people who are middle-aged and older.

Cause: Degenerative changes in one or more of the soft discs that cushion the vertebrae. The disc becomes narrowed and may squeeze out toward the side of the spine, pressing on the nerve roots coming out of the spinal canal (a herniated or slipped disc). There may be associated narrowing and inflammation of the joints nearby. When this occurs in the neck, there might be numbness or pain in the arm in addition to the pain and discomfort in the neck itself.

Severity of Problem: It is the hallmark of aging, with most people bothered by some disability but most able to function quite well. Can lead to slipped disc (herniated disc). Occasionally, pain can be debilitating.

Contagious? No.

Treatment: Depends on cause, but principles rely on common sense. Rest, avoidance of overstressing the back or neck but continuing to move in spite of pain are important. Sometimes bracing of the neck or back is necessary and, if pain continues, surgery.

Prevention: Probably not possible, since it is part of the normal aging process. Usually, disability can be prevented by assuring regular movement and avoiding stress on the back.

SPRAIN

Injury to a ligamnet (which connects bone to bone in a joint).

Symptoms: Rapid swelling and inflammation and some initial pain and stiffness around a joint. Swelling and pain seem worse 24 to 48 hours after the injury occurs. Discoloration and limitation in motion and function may also take place.

Cause: A ligament is like a rope, which, when stretched beyond resting length, a ligamnet is susceptible to injury; and with a severe enough force, it may be torn apart. Most often occurs when turning and twisting are involved, in particular very quick, sudden motions that twist the joint.

Severity of Problem: Disability depends on the degree of damage. Can be as minor as swelling and inflammation only, causing minimal discomfort, or as severe as a rupture of the ligament(s).

Contagious? No.

Treatment: Cold compresses after injury occurs (not heat) and elevation of the injured joint, if possible. The joint should be immobilized and a compression wrap used. If quite painful, inflamed or swollen, a physician should be consulted. Some sprains resolve themselves with rest and immobility, while others require splinting, casting or bracing. With very serious sprains, surgical repair may be required.

STOMATITIS—APHTHOUS (CANKER SORES)

Commonly called canker sores, the little ulcers that mark this mouth disease are very uncomfortable.

Symptoms: Tiny, grayish white ulcers on the lining of the mouth, usually along the teeth, especially in the groove at the base of the teeth. Very painful for first three to five days.

Cause: Unknown, but a virus related to the herpes virus has been suspected. Some people get them in reaction to certain foods, such as nuts, chocolate and citrus fruits, which suggests allergy or another kind of food sensitivity. Stress may be associated with flare-ups for some.

Severity of Problem: Very bothersome and uncomfortable, but no known threat.

Contagious? Not known, but probably not.

Treatment: Avoid foods and drinks that cause pain. Pain relief can sometimes be gotten from sprays and gels that contain local anesthetics. Nothing is known that will shorten the time the ulcers are present. Must run their course.

Prevention: Unknown.

STRAIN

Injury to the muscle-tendon unit because of excessive use or excessive effort. This injury can occur in several ways. Sometimes called a "pulled muscle."

Symptoms: Swelling, discomfort or pain in the injured area.

Cause: Excessive use; overtaxing; overstretching of muscle, tendon or muscle-tendon unit. Tears can occur in the muscle, tendon or both. Serious strains involve a complete rupture of the muscle or tendon unit.

Severity of Problem: From very mild to severe and incapacitating until it heals.

Contagious? No.

Treatment: Apply ice or cold packs, compression (firm dressing), and elevate. Recovery from a mild to moderate strain usually requires immobilization of area, rest and at times pain medication. Severe strains will need to be splinted, braced or placed in a cast. With serious strains, surgical repair is sometimes necessary.

Prevention: Do not overtax or overextend muscles. Lifting, pulling or pushing heavy objects can result in strains. Many strains are the result of athletic participation, but few people realize how easy it is to get a strain during everyday activities.

Discussion: In young people any swelling, pain, or inflammation around a joint should signal the need for medical evaluation. Adults, especially those who are highly susceptible to back strains, should seek a physician's opinion if pain over a muscle or tendon persists, or swelling does not reduce markedly.

STREP THROAT

Painful, inflamed throat (and/or tonsils and adenoids) caused by infection with group A beta hemolytic streptococcus bacteria.

Symptoms: Sudden onset of severe throat pain with swallowing, and nagging, dull pain when not swallowing. Fever, general weakness and aches and pains, nausea, headache and vomiting are common. Tender lymph nodes in the neck are most often present. The throat and tonsils are very red and swollen, and pus is usually visible on the tonsils.

Cause: Infection with the group A beta hemolytic streptococcus bacteria.

Severity of Problem: A serious infection that, if not treated appropriately, can lead to rheumatic fever. Some people with strep throat develop kidney problems as a reaction to the illness, even if antibiotics have been given. This kidney inflammation is called glomerulonephritis.

Contagious? The streptococcus is spread in the secretions of the nose and throat. Avoidance of unnecessary contact is important.

Treatment: Treatment with an appropriate antibiotic for at least 10 days, usually for two weeks. Penicillin and related drugs are usually used, with erythromycin a good substitute for people who are allergic to penicillin.

Discussion: Since it is nearly impossible to tell the difference between strep and the many possible viruses that can cause similar problems, a throat culture to look for beta streptococcus is important for confirming a suspicion of strep. The sole purpose of treatment with this disease is to relieve symptoms and to prevent rheumatic fever.

STRESS

Overloading of the physical and mental systems of an individual, brought about by inability to cope effectively with conditions and changes in his or her life.

Symptoms: Vary according to the individual. Typical symptoms include irritability, depression, insomnia, loss of appetite, fatigue, inability to function at work, headaches and an increasing incidence of health problems.

Cause: Change (e.g., new job, move to a new home or location, new personal relationships), poor health, death or sickness of a family member, breakup of a personal or family relationship, demands on the job, financial or legal problems, etc.

Severity of Problem: If not addressed and treated, the body's physiological response to the stress can result in high blood pressure, stroke, heart disease and other cardiovascular problems. Some medical specialists believe that stress is a significant factor in the development of cancer and even susceptibility to infection.

Contagious? No.

Treatment: Treatment of the underlying cause(s) is necessary. The most effective therapy is a "whole person" behavior modification, requiring the individual to address his or her physical, emotional and social needs. This includes a program of better diet and nutrition, fitness and the management of stress. Where depression is particularly pronounced, drug therapy may also be helpful. In all cases of severe stress, professional counseling is recommended.

Prevention: Stress can be prevented or minimized by an ongoing program of sound nutrition, exercise and use of relaxation techniques.

STRESS INCONTINENCE
Involuntary leakage of urine during activity that raises the pressure in the abdomen.

Symptoms: Sudden, unexpected loss of urine control during lifting, sneezing, coughing or other activity that puts pressure on the bladder.

Cause: Inability of the urinary sphincter (closure muscle) to remain closed under pressure. In women, happens with loss of muscle tone due to aging or having children. In men, may follow surgical removal of the prostate gland.

Severity of Problem: Not a health problem, but one of potential embarrassment.

Contagious? No.

Treatment: Some mild cases may be corrected by exercises of the pelvic muscles. Where the problem is severe, correction by surgery is recommended.

Prevention: None.

See also CYSTOCELE.

STROKE
Stroke, or cerebrovascular accident, is a nervous system disorder due to a localized defect or problem in a blood vessel. It produces a wide variety of symptoms and nervous system defects, depending on its location.

Symptoms: Sudden onset of a nervous system defect that can be minor or major. Common problems include slurred speech; weakness or paralysis of an extremity or a side of the body; loss of urine; confusion, stupor or coma; inability to speak; visual disturbances, including loss of sight in one side of the vision field, transient blindness or spots in front of the eyes; staggering walk; dizziness; and many more. Some people with impending stroke (sometimes called transient ischemic attacks—TIAs) have short, temporary episodes that quickly disappear. There might be headache, nausea, confusion, sleepiness and weakness associated.

Cause: Strokes can be caused by several disorders of a blood vessel leading to a certain area of the brain: thrombosis (blockage) of an artery, usually because of atherosclerosis and blood clot; embolism (traveling of a blood clot, fatty deposit or clump of debris from another area of the body to a brain artery, where it blocks the artery); or hemorrhage from a blood vessel in or on the surface of the brain. Any of these events leads to temporary or permanent loss of blood supply and oxygen to an area of the brain. Symptoms and defects in function depend on the affected area. When there is lack of oxygen supply to the brain, the cells of the brain die, leaving an area of dead tissue called an infarction. The size of the infarcted area determines to a certain extent the amount and type of permanent damage.

The most common underlying cause of stroke is atherosclerosis, with narrowing of the major arteries supplying the brain, followed by either obstruction or hemorrhage. In a few situations bleeding from a deformity of the blood vessels (an aneurysm) is the cause.

Severity of Problem: Extremely variable, from temporary, mild damage to permanent paralysis or loss of function and even death within hours.

Contagious? No.

Treatment: The basic treatment for stroke is supportive care (bed rest, oxygen when needed, good nutrition and prevention of complications like pneumonia). Sometimes medications are given to thin the blood, but this treatment is controversial. After the first few days following a stroke, intensive rehabilitation is started to help the stroke victim to regain as much function as possible and become independent. (It can take as long as two years before the permanent effects of a stroke can be determined, since recovery can be gradual but steady.)

Prevention: Prevention or treatment of the underlying disease, usually atherosclerosis. When there is known or suspected narrowing of the arteries supplying the brain (the carotid arteries in the neck), a surgical procedure to remove plaque and deposits from the inside of the blood vessels might be recommended. This surgery can be successful in preventing future strokes but is a risky procedure.

Discussion: Strokes usually affect people over the age of 40, whether cardiovascular disease is known or not. Use of oral contraceptive pills is associated with stroke in certain young women.

STY

Infection of one of the small glands of the eyelid.

Symptoms: Pain, redness and swelling over the eyelid, either at the margin or underneath. Formation of a pimple with pus, with an eyelash in the center is most common. There may be mild itching or burning of the eye, with some redness of the conjunctiva.

Cause: Infection of the hair follicle or small glands in the eyelid, usually with a staphylococcal bacteria.

Severity of Problem: Usually minor. However, some people have the tendency to have repeated problems with sty.

Contagious? Yes. Some forms are only mildly contagious, while others spread rather rapidly, especially among children.

Treatment: If early and mild, warm compresses to the eyelid, avoidance of rubbing and scratching. Antibiotic ointment or drops may be prescribed by a physician. If problem is recurrent, search for cause is important.

Prevention: Avoid contact with persons with known sty or staph infection. Avoid rubbing already infected eye to prevent spread to other eye.

SYPHILIS

Highly contagious, complicated disease that is transmitted by sexual contact. If not treated, it can persist for years and cause serious, life-threatening damage.

Symptoms: These occur in three stages: primary, secondary and tertiary. There is also a distinct set of symptoms (congenital syphilis) seen in infants whose mothers have syphilis.

Cause: Infection with the spirochete Treponema pallidum. The primary infection is usually on the genitals but can occur in other areas. Later stages (both secondary and tertiary) of the disease involve other areas of the body. After the secondary stage, the bacteria are able to become "latent"—hidden for many years—before producing the problems of tertiary syphilis.

Severity of Problem: A chronic infection with several stages. This disease can lead to serious disability (with damage to the heart and blood vessels and the nervous system) if not treated. It is equally severe in males and females.

Contagious? Yes, in the early stages (primary, secondary, probably latent). In the last (tertiary) stage, it is probably not contagious. The disease spreads by sexual contact with an infected person, and its incidence rises and falls with that of other sexually transmitted diseases and with the level of sexual activity and promiscuity in the population. Infants whose mothers have untreated syphilis can get this disease through the placenta (congenital syphilis).

Treatment: Antibiotic treatment, usually with penicillin, is very important to eradicate the bacteria and prevent late complications. The length of time required for treatment depends on the stage of the disease and its extent.

Prevention: Avoid sexual contact with persons in whom the disease is known or suspected. Screening of all people with other sexually transmitted diseases for syphilis (by a blood test called a VDRL) is very helpful in early detection and prevention of community outbreaks of syphilis.

Discussion: Measures to detect syphilis include routine blood testing of many groups of people for evidence of present or past infection with this bacteria. The usual blood test is called VDRL and, when positive, suggests present or past infection with syphilis. This test is known to give false values, however, so it must be followed by more specific tests if its results are positive.

One episode of syphilis, even if treated, does not make a person immune to the disease in the future. It is very possible to get this disease over and over again.

TEMPOROMANDIBULAR JOINT DISEASE

Problem in which there are symptoms related to opening and closing the mouth. There can be many causes.

Symptoms: Pain or discomfort and limitation of motion of the jaw are the most common complaints. There may be a sensation of cracking in the jaw with movement or a feeling that the jaw is stuck and unable to move or open.

Cause: Inflammation or degenerative changes in the jaw joint (temporo-mandibular joint) most often result from injury or aging, although the jaw can be involved with many forms of arthritis. Pain in the jaw without arthritis can be caused by muscle tension and strain due to continual or repeated jaw-clenching or tooth-grinding, as a result of anxiety or habit. Malocclusion of the teeth or dentures that fit badly can contribute to any jaw pain.

Severity of Problem: Usually uncomfortable and bothersome, although it can cause severe pain and difficulty with eating for a few people.

Contagious? No.

Treatment: In general, rest of the jaw by eating soft foods and use of medications that reduce inflammation and pain (for example, aspirin and aspirin substitutes or other anti-inflammatory medications that may be pre-scribed). A thorough evaluation of the teeth and jaw, with needed dental care, would be important. Sometimes, when jaw-clenching is a problem, devices that limit tooth-grinding and clenching can be used while sleeping. Stress management is important.

Prevention: Avoid excessive chewing damage to the jaw; prevent or con-trol jaw-clenching habits; and get regular dental evaluation and care. Some causes of TM joint disease cannot be prevented, but their discomfort can be reduced.

TETANUS (LOCKJAW)

Severe illness with muscle spasms caused by a toxin of the tetanus bacteria.

Symptoms: Usually, stiff neck and muscle spasms of the jaw are the first signs, along with difficulty swallowing and irritability. As the disease pro-gresses, stiffness and painful spasms of all the muscles of the trunk and extremities can occur, usually set off by minor irritations. Spasms cause inability to breathe and lack of oxygen. Occasionally, pain and tingling in a cut or wound, then muscle spasms in the area around the injury are the first symptoms, and the disease does not progress any further.

Cause: Infection of a wound or open sore with the Clostridium tetani bacteria, which are present everywhere, especially in the soil. The bacteria multiply in wounds with poor blood supply and produce a toxin that interferes with normal function of the nerve-muscle unit.

Severity of Problem: A life-threatening problem, with as many as 40 percent of victims dying. Muscle spasms are intensely painful, and spasms of the muscles of breathing lead to inability to breathe and lack of oxygen.

Contagious? Not in the usual sense of from person to person. However, the germ is contracted through contaminated soil.

Treatment: Intensive supportive medical care is a must. Quiet atmosphere, sedatives and muscle relaxants are used. There is an antitoxin available, but it is only partly effective after the disease has progressed. Respirator support is often needed. Penicillin and other antibiotics may be used if the wound infection is severe but will not reverse any spasms and toxin that have already been produced.

Prevention: Can be totally prevented by up-to-date immunizations for everyone, both children and adults. Immunization does not protect against getting the bacterial infection but does protect against the effects of the toxin. It is important that all people keep their tetanus immunity current by having booster injections at the recommended intervals.

Discussion: The disease is particularly threatening for the very young and the very old. It can occur in newborn infants through contamination of the umbilical cord and is very common in drug addicts who inject their drugs. If a person survives the disease, recovery is complete. The disease can occur from 5 to 15 days after a wound. The shorter the time between wound and spasms, the worse the outcome is likely to be.

THROMBOPHLEBITIS

Formation of a blood clot within a vein that is inflamed. (*Thrombo* refers to clot, *phlebitis* to *inflammation of a vein.*)

Symptoms: Pain, swelling and redness over a vein, usually in the leg. There may be known varicose veins, with pain, swelling or discomfort because of them.

Cause: Sluggish blood flow through a vein; inflammation of a vein due to irritation or pressure on it; tendency for infection in a clot that is in a blood vessel.

Severity of Problem: Potentially serious if not treated. Pieces of the clot (thrombi) can break off and travel through the bloodstream to other areas of the body (called embolism). They can cause serious problems, such as stroke, lung symptoms and heart compromise, depending on where they lodge.

Contagious? No.

Treatment: Bed rest in a hospital; elevation, heat to inflamed, clotted area. Drugs that inhibit blood clotting are often administered.

Prevention: Measures to prevent excessively slow blood flow through varicose veins; avoidance of prolonged pressure on legs (crossed legs, sitting in one position for a long time).

THROMBOSIS

Clot formation in a blood vessel, either artery or vein.

Symptoms: Depends on the location of the clot and the size of the blood vessel that is obstructed by the clot. Blockage of a large vessel produces severe symptoms, such as pain, discoloration of the body part served by the vessel, etc. Thrombosis of coronary vessels leads to symptoms of heart attack. Blockage of blood vessels to the brain leads to symptoms of stroke.

Cause: Irregularity of inner surfaces of blood vessels; clotting problems; sluggish blood flow.

Severity of Problem: Depends on location of clot. If in an artery to a major organ, very serious. Clots in smaller vessels are less serious.

Contagious? No.

Treatment: Depends on cause and location. Usually hospitalization, careful observation and medications that inhibit blood clotting.

Prevention: Depends on cause.

Discussion: Small or large pieces of blood clots (called thrombi) can potentially break off and travel through the bloodstream to other blood vessels and cause additional problems. A thrombus that travels through the body is called an embolus.

TIC

Involuntary, and sometimes painful, facial movement.

Symptoms: Uncontrollable blinking and/or grimacing, often involving both sides of the face. May also show up as involuntary contraction of muscles in shoulders or arms.

Cause: The cause ordinarily is not known. However, while usually attributed to neurological mechanisms, this condition can be worsened by emotional stress.

Severity of Problem: Some forms gradually increase in severity to include exaggerated spasms, grunting, shouting and loud barking-type noises.

Contagious? No.

Treatment: Maintenance of good, all-around health. Patients with severe tics may also respond to certain prescribed drugs, such as phenobarbital or diazepam (while under the care of a physician).

Prevention: None. Avoidance of stressful situations may lessen the severity of outbreaks.

Discussion: Tics generally begin during early childhood and then lessen in severity or disappear during maturity. One form of tic, if cured, may be replaced by another.

TINNITUS

Purely subjective sensation of sounds, such as ringing, roars or banging in the inner ear.

Symptoms: Hearing sounds, such as buzzing, roaring, banging, hissing or ringing, that do not actually exist in the nearby environment.

Cause: Common symptom of most ear disorders, including otosclerosis, tumor, presence of foreign body in the ear, organic ear obstruction and inner ear infection.

Severity of Problem: Tinnitus itself is not a severe or disabling problem, although it can be irritating or frustrating. However, a medical diagnosis is important in determining whether an underlying cause requires treatment.

Contagious? No.

Treatment: While there is no specific medical or surgical therapy for tinnitus itself, treatment may be required for those specific underlying causes that are potentially serious if left unattended (for example, otosclerosis, tumor, infection).

Prevention: Depends on the underlying cause. See entries for specific conditions for more information.

TONSILLITIS

Inflammation and infection of the tonsils (tissues located in the throat).

Symptoms: Soreness of the throat, with aching pain much of the time and more severe pain with swallowing. The tonsils and throat are usually very red and swollen, with pus on the tonsils. Usually fever, generalized aching, headache, nausea. Children may complain of abdominal pain and may vomit. Lymph nodes in the neck under the jaw are swollen and tender.

Cause: Usually a bacterial or viral infection. Strep throat—tonsillitis caused by group A beta hemolytic streptococcus—is one of the more serious infections.

Severity of Problem: Very uncomfortable. If caused by streptococcus, it can lead to the serious complications of rheumatic fever and glomerulonephritis (if not treated properly).

Contagious? Yes, by contact with an infected person.

Treatment: If cause of infection is streptococcus, antibiotic treatment for 10 to 14 days. Antibiotics do not cure viral infections, which will run their course in several days to a week. Aspirin or aspirin substitute for fever and pain, plenty of liquids, rest and gargling with a salt water solution may make the person feel better.

Prevention: Avoid contact with people known to have strep infection or viral sore throat. Otherwise, none.

Discussion: Sudden onset of a sore throat is most often an infection of the tonsils, with or without inflammation of the adenoids (adenoiditis). Diagnosis of strep is made by trying to grow (culture) the strep germ in the laboratory. It is generally impossible to tell the difference between strep throat and infections caused by a virus just by looking at the throat. If strep is the cause, it is imperative that *all* the prescribed medicine be taken.

While taking out the tonsils because of frequent sore throats was common in the past, it is not a popular form of treatment now (because the tonsils are a part of the body's immune system). People who have had their tonsils removed can still get throat infections (called pharyngitis) with strep.

TORTICOLLIS (WRY NECK)

Temporary or permanent deformity in which the head is tilted and twisted in its position on the neck.

Symptoms: Unusual position of the head noticed during the first few weeks after birth. The baby's head is tipped at an angle and the head turned to one side, and there is difficulty in turning the head to the other side. There may be a knotlike lump felt in the muscle at the side of the neck.

Cause: Often thought to be due to stretching and tearing of the large muscle at the side of the neck during a difficult delivery. The knot in the muscle is part of the healing of this kind of tear and represents a scar that tightens and pulls the head into the unusual position. Babies who have this problem tend to have been big babies who were crowded in the uterus, another factor that may be part of the cause. A few babies with wry neck deformity have underlying bony abnormalities of the spine and neck leading to this kind of deformity.

Severity of Problem: The deformity may become permanent if treatment is not done early in infancy. In babies with underlying spinal deformities, the condition is usually permanent.

Contagious? No.

Treatment: Involves stretching the tightened neck muscles regularly during infancy. In addition, the baby is encouraged to turn his or her head to stretch the muscle (for example, by putting toys or mobiles in a place where the baby must turn to look at them). Heat and massage of the lump in the neck might be helpful. If the condition is not helped by these measures, surgery to release the scar tissue in the muscles might be needed but not until after 1 year of age.

Prevention: None for the underlying condition, but permanent deformity can usually be prevented.

Discussion: Temporary wry neck ("stiff neck") can be seen later in life as a response to pain or injury to the neck muscles. In this case the position is one of comfort and is not a permanent deformity. For this type of problem heat to the sore muscles, gradual stretching of the muscles and avoiding further injury are helpful.

TOXEMIA OF PREGNANCY

General term that refers to the hypertensive diseases of pregnancy.

Symptoms: Depends on severity, but rapid weight gain, swelling, headaches and dizziness might occur. In late stages convulsions may occur. Elevated blood pressure, along with edema, protein in the urine and excessive weight gain, are symptoms found by the doctor.

Cause: Usually unknown. (See entries for HYPERTENSION; TOXEMIA OF PREGNANCY—PRE-ECLAMPSIA; ECLAMPSIA.)

Severity of Problem: Potentially very serious if not detected and controlled. For the baby, risk of growth retardation, stillbirth and placental abruption. For the mother, convulsions (eclampsia) plus all the risks of hypertension (heart disease, kidney disease, stroke, blindness).

Contagious? No.

Treatment: Depends on cause and severity and requires close medical supervision. General measures include rest, limited salt intake and drugs to control blood pressure if needed.

Prevention: Control of chronic hypertension. No prevention known for pre-eclampsia.

Discussion: Hypertension of pregnancy is divided into several categories. Some women have chronic hypertension before pregnancy. (Women over 35, blacks, those with diabetes and those with a family history of hypertension are at greatest risk.) This can be worsened by pre-eclampsia during the last three months. Conversely, some women have hypertension during the last three months of pregnancy, and their blood pressures return to normal after delivery. Detection and treatment of hypertension, regardless of cause, is important in reducing death and handicap in infants and long-term complications in hypertensive women.

TOXEMIA OF PREGNANCY—ECLAMPSIA

Hypertensive disorder of pregnancy—pre-eclampsia that has progressed to the point of convulsions and possibly coma.

Symptoms: All the symptoms of pre-eclampsia (edema, rapid weight gain, fatigue, dizziness, headaches) plus a convulsion. (See TOXEMIA OF PREG-NANCY—PRE-ECLAMPSIA.)

Cause: Convulsion probably results from the high blood pressure, but exact cause is not known.

Severity of Problem: Life-threatening to mother and baby. Lack of oxygen during convulsion leads to potential damage to the baby's brain and other organs. There is a potential for placental abruption. Mother is at risk because of low oxygen and questionable effect on the mother due to brain hemorrhages or blood vessel spasms.

Contagious? No.

Treatment: Rapid reduction in blood pressure with intravenous medications. Bed rest and sedation to keep mother calm. Delivery of the baby as soon as possible. (Fetal maturity needs to be assessed beforehand, if possible.)

Prevention: Control of pre-eclampsia.

Discussion: A complication of pre-eclampsia, this problem can usually be prevented by careful control of blood pressure during late pregnancy, labor and delivery.

TOXEMIA OF PREGNANCY—PRE-ECLAMPSIA

Hypertension that develops during the last three months of pregnancy.

Symptoms: Edema (swelling because of fluid retention) with rapid weight gain beginning during last three months of pregnancy. There may be fatigue, headaches, dizziness and blurred vision. The doctor finds elevated blood pressure and protein in the urine.

Cause: Unknown.

Severity of Problem: Can lead to problems with fetal growth and well-being if not controlled. Can lead to eclampsia. (See TOXEMIA OF PREG-NANCY—ECLAMPSIA.)

Contagious? No.

Treatment: Bed rest, often in a hospital, and dietary limitation of salt intake. Medications to reduce blood pressure if needed. If blood pressure cannot be controlled, prompt delivery of the baby may be necessary (its maturity is measured or estimated first).

Prevention: None known.

Discussion: Pre-eclampsia is most common in a woman's first pregnancy and occurs more often in the teen-age mother and the mother over 35 than in others. While it usually begins during the last three months of pregnancy, it can start during labor or even after the baby is delivered. If not associated with underlying hypertension, blood pressure returns to normal shortly after delivery of the baby.

TOXIC SHOCK SYNDROME
Very serious illness most commonly seen in (but not limited to) women who have used tampons.

Symptoms: Sudden high fever, generalized aches and pains, headache, vomiting and diarrhea. Collapse and shock may follow in hours or days. There is often a rash on the body that peels at the end of the illness. Palms of hands and soles of feet may also peel, even though rash may not have been visible there.

Cause: Not completely understood but believed to be caused by a toxic substance produced by a staphylococcus organism.

Severity of Problem: Potentially life-threatening, with death occurring in as few as 5 percent and as many as 15 percent of victims, with treatment.

Contagious? Not as such. Staphylococcus bacteria can be passed from one person to another but do not cause this or other problems very often, except in someone who is susceptible.

Treatment: Requires immediate medical treatment, with all possible measures to support blood pressure and treat shock. Antibiotics have been used to treat staphylococcal infection.

Prevention: Recommendations have included the avoidance of tampon use for women, especially use of the highly absorbent kind of tampon. This may be preventive. In other individuals there is no known prevention.

Discussion: A particularly devastating illness that affects women more than 90 percent of the time and often begins within three to five days of the start of a menstrual period for which the woman has used tampons. Has been seen in children and in a few adult men. Staphylococcus has not been proved as the cause, but it has been found in the nose and throat, the vagina and rectum of people with this disease. The germ has not, however, been found in the blood. (This is why the syndrome is thought to be due to a toxin.)

TOXOPLASMOSIS
Parasitic infection that usually produces a disease closely resembling infectious mononucleosis.

Symptoms: For the normal person who gets a mild form of this disease, generalized enlargement of the lymph nodes, with mild fever, listlessness, aches and pains, headache, sore throat and rash are common. Some people have symptoms of hepatitis, meningitis and uveitis as well. A few people develop slowly progressive inflammation and infection in the deep structures of the eye (uveitis, with involvement of the retina and choroid).

Another form of toxoplasmosis occurs in infants who were infected as developing fetuses when their mothers had active toxoplasmosis. These infants can be very ill at birth, with rash, fever, jaundice, hepatitis, seizures, small head and, later, mental retardation.

In people with poor immunity because of another disease, toxoplasmosis can be a life-threatening infection, with complications of hepatitis, encephalitis and general deterioration.

Cause: Infection with the parasite Toxoplasma gondii, which lives inside human cells. It is also found in many animals and birds but is especially common in the cat. The parasite can be carried in cat excrement.

Severity of Problem: The disease is usually mild and without complications in the normal person. The congenital form leads to lifelong handicap. The eye inflammation can cause partial or complete blindness. The infection can be fatal for people with suppressed immunity.

Contagious? Humans can get this infection through contact with cat excrement and by eating raw or partially cooked meat that contains cysts of the organism. It is transmitted to fetuses through the placenta and can be passed from one person to another through blood transfusions.

Treatment: Severe infection can be treated effectively, although treatment during pregnancy is controversial.

Prevention: Cook all meat thoroughly and wash hands after handling raw meat. Pregnant women should avoid contact with cat litter and should not eat raw meat.

TRAVELER'S DIARRHEA (MONTEZUMA'S REVENGE, LA TURISTA)

Diarrhea that occurs with a change in dietary habits and food during travel to other countries.

Symptoms: Diarrhea, mild to severe, with cramping of the abdomen, nausea, weakness and, occasionally, vomiting. Fever is rare. The diarrhea is loose to watery, but there is no blood or mucus present. Can last from one to five days usually, although a few people have difficulties for several weeks.

Cause: Not completely known but believed to be caused by exposure to different intestinal bacteria than people are accustomed to. These strains of bacteria (called E. coli) produce toxins that cause the diarrhea. There is rarely a true infection, as is the case with the usual bacterial causes of dysentery.

Severity of Problem: Seems to depend on the individual, from very mild to severe and bothersome. Some people seem not to be sensitive to changes in bowel bacteria in this way.

Contagious? Not really an infection, but exposure to the unusual bacteria is through eating and drinking—contact with water and foods that contain different strains of bacteria than those with which the person is normally in contact.

Treatment: Rest, adequate liquids to prevent dehydration. There is no specific cure, although there continue to be studies of drugs for this purpose. Medications that slow the diarrhea (such as Lomotil® or paragoric) are helpful. Recently there has been a suggestion that Pepto Bismol® in massive amounts will prevent or treat the problem. Antibiotic treatment is not effective and can aggravate the problem.

Prevention: May not be avoidable unless people carry their own supply of food and drink while traveling. People who are particularly susceptible might avoid all contact with local water and vegetables and fruits washed in local water. Use medications that diminish diarrhea if problems occur.

Discussion: One of the most common complaints of the traveling person, traveler's diarrhea is usually a mild to moderate but irritating problem. Travelers who have severe or persistent diarrhea should see a doctor to make sure there is not a more serious intestinal infection present.

TRICHOMONIASIS ("TRIC")

Sexually transmitted infection of the vagina (female) or urethra (male).

Symptoms: In women: frothy, foul-smelling vaginal discharge; pain in the genital area; irritation and soreness of genitals and upper thighs; pain with intercourse; burning on urination. In men: usually without any symptoms; however, if present, burning and pain on urination; mild morning urethral discharge; mild discomfort in genital area or pelvis.

Cause: Infection with the organism Trichomonas vaginalis. Sexually transmitted from infected partner.

Severity of Problem: Bothersome but no serious complications.

Contagious? Yes, by sexual contact. Male carriers who have no symptoms may not know they have the organism.

Treatment: Requires medical attention: treatment of *both* partners, using oral medication. In women vaginal suppositories can be used, and douches with vinegar solution can be helpful with discomfort but do not eliminate the infection.

Prevention: Avoid sexual contact with infected partners.

Discussion: Failing to treat male partner can result in reinfection of woman after treatment.

TUBERCULOSIS (TB, CONSUMPTION)

Infectious illness that can be very slow and silent in appearing. Most often involves lungs (pulmonary tuberculosis), but can occasionally involve other organs (kidney, brain, bone, lymph nodes, skin).

Symptoms: There may be no symptoms at first, then gradual start of cough, fatigue, loss of both appetite and weight. Cough may produce bloody sputum. Low-grade fevers, especially in the afternoon, and night sweats may occur later. General feeling of not being well.

Cause: Infection with the bacteria called Mycobacterium tuberculosis. Occasionally "atypical tuberculosis," with infection by other types of mycobacteria.

Severity of Problem: Potentially progressive and severe if not recognized and treated. If treated, can most often be cured; can be controlled in other cases. Severe forms leave lung scars and chronic progressive lung disease.

Contagious? Yes, by contact with sputum and secretions of a person with untreated TB. People with TB who are not coughing and have been taking anti-TB medication for over two weeks are not contagious.

Treatment: Depends on type and severity of disease but consists of drug treatment for at least one year, often longer. Depending on location and severity of disease, one to three anti-TB drugs are used. Hospitalization may or may not be needed. Rest and good, balanced nutrition are very important. People in contact with persons with untreated TB or those who show a positive TB skin test but no other signs of disease are treated preventively for at least one year with the drug isoniazid (INH).

Prevention: Depends on recognition and treatment of disease in people at risk. Screening of all children periodically to detect and treat those with positive tests is important. Adults with positive skin tests or those who have contact with people likely to have TB need routine chest X rays to detect TB lung disease. A vaccination called BCG is available but is used only in areas where risk of TB is very high.

Discussion: The first exposure to TB is often in childhood, and the infection (so-called primary tuberculosis) is a mild disease that is usually not serious enough to be noticed. However, the bacteria lie dormant in the body, able to produce active TB later. This first infection causes the TB skin test to become positive. Pulmonary TB is a reactivation of that dormant bacteria and usually affects the very top portions of the lungs (the apices). Without treatment, the patch of infection forms a cavity of pus in the lung. Certain factors can make a person susceptible to reactivation of TB: general weakness and illness; malnutrition; alcoholism (probably at least partly related to poor nutrition); measles; diabetes; the occupational disease silicosis; and chronic use of steroid (cortisone-related) drugs. Children and very debilitated, chronically ill adults are at risk for TB meningitis especially, and for TB in sites other than the lungs.

ULCER DISEASE—MASSIVE HEMORRHAGE

Bleeding from an ulcer because of erosion through a blood vessel.

Symptoms: Vomiting of fresh blood or dark, grainy material; sometimes passage of blood or dark, tarlike stools. Blood loss may result in weakness, dizziness, intense sweating and shock.

Cause: Peptic ulcer.

Severity of Problem: If not treated, pulse rate and blood pressure deteriorate; shock may lead to cardiopulmonary arrest and death.

Contagious? No.

Treatment: Major blood loss is treated by transfusions of fresh blood. When pulse rate, blood pressure and blood loss indicate a deterioration in patient's condition, emergency surgery may be required.

Prevention: Hemorrhaging is a common complication of ulcers. A diet of generally bland foods, taken in a regular, unrushed schedule is recommended. Stressful situations should be avoided, or behavior modification to cope with stress should be considered. No smoking. No alcohol consumption. Eliminate coffee and tea.

Discussion: Ulcers are more commonly found in men. Symptoms may vary with the age of the patient and the location of the ulcer.

ULCER DISEASE—PERFORATION

Rupture or bursting of wall of stomach or duodenum resulting from erosion by an ulcer.

Symptoms: A sudden pain in the abdominal area, steady and of great intensity. Pain may spread quickly throughout the abdomen, which becomes tender, with abdominal muscles rigid. Pain may radiate to one or both shoulders.

Cause: Erosion of the wall of the stomach or duodenum by an ulcer.

Severity of Problem: Acute emergency requiring immediate medical attention. Condition may deteriorate, with chance of shock.

Contagious? No.

Treatment: Immediate surgical repair required; long delay prior to surgery can hinder chances of recovery. If surgery cannot be performed, continuous stomach suction may be a possible alternative treatment.

Prevention: Medical treatment of ulcer disease.

ULCER DISEASE—PYLORIC OBSTRUCTION

Blockage of the pylorus (the opening of the stomach into the duodenum) as a result of scarring due to ulcer disease.

Symptoms: Feeling of fullness after meals, bloating, loss of appetite and vomiting. Pain in upper abdomen may or may not be present, depending on whether or not ulcer is acute. As blockage becomes more complete, less and less food passes through, and vomiting increases.

Cause: Swelling and spasm, then scarring due to ulcer near or at the pylorus.

Severity of Problem: Can progress to complete blockage, requiring surgical correction.

Contagious? No.

Treatment: Treatment of ulcer disease (bland diet, antacids, medications that reduce acid secretion, elimination of alcohol and smoking) if obstruction is mild or partial. Surgery is required to completely correct problem. Several types of surgery are possible, depending on exact location and extent of scarring.

Prevention: Prompt, vigorous treatment of ulcer disease.

ULCER—PEPTIC (DUODENAL)

Break or wound of the surface tissue of the first part of the small intestine (duodenum).

Symptoms: Most often a fairly constant burning, aching and gnawing pain in the stomach (generally after eating). Other symptoms may include heartburn; vomiting; blood in stools (looks black, not red); and usually no loss of appetite, but a sense of fullness after meals.

Cause: Stress, anxiety, tension, and certain foods and drugs may essentially produce a breakdown in the stomach's and small intestine's natural protection against acids, and/or this may occur because of an oversecretion of hydrochloric acid (a gastric acid).

Severity of Problem: Peptic ulcers can cause extremely incapacitating pain. If serious complications occur, such as obstruction, hemorrhage or perforation, death can take place without immediate medical intervention. Also, cardiovascular disease is not uncommon in those with peptic ulcer.

Contagious? No.

Treatment: A physician's evaluation and care are necessary. Bland foods, the use of antacids, more frequent but smaller meals, and the management or reduction of stress help to control the problem if it is diagnosed and treated early. Medications to reduce the production of stomach acid are often used. At times sedatives may be prescribed to control the stress and anxiety. Surgery is necessary if obstruction, perforation or hemorrhage occur.

Prevention: Avoidance of stressful situations; stress management; proper dietary habits; prudent use of caffeine and other stimulants found in food or drink; adequate exercise and overall fitness/wellness. Also, the early recognition of symptoms of possible peptic ulcer and prompt medical attention to avoid serious complications.

Discussion: Occasionally, an ulcer may occur in the stomach itself (called a gastric ulcer). This type of ulcer may have other causes, including cancer and pernicious anemia. Its medical evaluation is also essential.

ULCER—STOMACH (GASTRIC)

Eroded area with a ccraterlike center and inflamed, raised margins located on the lining of the stomach.

Symptoms: Very similar to those of duodenal ulcer, with a feeling of fullness and burning or dull pain in the upper part of the abdomen. Pain is often most pronounced between meals and is relieved by eating, taking antacids or vomiting. There is often nausea and loss of appetite. The pain may feel like "hunger pangs." When the symptoms have been present for some time, there may be weight loss and fatigue. If vomiting occurs, there may be blood streaking.

Cause: Excessive acid secretion by the stomach is associated, but the exact cause for this is unknown. Such factors as alcohol intake, smoking and caffeine, which stimulate acid secretion, tend to make it worse.

Severity of Problem: If untreate, the ulcer may bleed or perforate or cause enough inflammation to obstruct the outlet of the stomach. While most gastric ulcers are benign, some are cancerous, so thorough evaluation is a must.

Contagious? Avoidance of foods and substances that stimulate gastic acid secretion (alcohol, caffeine, tobaccco, spices) or irritate the stomach (aspirin and related medications); use of antacids or newer medications that reduce the secretion of stomach acid; stress reduction; small, frequent meals.

Prevention: Probably not possible.

Discussion: Because of the possibility of gastic ulcers' being malignant, the doctor will want to evaluate a person with a gastric ulcer frequently to verify that healing has occurred and that the ulcer does not recur or get worse. When gastic cancer is a possibility, the doctor may recommend a procedure in which the ulcer can be biopsied (have a tissue sample analyzed in the laboratory).

UPPER RESPIRATORY INFECTION (URI, COMMON COLD)

Very common virus infection that affects primarily the nose and other mucous membranes of the head and upper respiratory tract.

Symptoms: Well known to all, the first symptoms are usually a scratchy sensation in the nose and throat, followed by congestion of the nose, sneezing, watery eyes and a hacking cough. There may be slight fever, especially in children, for the first day or so. The congestion of the nose and sore throat increases for several days, then the cough becomes more of a problem, loosening and producing a small amount of clear or white mucus. Appetite is poor, with general fatigue, aches and pains. In infants and children mild diarrhea and vomiting may be noticed, along with fussiness.

Cause: Infection with one of the several hundred viruses that can infect the respiratory tract. Each infection produces immunity to *one* of the viruses but not to the others.

Severity of Problem: Mildly uncomfortable and goes away in 7 to 10 days without treatment. Complications are unusual in healthy children and adults but may include ear infection, bronchitis and pneumonia.

Contagious? Yes, very. URIs spread by contact with secretions scattered through the air by sneezing and coughing, for about one day before the cold symptoms appear and for several days afterward.

Treatment: Rest, liquids and medications (aspirin or aspirin substitute) for fever and general aches and pains. While certain people seem to get some relief from various types of nonprescription cold remedies, these usually do not help a great deal. Cough can be suppressed by a cough medicine if it interferes with sleep. Antibiotics are not useful unless a complicating bacterial infection has occurred.

Prevention: Avoidance of exposure to persons with colds, although this is nearly impossible.

Discussion: Without question, the most common of human infections. No specific cure has been discovered, and a preventive vaccine is unlikely. Is more uncomfortable than dangerous.

UREMIA

End stage of kidney failure when the inability of the kidneys to function allows toxins to circulate in the blood.

Symptoms: Weakness, fatigue and decreased mental activity. Muscular twitches and cramps. Gastrointestinal symptoms, including vomiting, nausea, foul taste in mouth. Excessive or minimal urine production. Respiratory distress, general swelling and water retention at times.

Cause: Can result from several factors, including structural abnormalities of the kidneys, chronic kidney infection, severe hypertension and diabetes, among others.

Severity of Problem: Advanced stages of acute uremia are indicated by gastrointestinal ulceration and bleeding, infections, discoloration of the skin, intense itching and severe testicular pain. Advanced uremia, if not controlled, can lead to total renal failure and death.

Contagious? No.

Treatment: Requires intensive medical care, usually hospitalization. The specific causes of the kidney failure, if correctable, must be treated first. If the kidney disease is non-correctable, a program of kidney treatment—which might include dialysis (artificial kidney), special diet, drugs, etc.—is indicated. Beyond dialysis, kidney transplant may be the only means of sustaining life.

Prevention: Depends on cause of kidney failure. Early recognition of signs of uremia allows it to be treated and controlled more successfully.

URETHRITIS

Inflammation of the passage that carries urine from the kidneys to the bladder.

Symptoms: Pus or mucus-filled discharge from the penis in males, accompanied by burning sensation during urination. Sense of urgency and frequency of urination. In females symptoms similar to those of bladder infection: burning and pain on urination, urgency and frequency.

Cause: Infection of the channel through which the urine is ejected, brought about by microorganisms that colonize the glands lining the urethra, producing acute and chronic infection. Most commonly caused by contact with infected sexual partner.

Severity of Problem: While not in itself an emergency condition, urethritis requires medical attention. Lack of treatment can result in a worsening condition. Very uncomfortable.

Contagious? Yes, by sexual contact.

Treatment: Appropriate antibiotic therapy after identification of the offending organism.

Prevention: Use of prophylactics during sexual intercourse.

Discussion: Gonorrhea is the most common infection causing urethritis in men. A condition called "nonspecific urethritis" is now known to usually be caused by chlamydia infection, another sexually transmitted disease. Occasionally other bacteria might be responsible. "Nonspecific urethritis" in the male might be associated with "nonspecific vaginitis" in the female sexual partner.

URINARY TRACT INFECTION

Infection of any of the parts of the urine-collecting system, extending from the kidney, through the bladder and to the outside. May include structures in and around the kidney (pyelonephritis), the ureters (tubes leading from the kidney to the bladder), the bladder (cystitis) and urethra (tube leading from the bladder to the outside—urethritis).

Symptoms: Depends on the severity and location of the infection. May be mild to severe, from burning and discomfort on urination to severe chills and fever with backache. (See URINARY TRACT INFECTION—ACUTE PYELONEPHRITIS; URINARY TRACT INFECTION—CYSTITIS.)

Cause: Invasion of the urine-collecting system by bacteria, causing infection. Risk factors include any stagnation of urine or blockage of urine flow.

Severity of Problem: Depends on site and cause. There is always the potential for progressing to severe kidney damage.

Contagious? No.

Treatment: Depends on severity and cause.

Prevention: Depends on cause.

Discussion: Can be very difficult to tell where a urinary infection is located. All require medical attention and vigorous treatment if long-term damage is to be prevented.

URINARY TRACT INFECTION—ACUTE PYELONEPHRITIS

Acute infection of the kidney's collecting system and the upper urinary tract.

Symptoms: Rapid development of fever, chills, nausea, vomiting and pain the back or deep abdomen. Bladder irritation resulting from the infected urine may cause a sense of urgency and frequency of urination. Some abdominal tenderness.

Cause: Almost any bacteria that enter the urinary tract can cause infection. Sometimes an underlying abnormality of the urinary tract leads to susceptibility to upper urinary infection.

Severity of Problem: Can be effectively treated. However, if it goes untreated, can leave kidney damage and lead to chronic pyelonephritis

Contagious? No.

Treatment: Antibiotic therapy recommeded after causative bacteria are identified. Hospitalization and intravenous medicaion usually needed. Analgesics may be required briefely for pain. Surgery may be required if obstruction is present.

Prevention: Prompt treatment of lower urinary tract infections (see URINARY TRACT INFECTION—CYSTITIS) to prevent extension up to the kidney. Surgery to correct abnormalities when indicated. Women who get urinary infections afer sexual intercours shoudl drink much liquid an dlearn to empty the bladder immediately after intercourse.

Discussion: Acute pyelonephritis may happen as a result of spread of an infection from the bladder upward to the kideny or, less commonly, as an infection carried in the blood. People with conditions that result in incomplete emptying of the bladder or tendency of urine to back up to the kidney are at special risk. These include: infants and children with congenital abnormalties; older men with prostate enlargement; females of any age, including some women in whom it is expecially related to sexual activity

URINARY TRACT INFECTION—CYSTITIS

Inflammation and infection of the bladder.

Symptoms: Pain or burning with urination. Sensation of having to urinate constantly; tendency to lose urine. Pain or discomfort in the lower abdomen. Urinary frequency. Blood may be noticed in the urine.

Cause: Most commonly, infection of the bladder and lower urinary tract. Rarely caused by irritation of the bladder from chemicals or drugs.

Severity of Problem: Of itself not severe. However, can lead to more serious infection of the upper urinary tract and to damage to the urinary tubes, with backflow of urine to the kidneys. Rarely leads to generalized infection (sepsis).

Contagious? No.

Treatment: Requires doctor's evaluation and treatment. Antibacterial medications after infection is identified. Plenty of liquids, frequent emptying of the bladder, relief of blockage to urination if this is a cause.

Prevention: Prevention or treatment of obstruction to urine flow, if present. Good genital hygiene for women and young girls.

Discussion: Cystitis is a common problem of women and girls of any age because of the shortness of the urethra (the tube that leads from the bladder to the outside). Infection enters the bladder through this short tube, and the risk for problems is increased by poor hygiene habits.

Some women are particularly prone to urinary tract infection after sexual intercourse. Regularly emptying the bladder immediately after intercourse and drinking plenty of liquids may prevent infection.

Anything that allows urine to stagnate in the bladder will also increase the risk of infection. Examples of this type of problem include some congenital malformations of the urinary tract in both boys and girls; prostate enlargement in older men; and paralysis with inability to urinate or completely empty the bladder (for example, in spina bifida or spinal cord injury). Women with cystocele and pelvic relaxation also have a tendency to urinary infection. Treatment for all these includes relieving blockage if possible and any measures to allow the bladder to empty completely.

VAGINITIS

Inflammation of the vagina. Vaginitis is often associated with inflammation of the vulva (the external genitalia) as well and is then called vulvovaginitis.

Symptoms: Vaginal and genital itching, burning or soreness, often with a sensation of needing to urinate frequently. Vaginal discharge is frequent and can be thick or thin, white or colored, blood-tinged or not. Burning with urination, pain with sexual intercourse are not uncommon. There may be bleeding with intercourse as well, especially with atrophic vaginitis.

Cause: There are many possible causes. Infections that cause it include: candidiasis (yeast infection), often seen after antibiotic treatment, during pregnancy or in people with diabetes mellitus; sexually transmitted infections, such as trichomoniasis, herpes simplex 2, chlamydia infection and gonorrhea; and pinworms in young girls. Atrophic vaginitis, caused by lack of estrogen hormone, is seen after menopause. Use of vaginal creams, douches and sprays can cause a contact dermatitis or allergic reaction.

Severity of Problem: Varies depending on the cause but is very uncomfortable. Can recur frequently, depending on the cause.

Contagious? The infectious causes are.

Treatment: Specific treatment depends on identifying and treating the underlying cause. However, certain things are helpful in making a person more comfortable: sitz baths in warm or cool water; avoidance of scratching and other forms of irritation (douching, suppositories other than those prescribed to treat the cause); frequent changes of underwear and wearing cotton underwear to absorb moisture. If infection is the cause, specific treatment is important and often includes the sexual partner(s) as well. Atrophic vaginitis can be treated using estrogen cream applied to the vagina.

Prevention: Depends on the underlying cause.

VARICES OF THE ESOPHAGUS

Enlargement of the veins that encircle the esophagus just as it enters the stomach, a condition that is the same as varicose veins in the legs.

Symptoms: Usually no specific symptoms until the varices bleed, causing vomiting of large amounts of bright red blood or the passage of black, tarry stools. There are usually signs and symptoms of the underlying disease, which is often cirrhosis of the liver.

Cause: Back pressure on the veins of the esophagus because of obstruction or blockage of blood flow in the liver. This is most often caused by cirrhosis of the liver but can result from a problem called portal hypertension (rise in pressure in the portal vein in the liver).

Severity of Problem: Potentially life-threatening if the varices rupture and bleed. This can happen without warning or as a result of vomiting from another cause.

Contagious? No.

Treatment: Requires immediate emergency medical care to stop the bleeding and treat shock and anemia. This may involve use of medications, special procedures to apply pressure to the inside of the esophagus and emergency surgery in some cases. Control of the underlying problem, if possible, is important.

Prevention: Prevention of the underlying cause. Prevention or control of vomiting in people who have known varices.

VARICOSE VEINS

Enlarged, irregular veins, most often seen on the surface of the legs.

Symptoms: Enlargement and irregularity of the surface veins of the lower leg, often during and after a pregnancy in women, and in older individuals. There might be dull, aching pain in the legs after standing, swelling of the ankles and leg cramps, especially at night. Some very large varicose veins cause no discomfort, while others that do not look as bad are very uncomfortable.

Cause: Dilatation and enlargement of the veins of the lower legs is usually caused by backward pressure on the veins and sluggish circulation back to the heart, in combination with a defect in the valves of the veins, which usually help move blood back to the heart. The veins that are on the surface of the leg do not have muscle around them, so there is no help by muscle activity to move blood back to the heart. Blockage of the veins of the legs from clotting (thrombosis) or inflammation (thrombophlebitis) may also be a factor. There is a family tendency to develop varicose veins, which are almost always worsened in women by pregnancy.

Severity of Problem: Discomfort and appearance are bothersome for some people. There is a risk of developing thrombophlebitis (blood clot with inflammation of the vein) and resultant embolism (distant movement of a blood clot) with prolonged sitting. Varicose ulcers and eczema, along with persistent swelling, are complications of severe varicose veins with poor circulation.

Contagious? No.

Treatment: For mild to moderate problems, wearing of elastic stockings, along with avoidance of tight bands at the tops of the legs or around the knees will relieve some discomfort. Elevation of the legs reduces swelling of the ankles. Surgery to remove dilated veins (called vein stripping) is usually successful in correcting the problem.

Prevention: Not completely successful, but wearing of elastic stockings by people who are at risk for varicose veins, especially women who are pregnant, may prevent severe dilation of the veins. Avoid any tight bands (for example, tight stockings) around the knees or at the tops of the thighs (tight elastic at legs of underwear).

VINCENT'S INFECTION (TRENCHMOUTH)

Acute, severe infection of the gums.

Symptoms: Sudden onset of painful, swollen gums, with bleeding of the gums, fever and swollen lymph nodes under the jaw. As the problem progresses, there may be some pus formation and ulcers on the gums. This problem does not usually involve the lining of the cheeks to any great extent, nor the tongue.

Cause: Not certain. Thought to be an infection with some of the bacteria that are usually found in the mouth, but this is not a clear cause. Can be brought on by stress, poor dental hygiene, poor diet and sleep, chronic illness (such as alcoholism, chronic malnutrition) or acute infection (such as infectious mononucleosis, candidiasis, viral infection). Can occur in diabetics and in others who have poor immunity.

Severity of Problem: Very painful disease that usually resolves with good mouth care and antibiotics.

Contagious? Probably not. (Previously believed to be contagious, but many people normally carry the bacteria that were thought responsible. It is important to distinguish this kind of mouth inflammation from others that are contagious, such as herpetic stomatitis.)

Treatment: Good mouth care, with toothbrushing and rinsing the mouth often with hydrogen peroxide. Pain relief, good nutrition are important. Antibiotics are usually given by mouth.

Prevention: Many cases can be prevented by good dental hygiene and nutrition, and control of underlying infection or chronic disease.

Discussion: Trenchmouth is a term commonly used to mean all kinds of inflammation and infection of the mouth. It is important that Vincent's infection be distinguished from the other forms of stomatitis and gingivitis.

VITAMIN DEFICIENCIES

Lack of one or more vitamins in the body. Vitamins are chemicals that help with certain metabolic functions in the body.

Most often vitamin deficiency occurs because of imbalance in the diet, so certain vitamins are not supplied in the amounts needed. Other causes include factors that increase the demand for vitamins (for example, smoking or pregnancy) or interefere with the body's absorbing them from the diet. Vitamin deficiencies usually involve more than one vitamin, and replacement or supplementation of just one of the missing or inadequate vitamins may do more harm than good.

While vitamin deficiency certainly occurs, many people with diets that are completely adequate in vitamins take extra vitamins each day. As long as these are taken sensibly, there is probably no harm, although the supplementation may not be needed. However, certain vitamins can be dangerous if taken in excess. These are vitamins A, D, K and niacin. There is no good evidence that "megavitamin" therapy is beneficial to healthy people, and it may be harmful if it involves taking large doses of these vitamins over a prolonged period of time.

VITAMIN DEFICIENCIES—VITAMIN A DEFICIENCY

Lack of carotene, which is needed for production of vitamin A in the body, or lack of vitamin A in the diet.

Symptoms: Dry skin, with thickening and bumpiness, especially around the hair follicle. Night blindness, tunnel vision and, later, dry eyes.

Cause: Lack of carotene or vitamin A in the diet. Carotene is the yellow pigment found in yellow and red vegetables and is converted to vitamin A in the body. Vitamin A is found in milk and milk products, eggs and fish. Vitamin A is needed for development of the cells in the retina responsible for certain parts of vision and for cells that form skin and mucous linings.

Severity of Problem: Varies with the degree of lack.

Contagious? No.

Treatment: Administration of vitamin A supplement. Balanced diet that includes both carotene and vitamin A.

Prevention: Balanced diet that contains adequate sources of carotene and vitamin A.

Discussion: Higher vitamin A needs are found during childhood and during pregnancy and breast-feeding. Excessive vitamin A supplementation produces a severe disease with loss of weight, loss of appetite, sore mouth and tongue, excessive blood calcium, cirrhosis of the liver, anemia and nervous system damage.

VITAMIN DEFICIENCIES—VITAMIN B COMPLEX DEFICIENCY

Deficiency of the B vitamins (B complex—B_1, called thiamine; B_2, called riboflavin; B_6, called pyridoxine; and niacin), usually involving more than one of them.

Symptoms: Depends to a certain extent on which vitamin is missing. However, the symptoms of all of the deficiencies are similar. For thiamine deficiency, lack of appetite, numbness and tingling of the skin, muscle cramps and, later, symptoms of heart failure are prominent. For B_2 deficiency, paleness of the mouth, sore tongue, generalized rash, fissures and sores at the corners of the mouth, eye inflammation and weakness are prominent. For niacin deficiency (called pellagra), symptoms include red, irritated skin; sore tongue; diarrhea; depression; and sore mouth. Pyridoxine deficiency may involve sore tongue and fissures at the corners of the mouth; it can also cause anemia. Certain individuals have a higher than usual need for pyridoxine and have seizures if this need is not met.

Cause: Deficiency in the diet of the B complex group of vitamins or an increased need for them. This often occurs in people who generally eat an unbalanced diet, those who eat only certain foods to the exclusion of others, alcoholics, people with certain chronic diseases, and those who have intestinal problems that prevent the absorption of the vitamins from food. Particular individuals have an increased need for certain of these vitamins, based on hereditary factors.

Severity of Problem: Can vary from mild, unrecognized deficiency to full-blown deficiency diseases. Extreme deficiency of these vitamins ultimately leads to death or heart and nervous system damage.

Contagious? No.

Treatment: Supplementation of the diet with B complex vitamins. Usually when a deficiency actually exists, dosage is between 5 and 10 times the minimum requirement. Providing a well-balanced diet is a cornerstone of treatment. People with excessive pyridoxine need (pyridoxine dependency) require additional B_6.

Prevention: A well-balanced diet, which supplies the needed requirements of these vitamins.

VITAMIN DEFICIENCIES—VITAMIN C DEFICIENCY

Deficiency of vitamin C produces a disease called scurvy.

Symptoms: Early in scurvy, there is gingivitis (inflammation of the gums) and sore mouth, with bleeding from the gums. There are also skin changes, with dryness and bumpy enlargement of the hair follicles. Later, teeth loosen, the muscles become weak and there is bleeding into the skin and joints. Healing of wounds is poor.

Cause: Dietary lack of vitaimin C, usually because of failure to eat fruits and vegetables. This can be seen in the elderly and food faddists, and in babies who drink unfortified milk without added vitamins.

Severity of Problem: Varies with the degree of lack and how long the vitamin has been deficient.

Contagious? No.

Treatment: Balanced diet that contains citrus fruits and vegetables. Addition of vitamin C (ascorbic acid) supplements.

Prevention: Balanced diet that contains vitamin C.

Discussion: Recently vitamin C in very large doses has been recommended to prevent colds. Scientific studies show that this is not effective.

VITAMIN DEFICIENCIES—VITAMIN D DEFICIENCY

Deficiency of vitamin D produces a disease called rickets.

Symptoms: Muscle weakness and soreness, aching and pain in the bones, especially of the ribs. Bowing of the bones develops because of softening and loss of calcium.

Cause: While rickets may develop in children as a result of dietary deficiency of vitamin D, it may also result from other defects, such as renal diseases, which waste phosphorus; osteomalacia, where there is resistance of the bones to vitamin D; inability to absorb vitamin D and calcium from the intestine; and defects in calcium metabolism. Lack of sunlight, especially for children, prevents the body from making its own vitamin D.

Severity of Problem: In children permanent bowing of the arms and legs and tender nodules on the ribs result from rickets. In adults with osteomalacia, weakness and bowing of the legs occur.

Contagious? No.

Treatment: Depends on the cause. If there is pure dietary deficiency of vitamin D, or there is an increased need for it, vitamin D supplied in the diet or as a supplement is needed. Treatment of the other causes of rickets and osteomalacia is very complicated.

Prevention: Depends on the cause. Adequate vitamin D in the diet (fish liver, egg yolks, butter) and sunlight, fortified milk when available.

Discussion: Rickets usually does not occur in developed countries, except when there is another disease, such as intestinal problems that prevent absorption or kidney disease. It is seen in premature infants, however, based on nutritional deficiency. Excessive doses of vitamin D over a prolonged period of time are dangerous, and lead to elevation of calcium in the blood, with cardiac arrhythmias and formation of kidney stones.

WART

Small growth or cluster of growths on the skin or mucous membranes.

Symptoms: Development of small, firm lumps on the skin or various mucous membranes. These are usually less than ¼ inch in size and do not hurt. May appear as single lesion or as clusters.

Cause: Infection with one of several wart viruses.

Severity of Problem: A mild problem but lasts a long time and can be unsightly if warts are multiple.

Contagious? Yes. It takes from about 2 to 18 months to develop infection after exposure.

Treatment: Depends on type and location but includes removal by any of a number of methods: surgical removal; application of liquid nitrogen to freeze the abnormal growths; use of peeling medications such as salicylic acid; and treatment with more elaborate methods if warts are particularly severe or extensive. X-ray treatments previously used for plantar warts are no longer recommended.

Prevention: Avoid direct contact with warts. Do not pick at or scratch warts, because this may cause new warts to appear in the areas of damaged skin.

Discussion: Most common in children and young adults, warts have many shapes and characteristics. They may disappear without treatment after months to years or continue to crop up in new areas. Many of the treatments will eliminate warts, but new ones often appear either in the same area or nearby.

WART—COMMON

Rough-surfaced, irregular growth that is most often located on the fingers and hands but can occur either alone or in clusters anywhere on the skin.

Symptoms: Rough skin growth, sometimes with tenderness to pressure. Commonly is bothersome, so there is a tendency to pick and scratch at the wart.

Cause: Infection of the cells with a wart virus.

Severity of Problem: Minor but bothersome.

Contagious? Yes, by direct contact with warts.

Treatment: Frequent application of wart treatments with over-the-counter medications as directed on the package may be effective for some. Others need treatment with a salicylic acid preparation (see a doctor) to cause the skin to be irritated and peel. Application of liquid nitrogen may be done every two to three weeks and is quite effective in eliminating existing warts. Surgical removal may also be effective.

Prevention: Avoid contact with warts.

WART—PLANTAR

Growth on the bottom (plantar surface) of the foot.

Symptoms: Tender, painful lump on the bottom of the foot, as a single growth or several in clumps. Looks a lot like a "corn" that is in the wrong place—a firm, flesh-colored tender lump.

Cause: Infection with a wart virus.

Severity of Problem: A very uncomfortable problem but not serious.

Contagious? Yes, by contact with warts. Public showers, locker rooms, etc., where many people have bare feet, may be a source of possible infection.

Treatment: Pain can be helped by padding the foot to keep pressure off the wart. Liquid nitrogen applied to the wart (see a physician), surgical removal or electrical cautery (burning the wart with a special tool) followed by surgically removing fragments may be effective.

Prevention: Avoid contact with warts. Wear shoes or sandals in public showers and locker rooms.

Discussion: Previously used X-ray treatment of plantar warts is no longer recommended. These, like other warts, may be responsive to treatment but may come back again in the same area or nearby. Most warts, if not treated, will disappear spontaneously in months to years.

WHIPLASH

A form of neck injury resulting when the head is rapidly shaken back and forth.

Symptoms: Pain and stiffness in the neck, with inability to bend the neck forward, backward or to the side without pain. There may be headache, usually dull.

Cause: Rapid shaking of the head back and forth causes stretching of the ligaments and muscles of the neck. This stretching results in stiffness and limitation of the motion of the head. The pain may last for several days to weeks, depending on the extent of the injury. Small infants who are shaken vigorously can get this kind of injury and often have intracranial bleeding as well.

Severity of Problem: Variable and can be worsened if there is already degenerative joint disease in the cervical spine.

Contagious? No.

Treatment: Rest, prevention of excessive movement at the neck. Often a soft cervical collar is recommended for two to three weeks, in order to provide rest for the neck and prevent further muscle and ligament damage.

Prevention: Avoidance of activities in which there is a possibility of neck injury, especially through jarring against another, as in certain sports. Wearing of automobile seat belts and shoulder harnesses.

WHOOPING COUGH (PERTUSSIS)

Long, contagious preventable respiratory infection with characteristic cough. Usually affects infants and children who are not immunized against it, but can affect adults who are no longer immune.

Symptoms: This disease lasts approximately six weeks and is marked by three stages, each with different symptoms.

Catarrhal stage: slow onset of nasal congestion, watery eyes, sneezing and a hacking night cough. Appetite is usually suppressed, and child is listless. This stage lasts about two weeks and usually cannot be told apart from a cold.

Paroxysmal stage: Coughing of the previous stage gradually worsens and begins to be characteristic of whooping cough. There are bursts of continuous, rapid coughs, often as many as 10 to 15 in a row, followed by a characteristic "whoop," which is a deep breath at the end of the coughing spell. There is much mucus with the cough, and vomiting is very common. These spells can happen as often as every few minutes throughout the day at the height of the illness. They are set off by crying, eating, sneezing, anger and inhaling irritating substances. This stage lasts about two weeks.

Convalescent stage: Gradual reduction in the number and length of the coughing paroxysms, increasing ability to eat and drink necessary amounts.

There is little or no fever with this disease unless a complication occurs.

Cause: Infection with the bacteria Bordetella pertussis. Occasionally an infection with a related bacteria, Parapertussis, will look like this disease, as will infections with certain viruses.

Severity of Problem: A very serious disease for infants under 1 year of age. There is still a risk of death, although it is only about 1 percent to 2 percent with careful hospital treatment. Complications, which are most severe in infants less than 1 year of age, include bacterial pneumonia, chronic collection of pus in the lung (called bronchiectasis), lack of oxygen to the brain and ear infection. In older children and adults, is less serious.

Contagious: Yes, very contagious by contact with respiratory secretions. Young infants and others who are not immunized are at particular risk. Adults seem to lose part of their immunity and may be at risk for the disease if in close contact with an infected infant.

Treatment: Treatment with erythromycin or ampicillin is given to kill the bacteria and reduce the risk to others. (This does not shorten the disease.) General support, including oxygen, and adequate nutrition by whatever means are very important. Feeding usually has to be done in small amounts and just after a paroxysm.

Prevention: The disease can be nearly completely prevented by careful administration of vaccine. This killed bacterial vaccine is given in combination with diphtheria and tetanus vaccine most of the time. Three doses are given in infancy, followed by a booster a year later and again at 5 years.

Discussion: There has recently been a controversy about the use of this vaccine. In general, disorders that follow administration of the vaccine (vaccine-associated complications) have a lower risk than the risk to young infants of getting this disease in their first few months.

SECTION THREE

QUICK-REFERENCE SYMPTOMS GUIDE

This section presents a group of major symptoms that are common to many diseases. Under each major symptom is a general discussion of that symptom—what it is, what it could mean. This description is followed by groupings of the major symptom with other related symptoms, followed by a list of diseases or problems in which that grouping of symptoms is often found.

In order to use this section, first locate your major symptom—the one that bothers you the most. Then, after reading about what it might mean, go through the more detailed listings and find the group of symptoms that most closely matches yours (or look at several groupings if they don't match exactly). Then look up the diseases or problems that correspond to your symptoms and read about them. (With certain entries, for example, see HEP-ATITIS, ALL TYPES, you will be referred to "all types" of that disease. In other situations, you will be referred to only one type of a disease. Be sure to read about the individual types specified.) After reading about each possibility, you will have a better idea of which problem(s) you might have that would account for your symptoms and which ones might be unlikely, by process of elimination.

The following is a list of the major symptom headings to be found in this section. A word of caution: The symptoms list here is presented in alphabetical order, for ease of use. *The symptoms are not presented in the order of seriousness.* And as mentioned before, this is not a complete list of *all* possible symptoms or all possible diseases or problems that cause them.

APPETITE, DECREASE IN
APPETITE, INCREASE IN
BEHAVIOR CHANGES
BLEEDING
BLISTERS OR SORES
BLUE COLOR (CYANOSIS)
BREATHING DIFFICULTY
COLLAPSE
CONGESTION
COUGH
DEFORMITY
DIARRHEA
DISCHARGE
DIZZINESS
FAINTING, LOSS OF CONSCIOUSNESS
FATIGUE
FEVER
HEARING LOSS
HEART RATE CHANGES
HOARSENESS
INFECTION
INFLAMMATION
ITCHING
JAUNDICE

LUMP, TUMOR, GROWTH, THICKNESS
MOVEMENTS, ABNORMAL
NAUSEA
NUMBNESS
PAIN
PARALYSIS
PEELING OF SKIN
PROTRUDING (see DEFORMITY)
RASH
SEIZURE
SEXUAL FUNCTION,
    PROBLEMS OF
SHOCK
SLEEP DISTURBANCE
STIFFNESS
SWALLOWING DIFFICULTY
SWELLING
URINARY DISTURBANCES
VISUAL DISTURBANCES
VOMITING
WEAKNESS (MALAISE)
WEIGHT GAIN
WEIGHT LOSS
MISCELLANEOUS

TABLE 1 · APPETITE, DECREASE IN

Many factors can influence how much food a person eats. One of the most common symptoms of illness—no matter what kind—is loss of appetite. Whenever a person does not feel well, he or she usually eats less than when things are at their normal state. However, the loss of appetite may be more pronounced with certain diseases and conditions than with others.

Appetite, Decrease in

See also: INFECTION (this section)

Loss of Appetite with Severe Abdominal Pain

See: APPENDICITIS; CHOLECYSTITIS—ACUTE; PANCREATITIS—ACUTE; PELVIC INFLAMMATORY DISEASE

Loss of Appetite with Fever and General Aches and Pains

See: CYTOMEGALOVIRUS INFECTION; HEPATITIS (ALL TYPES); MONONUCLEOSIS, INFECTIOUS; TOXOPLASMOSIS

Loss of Appetite with Weight Loss

See: ALCOHOLISM; ANOREXIA NERVOSA; CANCER (ALL TYPES); HEPATITIS (ALL TYPES); MONONUCLEOSIS, INFECTIOUS

Loss of Appetite with Irritability and Weight Loss
See: HYPERTHYROIDISM; STRESS
Loss of Appetite with Pain and Indigestion/Upset Stomach
See: APPENDICITIS; CANCER—STOMACH; ULCER—PEPTIC

TABLE 2 • APPETITE, INCREASE IN

Appetite refers to one's desire for food, a characteristic that is dependent on several factors. Appetite is usually determined by the body's need for food and therefore for energy. When the energy needs are increased, the appetite increases also. When the energy needs decrease, appetite follows. Emotions can also play a part. Certain individuals react to stress and anxiety by reducing their intake of food just because of being upset. Others learn as children that food is satisfying when they are upset—so they overeat when stressed.
Appetite, Increase in
See: DIABETES MELLITUS; HYPERTHYROIDISM; HYPOGLYCEMIA

TABLE 3 • BEHAVIOR CHANGES

Many diseases and conditions lead to changes in behavior for the people who suffer from them. These vary from changes in mood (sadness or depression is common in all people who are ill) to irritability, which can result from either mental or physical illness.
Behavior Changes—Abnormal Mood and/or Abnormal Thought Processes
See: ALCOHOLISM; MENOPAUSE
Behavior changes—Confusion and/or Drowsiness
See: HYPOTHERMIA; STROKE
Behavior Changes—Depression with or Without Other Symptoms
See: MENOPAUSE; MULTIPLE SCLEROSIS; PARKINSON'S DISEASE; STRESS
Behavior Changes—Fear and/or Anxiety
See: STRESS
Behavior Changes—Irritability
See: CROUP OTITIS MEDIA—ACUTE; PREMENSTRUAL SYNDROME; STRESS; VITAMIN DEFICIENCIES—VITAMIN B COMPLEX DEFICIENCY
Behavior Changes—Memory Loss
See: CONCUSSION; SYPHILIS; VITAMIN DEFICIENCIES—VITAMIN B COMPLEX DEFICIENCY

TABLE 4 • BLEEDING

Bleeding is potentially one of the most serious symptoms of any illness and can result in either major or minor loss of blood. Bleeding results from a break in a blood vessel—from a large artery to a tiny capillary. It may be seen at the outside or may be hidden as internal bleeding. While the start of bleeding requires a break in a blood vessel, some disorders of clotting make hemorrhage more likely in some people than in others. In certain people with bleeding tendency, spontaneous bleeding, without apparent injury or cause, may occur.

Bleeding on the surface of the body is the easiest to see and evaluate. It may result from a cut or tear in the skin and tissues, or it may occur as a "hematoma"—a collection of blood under the skin, commonly called a bruise. Bleeding into a muscle or joint can also occur, producing pain and swelling, as well as increased warmth over the bleeding area. This kind of bleeding usually stops over a period of minutes to hours, although slight oozing may continue for a day or so.

Deeper, internal bleeding can be more difficult to recognize and so can present a more serious situation. The amount of bleeding may be small, but this is still important, because a reason must be found. Sometimes massive internal bleeding results in shock and death before the cause can be accurately determined.

Internal bleeding can result from trauma or injury to the body—for example, to the abdomen or chest—or from diseases of the various organs. Most of the time, bleeding or hemorrhage into the brain and skull is very serious, because it raises the pressure on the brain and causes damage in that way rather than by direct blood loss.

Bleeding in the digestive tract can be hidden or obvious. Bleeding in the esophagus or stomach often results in vomiting, because the blood is irritating to the stomach. The blood may appear bright red, indicating that the bleeding is fresh, or dark black (often called "coffee grounds"), indicating that the blood has been in the stomach for some time. Sometimes, bleeding in the stomach or upper intestine—for example, the kind seen with an ulcer—is slow and continuous, not enough to cause vomiting. When this happens, the bowel movement may be darker than usual, but no blood is actually seen. However, when the doctor tests the stool, there is hidden (called occult) blood present. When lower digestive tract bleeding is vigorous, or blood from the stomach and upper intestine is transported down the digestive tract, it is converted into very dark black stool, so-called tarry stools, or melena. Black tarry stools most often indicate rather significant amounts of bleeding.

Other internal bleeding may result from damage to the kidneys or other internal organs. Cancers and other diseases, such as ulcerative colitis or diverticulitis, also cause bleeding. Or anal fissures and hemorrhoids—a minor cause of bleeding—can lead to bright red bleeding.

Any bleeding, whether minor or severe, warrants a thorough medical investigation to determine the cause and stop it. Prolonged minor bleeding or severe bleeding can lead to anemia from the blood loss and to further weakness.

Anal (Rectal) Bleeding

See: BLACK STOOLS (MELENA); CANCER—COLON AND RECTUM; COLITIS—ULCERATIVE; DIVERTICULAR DISEASE—DIVERTICULITIS; DIVERTICULAR DIS-EASE—DIVERTICULOSIS OF THE COLON; DYSENTERY—AMEBIC; DYSENTERY—BACILLARY; FISSURE, ANAL; HEMORRHOIDS; POLYPS—COLON AND RECTAL; UL-

CER DISEASE—MASSIVE HEMORRHAGE; ULCER—PEPTIC; VARICES OF THE ESOPH-
AGUS

Anal (Rectal) Bleeding with Constipation

See: CANCER—COLON AND RECTUM; DIVERTICULAR DISEASE—DIVERTICU-
LOSIS OF THE COLON; FISSURE—ANAL; POLYPS—COLON AND RECTAL; HEMOR-
RHOIDS

Anal (Rectal) Bleeding with Diarrhea

See: CANCER—COLON AND RECTUM; COLITIS—ULCERATIVE; CROHN'S DI-
SEEASE DIVERTICULAR DISEASE—DIVERTICULITIS; DIVERTICULAR DISEASE—
DIVERTICULOSIS OF THE COLON; DYSENTERY—AMEBIC; DYSENTERY—BACIL-
LARY

Black Stools (Melena)—Gastrointestinal Bleeding

See: BLACK STOOLS; CANCER—COLON AND RECTUM; CANCER—ESOPHAGUS;
CANCER—STOMACH; CIRRHOSIS OF THE LIVER; ESOPHAGITIS (PEPTIC OR RE-
FLUX); NOSEBLEED; ULCER DISEASE—MASSIVE HEMORRHAGE; ULCER DISEASE—
PERFORATION; ULCER—PEPTIC

Coughing up Blood

See: BRONCHIECTASIS; CANCER—LARYNX; CANCER—LUNG; NOSE-BLEED;
TUBERCULOSIS

Bleeding from the Ear

See: OTITIS MEDIA—ACUTE

Bleeding from the Gums

See: GINGIVITIS (ALL TYPES); VITAMIN DEFICIENCIES—VITAMIN C DEFI-
CIENCY

Bleeding from the Nose

See: NOSEBLEED; POLYPS—NASAL

Bleeding into the Skin

See: ANEMIA—APLASTIC ANEMIA; SYPHILIS; VITAMIN DEFICIENCIES—VI-
TAMIN C DEFICIENCY

Blood in the Urine

See: CANCER—BLADDER; KIDNEY STONES; NEPHRITIS—ACUTE AND CHRONIC;
URINARY TRACT INFECTION—ACUTE PYELONEPHRITIS; URINARY TRACT INFEC-
TION—CYSTITIS

Vaginal Bleeding, Abnormal

See: ABORTION—INDUCED, COMPLICATIONS OF; AMENORRHEA; CANCER—
CERVICAL; CANCER—OVARY; CANCER—UTERUS (AND ENDOMETRIUM); CERVI-
CITIS; FIBROID TUMOR—UTERUS; MENORRHAGIA; METRORRHAGIA; PELVIC IN-
FLAMMATORY DISEASE; VAGINITIS

Vaginal Bleeding, Abnormal—During Pregnancy

See: ABORTION—SPONTANEOUS; PLACENTA PREVIA; PLACENTAL ABRUP-
TION; PREGNANCY—ECTOPIC

Vomiting Blood

See: CANCER—STOMACH; ESOPHAGITIS (PEPTIC OR REFLUX); NOSE-BLEED;
ULCER DISEASE—MASSIVE HEMORRHAGE; ULCER DISEASE—PERFORATION;
VARICES OF THE ESOPHAGUS

TABLE 5 • BLISTERS OR SORES

Blisters are spots that are filled with fluid and located on the skin or mucous membranes. They can arise because of injury to the skin or mucous membranes, from infection or occasionally from other causes. They can be found in only one area of the body or may be generalized to many areas. Their appearance and location can often point to the cause.

When blisters break, they often lead to the formation of ulcers or sores. Sores can be either deep or right on the surface and can heal quickly or very slowly, depending on their cause. They can result from inflammation, lack of blood supply and infection.

Blisters or Sores on or Around the Anal Opening
See: IMPETIGO; SYPHILIS

Blisters or Sores on Genitals
See: BALANITIS; HERPES SIMPLEX TYPE 2; IMPETIGO; SYPHILIS

Blisters or Sores of the Mouth, with Inflammation
See: CANCER—MOUTH; HERPES SIMPLEX TYPE 1; LEUKOPLAKIA; STOMATITIS—APHTHOUS; SYPHILIS

Blisters or Sores on the Skin
See: BEDSORE (DECUBITUS ULCER); CANCER—SKIN; CHICKENPOX, HERPES ZOSTER; IMPETIGO; LEPROSY; RAYNAUD'S DISEASE; WART (ALL TYPES)

TABLE 6 • BLUE COLOR (CYANOSIS)

A blue color to the skin means lack of oxygen in the tissues. Lack of oxygen (called hypoxia) can occur for a variety of reasons, including lung problems, heart problems or circulation problems. When hypoxia is moderately severe, blue color can be limited to the lips, the fingers and toes. Severe hypoxia causes a blue or gray color to appear over the entire body. Cyanosis should always lead to an evaluation by a doctor and often means an emergency situation. If it develops suddenly, call paramedics if the person seems very ill or go to an emergency facility.

Blue Color (Cyanosis)
See: BRONCHIECTASIS; EMPHYSEMA; HEART FAILURE
See also:
BREATHING DIFFICULTY (this section); PNEUMONIA (ALL TYPES)

TABLE 7 • BREATHING DIFFICULTY

One of the most distressing, frightening symptoms for a person to have is difficulty breathing. And this can indeed signal a serious problem. However, as with other symptoms, the seriousness of this symptom depends on what its underlying causes are and on what other symptoms are present.

Difficulty breathing can result from a variety of problems. Among the most serious is that caused by obstruction or blockage of the upper airway. This prevents air from entering the lungs at all and must be relieved immediately if a person is to survive. This can be recognized by a choking episode followed by inability to breathe or turning blue. The person is usually struggling to breathe, but no air can be heard moving in and out of the lungs. With only partial obstruction, there may be a whistling or crowing sound as air passes the obstruction. If there is complete blockage, take steps to relieve the obstruction by performing the Heimlich maneuver (take a class in CPR to learn this and other life-saving measures).

Other causes of breathing difficulty include other types of blockage of the upper airway (usually infection); partial blockage of the lower airways because of inflammation or spasm of the airways; fluid or infection in the lungs themselves; several types of heart problems; pressure on the lungs from the outside (enlargement of the abdomen, for example); and even emotions.

Breathing difficulty may involve true difficulty moving air into and out of the lung or may be seen as rapid, but shallow breathing. The person is usually able to report that there is a sensation of shortness of breath or inability to get enough air. When there is serious difficulty, the chest moves in an abnormal way, with sucking in of the tissues at the neck and between the ribs. When oxygen is not adequate, the skin may turn pale, slightly gray or blue.

Anyone who has shortness of breath, with or without other symptoms, should be evaluated by a doctor.

Breathing Difficulty
See also: CONGESTION (this section)
Breathing Difficulty with Abdominal Swelling
See: ASCITES; HEART FAILURE; RENAL FAILURE—ACUTE; UREMIA
Breathing Difficulty (Shortness of Breath) with Chest Pain or Discomfort
See: EMBOLISM; EMPHYSEMA; HEART FAILURE; PERICARDITIS; PLEURISY; PNEUMONIA (ALL TYPES); PNEUMOTHORAX; RHEUMATIC HEART DISEASE
Breathing Difficulty with Cough
See: ALLERGIC REACTIONS AND DISORDERS (ATOPY)—ASTHMA; ANAPHYLACTIC SHOCK; BRONCHIECTASIS; BRONCHIOLITIS; BRONCHITIS—ACUTE AND CHRONIC; GROUP EMPHYSEMA; FOREIGN BODY—IN THE AIRWAY; HEART FAILURE; PLEURISY; PNEUMOCONIOSIS; PNEUMONIA (ALL TYPES); PNEUMOTHORAX; TUBERCULOSIS
Breathing Difficulty with Cough and Cyanosis (Blueness)
See: Same as for "Breathing Difficulty with Cough."
Breathing Difficulty with Fever and Sore Throat
See: CROUP DIPHTHERIA; MONONUCLEOSIS, INFECTIOUS
Shortness of Breath with Headache and Nausea
See: INFLUENZA
Breathing Difficulty with Skin Rash or Hives
See: ANAPHYLACTIC SHOCK
Breathing Difficulty with Wheezing
See: ALLERGIC REACTIONS AND DISORDERS (ATOPY)—ASTHMA; ANAPHYLACTIC SHOCK; BRONCHIOLITIS; BRONCHITIS—ACUTE AND CHRONIC; EMPHYSEMA; FOREIGN BODY—ESOPHAGUS; FOREIGN BODY—IN THE AIRWAY

TABLE 8 · COLLAPSE

Collapse (emergency problems that lead to the sudden inability of a person to function) can involve problems that cause sudden shock and loss of consciousness or weakness or paralysis. Similar to collapse is loss of consciousness, often called fainting, which is listed separately in this section. Be sure to refer also to the listing in this section for shock. Any episode in which a person collapses should be looked upon as a serious emergency. Seek medical care as soon as possible.

Collapse

See also: FAINTING, LOSS OF CONSCIOUSNESS (this section); SHOCK (this section)

Collapse with Severe, Sudden Abdominal Pain

See: ANEURYSM; PLACENTAL ABRUPTION; PREGNANCY—ECTOPIC; ULCER DISEASE—PERFORATION

Collapse with Inability or Failure to Breathe

See: ANAPHYLACTIC SHOCK; FOREIGN BODY—IN THE AIRWAY; STROKE

Collapse with Faintness, Fluttering in Chest

See: CARDIAC ARRHYTHMIA—VENTRICULAR FIBRILLATION; CORONARY ARTERY DISEASE

Collapse with Severe, Sudden Chest Pain

See: ANEURYSM; CORONARY ARTERY DISEASE

Collapse with Severe Diarrhea

See: CHOLERA; DYSENTERY—BACILLARY; FOOD POISONING

Collapse with Severe, Sudden Head Pain

See: ANEURYSM; STROKE

Collapse with Headache and Dizziness

See: BOTULISM (with weakness, double vision); CONCUSSION; HEATSTROKE

Collapse with Sudden High Fever

See: SEPTICEMIA; TOXIC SHOCK SYNDROME

TABLE 9 · CONGESTION

The term *congestion* is usually used to mean swelling and blockage, with the formation of excessive mucus. Congestion can be due to infection or allergy and irritation, and can lead to a variety of other symptoms. Nasal congestion can affect not only the nose but also the sinuses, the eyes and the Eustachian tube into the middle ear. So-called chest congestion usually refers to a problem in which there is chest discomfort or difficulty breathing along with the production of much mucus. "Chest congestion" is often not chest congestion at all (especially in infants and children) but rather mucus in the upper airways.

Congestion

See also: BREATHING DIFFICULTY (this section); COUGH (this section)

Nasal Congestion

See: ALLERGIC REACTIONS AND DISORDERS (ATOPY)—ALLERGIC RHINITIS; POLYPS—NASAL; POSTNASAL DRIP; SINUSITIS—ACUTE AND CHRONIC; SYPHILIS; UPPER RESPIRATORY INFECTION

Chest Congestion
See: ALLERGIC REACTIONS AND DISORDERS (ATOPY)—ASTHMA; BRONCHIECTASIS; BRONCHITIS—ACUTE AND CHRONIC; PNEUMONIA (ALL TYPES)

TABLE 10 • COUGH

Cough is a sudden, explosive sound produced when air is forcefully pushed out of the lungs past the partially closed vocal cords. It is a reflex that is designed to allow us to clear out foreign matter from the breathing passages. The reflex can be set off by a variety of things that irritate the airways: dust or particles that enter the nose and upper airways, fumes and pollens. It can also be stimulated by inflammations and infections that produce mucus and secretions that have to be coughed out. Mucus that stimulates a cough can be from the nose, sinuses, voice box area, trachea, bronchi or lower airways.

The type of cough present can be of some help in determining what the problem might be. Dry coughs tend to be caused by problems in the nose, throat and upper airways. This kind of cough is seen with irritation of the lining of the respiratory tract and at the first stages of infections. Barking, harsh coughs tend to come from the voice box area and the trachea, while wet coughs are useful in bringing up mucus and secretions from the bronchi and lungs.

Because it is a protective reflex, cough should usually not be suppressed by medication. Only when it is itself irritating (the dry kind that comes from the upper part of the respiratory tract) or is interrupting sleep is it reasonable to try to eliminate cough. Persistent coughs or those that have other symptoms associated should be evaluated by a doctor.

Cough with Difficult or Rapid Breathing
See: CROUP; DIPHTHERIA; EMPHYSEMA; FOREIGN BODY—IN THE AIRWAY; PNEUMOCONIOSIS; PNEUMONIA (ALL TYPES); WHOOPING COUGH

Cough with Chest Pain or Discomfort
See: PLEURISY; PNEUMONIA (ALL TYPES)

Cough with Congestion
See: ALLERGIC REACTIONS AND DISORDERS (ATOPY)—ALLERGIC RHINITIS; BRONCHITIS—ACUTE AND CHRONIC; CROUP; PNEUMONIA—BACTERIAL; PNEUMONIA—VIRAL; POSTNASAL DRIP; SINUSITIS—ACUTE AND CHRONIC; UPPER RESPIRATORY INFECTION

Cough with Cyanosis (Blue Color)
See: CROUP; DIPHTHERIA; FOREIGN BODY—IN THE AIRWAY; PNEUMONIA (ALL TYPES); WHOOPING COUGH

Cough with Fever and Difficulty Breathing
See: BRONCHITIS—ACUTE; CROUP; LARYNGITIS; MEASLES; PNEUMONIA (ALL TYPES); TUBERCULOSIS

Cough with Hoarseness
See: CANCER—LARYNX; CROUP; LARYNGITIS
Cough with Wheezing and Shortness of Breath
See: ALLERGIC REACTIONS AND DISORDERS (ATOPY)—ASTHMA; BRONCHITIS; EMPHYSEMA
Chronic Cough with Weight Loss, with or Without Night Sweats
See: CANCER—LUNG; BRONCHIECTASIS; TUBERCULOSIS

TABLE 11 • DEFORMITY

A deformity is a malformation that can be present from birth or develop at any point during the lifetime. While only a few of the many hundreds of possible deformities are listed here, these are common and associated with other symptoms and illnesses. A deformity can be inherited, can result from stresses and damage during fetal life or can be a result of illness or injury at any time after birth.

Crooked Teeth
See: MALOCCLUSION
Deformity of the Genitals
See: HERNIA—INGUINAL; HYDROCELE
Deformity of Hands
See: ARTHRITIS—DEGENERATIVE JOINT DISEASE; ARTHRITIS—RHEUMATOID; LEPROSY
Deformity of a Joint or Bone
See: BUNION; CONGENITAL HIP DISLOCATION (DYSPLASIA); CURVATIVE OF THE SPINE—KYPHOSIS; CURVATURE OF THE SPINE—SCOLIOSIS; FLAT FOOT; (DYSPLASIA); OSTEOPOROSIS; PAGET'S DISEASE OF BONE
Deformity of the Neck or Back
See: CURVATURE OF THE SPINE—KYPHOSIS; CURVATURE OF THE SPINE—SCOLIOSIS; TORTICOLLIS (WRY NECK)

TABLE 12 • DIARRHEA

Diarrhea is an increase in number or frequency of bowel movements (stools). It also includes a loosening of the consistency of the bowel movement to soft, liquid or even watery. As the stools become looser, they change in color from brown to yellow to greenish or clear. Diarrhea can be associated with increased mucus in the intestine if it is caused by inflammation, and blood may also be present.

As with other symptoms, diarrhea must be looked at as one of many indicators of things that could be wrong. Therefore, it is important to look at other associated symptoms in order to determine what the possible causes are. Severity is also important—severe diarrhea, especially in infants and young children, can lead to serious dehydration and imbalance of the salts in the body. If severe enough, this can lead to shock and collapse. Severe diarrhea, or that which persists for more than several days, should be medically evaluated.

Diarrhea

See: COLITIS—IRRITABLE COLON SYNDROME; GASTROENTERITIS—ACUTE; HYPERTHYROIDISM

Severe Diarrhea with Mild to Severe Abdominal Cramps

See: CHOLERA; DIVERTICULAR DISEASE—DIVERTICULOSIS; DYSENTERY—AMEBIC; DYSENTERY—BACILLARY; FOOD POISONING; GIARDIASIS; GASTROENTERITIS—ACUTE; SALMONELLOSIS—SALMONELLA GASTROENTERITIS; TRAVELER'S DIARRHEA

Severe Diarrhea with Fever and Cramps

See: DIVERTICULAR DISEASE—DIVERTICULITIS; DYSENTERY—AMEBIC; DYSENTERY—BACILLARY; GASTROENTERITIS—ACUTE; SALMONELLOSIS—SALMONELLA GASTROENTERITIS

Diarrhea with Vomiting, with or without Fever or Cramps

See: FOOD POISONING; GASTROENTERITIS—ACUTE

TABLE 13 • DISCHARGE

Most of the time, discharge from a sore or body opening results from inflammation of the tissues, with pus or fluid formation. A discharge can be thin and watery or thick and purulent, and there can be blood or blood tinging present. Sometimes the color of the discharge can help in determining what its cause is: Yellow and greenish discharge suggest some of the more common bacteria; brownish discharge usually has some blood mixed with it; clear yellow discharge is made up of tissue fluid and may not be an indication of an infection.

Breast Discharge (Nipple)

See: BREAST—FIBROCYSTIC DISEASE; BREAST—MASTITIS; CANCER—BREAST

Ear Discharge

See: OTITIS, EXTERNAL (SWIMMER'S EAR); OTITIS MEDIA, ACUTE–WITH PERFORATION

Discharge from the Eye, with Itching or Pain

See: CONJUNCTIVITIS; CONJUNCTIVITIS—ALLERGIC; CONJUNCTIVITIS—INFECTIOUS; DACRYOCYSTITIS; STY

Nasal Discharge

See: ALLERGIC REACTIONS AND DISORDERS (ATOPY)—ALLERGIC RHINITIS; POLYPS—NASAL; SINUSITIS—ACUTE AND CHRONIC

Discharge from Penis

See: "Urethral discharge" (below)

Urethral Discharge

See: CHLAMYDIA INFECTION; BALANITIS; GONORRHEA; PROSTATIS—ACUTE; TRICHOMONIASIS; URETHRITIS

Vaginal Discharge with or without Bleeding/Spotting

See: CANCER—CERVICAL; CANDIDIASIS; CERVICITIS; CERVICAL; VAGINA; GONORRHEA; HERPES SIMPLEX TYPE 2; TRICHOMONIASIS; VAGINITIS

TABLE 14 • DIZZINESS

Dizziness can mean several things to people. Some refer to a light-headed or "fuzzy" feeling as dizziness, while others mean a feeling of spinning or reeling (which is more properly called vertigo). Light-headedness or giddiness often results from a decrease in blood flow to the brain. Vertigo, on the other hand, originates in the inner ear, which controls balance. Listed below are diseases and problems that can cause either light-headedness or vertigo.

Dizziness with Loss of Consciousness or Fainting
See: CANCER—BRAIN; CARDIAC ARRHYTHMIA—VENTRICULAR FIBRILLA-TION; CONCUSSION; FAINTING; HEATSTROKE; HYPOGLYCEMIA; HYPOTHERMIA; RHEUMATIC HEART DISEASE; STRESS; STROKE

Dizziness with Headache
See: ANEURYSM; CANCER—BRAIN; CONCUSSION; HEADACHE; HEATSTROKE; STRESS

Dizziness with Hearing Loss
See: ACOUSTIC NEURINOMA; MENIERE'S DISEASE OR SYNDROME

Dizziness with Nausea and Vomiting
See: CANCER—BRAIN; CONCUSSION; GASTROENTERITIS—ACUTE; HEAT EX-HAUSTION; INFLUENZA; MENIERE'S DISEASE OR SYNDROME; STRESS

Dizziness in Pregnancy
See: PREGNANCY—MINOR DISORDERS; TOXEMIA OF PREGNANCY—PRE-ECLAMPSIA

Dizziness with Shortness of Breath
See: HEART FAILURE; RHEUMATIC HEART DISEASE

TABLE 15 • FAINTING, LOSS OF CONSCIOUSNESS

Fainting or loss of consciousness occurs when there is disruption in the normal functioning of the central nervous system. This kind of temporary problem can result from a mild insult to the brain or can be an indicator of a serious underlying problem. Loss of consciousness that lasts for longer than a few seconds requires medical evaluation promptly in order to find out the cause. If there has been an injury to the head, even a brief period of uncon-sciousness should mandate a trip to a medical facility.

Fainting (Loss of Consciousness) with Abnormal Movements
See: CONCUSSION; SEIZURE; SEIZURE, FEBRILE

Fainting with Chest Pain
See: CARDIAC ARRHYTHMIA (ALL TYPES); CORONARY ARTERY DISEASE

Fainting with Dizziness
See: CARDIAC ARRHYTHMIA (ALL TYPES); CONCUSSION; EMBOLISM; HYPOG-LYCEMIA; HYPOTHERMIA; STRESS; STROKE; THROMBOSIS

Fainting (Loss of Consciousness) with Fever, Headache and Vomiting
See: ENCEPHALITIS; MENINGITIS—BACTERIAL

Fainting with Headache
See: CONCUSSION; HEADACHE; STROKE

Fainting with Irregular or Abnormal Heartbeat
See: BRADYCARDIA; CARDIAC ARRHYTHMIA (ALL TYPES); HEART BLOCK

TABLE 16 • FATIGUE

Excessive tiring and a feeling of weakness or sleepiness can be a symptom of many disorders, or it can be a normal reaction to exercise and exertion. As a symptom of illness, it accompanies nearly all illnesses. The problems listed here have fatigue as a very prominent symptom, one that is usually recognized as excessive by the person who is ill. As with other symptoms, it is very important to determine what additional symptoms are associated and how bothersome they are.

Fatigue
See: ANEMIA—APLASTIC ANEMIA; CANCER (ALL TYPES); PREGNANCY—MINOR DISORDERS

Fatigue and Fever, with or Without Other Symptoms
See: ARTHRITIS—JUVENILE RHEUMATOID; ARTHRITIS—RHEUMATOID; CANCER—LEUKEMIA; CYTOMEGALOVIRUS INFECTION; MONONUCLEOSIS, INFECTIOUS; INFLUENZA; ROCKY MOUNTAIN SPOTTED FEVER; TOXOPLASMOSIS; TUBERCULOSIS

Fatigue with Excessive Sweating, Dizziness
See: HEAT EXHAUSTION; STRESS

Fatigue with Shortness of Breath
See: CORONARY ARTERY DISEASE; EMPHYSEMA; HEART FAILURE

Fatigue with Weakness and Blurred Vision
See: BOTULISM; DIABETES MELLITUS; MULTIPLE SCLEROSIS

Fatigue with Weakness and Weight Loss
See: CANCER (ALL TYPES); CIRRHOSIS OF THE LIVER; HEPATITIS (ALL TYPES); HYPERTHYROIDISM; STRESS

TABLE 17 • FEVER

Fever is an abnormal elevation of body temperature and is usually a sign of illness. But remember—fever, no matter how high or low, *is not* a disease of itself. It is, in fact, just one of many indicators of the potential cause and seriousness of a problem.

While most often fever signals an infection, the body temperature can rise to as high as 103° F with something as normal as vigorous exercise on a hot day. Other noninfectious causes of fever include several forms of arthritis, some cancers, hyperthyroidism and inflammatory bowel disease. The body temperature varies during the day, with a high in the late afternoon and evening and a low in the early morning hours. Fever is apt to be highest in the evening.

Fever is, in reality, the result of the body thermostat's readjusting to a new level. When that happens, the temperature rises. A fast rise will be associated with a "chill"—the body's attempt to raise the temperature quickly.

Blood is shunted from the hands and feet to the center of the body to keep the temperature up—so the hands and feet are cold, while the body is hot. When the temperature rises more slowly, there is less discomfort, but headache, general aches and pains, and a sensitive or painful feel to the skin are usual. When a fever breaks, the body sweats in an attempt to cool down—as the thermostat is readjusted downward again.

The following factors are helpful in evaluating the potential seriousness of the problem a fever signals:

1. The height of the fever and the age of the ill person. Mild fevers, under 101°F, do not usually represent serious illness in children, unless the child also looks *very* sick. In an adult this can be a moderate fever and requires investigation. (Children tend to run higher fevers than adults, but the illnesses are not any worse.) In infants under 4 months old, a fever of 101°F or above warrants a call to the doctor.
2. How long the fever has lasted. A fever that has lasted under three days, in the absence of other serious symptoms, most often does not mean serious disease.
3. The other symptoms associated with the fever. These are often more important than how high the fever is.

Whether or not to treat a person with fever with a medication to reduce the fever is controversial. In general, treatment for a fever should be based on how uncomfortable the person is. If he or she is very uncomfortable, then treat the fever. If not, let the body handle the problem. In general, fevers over 103°F should be treated. Fever medications include aspirin or an aspirin substitute, with acetaminophen (aspirin substitute) recommended if chickenpox or influenza is suspected or possible. Check the package label for dosage or check with your physician for the dosage for young infants.

Fever Without Other Symptoms

See: ARTHRITIS—JUVENILE RHEUMATOID; ENDOCARDITIS; ROSEOLA; SEIZURE—FEBRILE

Fever with Abdominal Pain

See: ABORTION—INDUCED, COMPLICATIONS OF; APPENDICITIS; CHOLECYSTITIS—ACUTE; COLITIS—ULCERATIVE; DIVERTICULAR EASE—DIVERTICULITIS; GALLSTONES; GASTROENTERITIS—ACUTE; SALMONELLOSIS—TYPHOID FEVER; URINARY TRACT INFECTION—ACUTE PYELONEPHRITIS

Fever with Back Pain

See: URINARY TRACT INFECTION—ACUTE PYELONEPHRITIS

Fever with Bone Pain

See: CANCER—BONE; CANCER—LEUKEMIA; CANCER—MULTIPLE MYELOMA; OSTEOMYELITIS

Fever, Chills and Collapse

See: SEPTICEMIA; TOXIC SHOCK SYNDROME

Fever with Congestion and/or Cough

See: CROUP MEASLES; UPPER RESPIRATORY INFECTION; WHOOPING COUGH

Fever with Shortness of Breath, Difficulty Breathing
See: CROUP ENDOCARDITIS; PLEURISY; PNEUMONIA (ALL TYPES)
Fever, Congestion and Rash
See: CROUP; RUBELLA—GERMAN MEASLES, "THREE-DAY MEASLES"
Fever with Convulsion
See: DYSENTERY—BACILLARY; ROSEOLA; SEIZURE, FEBRILE
Fever with Cough, Sweats and Weight Loss
See: BRONCHIECTASIS; TUBERCULOSIS
Fever with Earache
See: MUMPS; OTITIS MEDIA—ACUTE
Fever with Facial Swelling
See: ABCESS—TOOTH; MUMPS; NEPHRITIS—ACUTE; SINUSITIS—ACUTE
Fever, Headache and Stiff Neck
See: ENCEPHALITIS; MENINGITIS
Fever with Severe Headache
See: ENCEPHALITIS; INFLUENZA; MENINGITIS; SALMONELLOSIS—TYPHOID
FEVER; SINUSITIS—ACUTE; TOXIC SHOCK SYNDROME
Fever with Headache, Dizziness
See: HEATSTROKE; INFLUENZA
Fever with Heart Failure
See: ENDOCARDITIS; RHEUMATIC FEVER
Fever with Joint Pain, with or Without Swelling
See: ARTHRITIS—JUVENILE RHEUMATOID; ARTHRITIS—RHEUMATOID; AR-
THRITIS—SEPTIC; RHEUMATIC FEVER
Fever with Enlargement of One Lymph Node
See: CANCER (ALL TYPES); GONORRHEA; HERPES SIMPLEX TYPE 2
Fever with Enlargement of Lymph Nodes
See: CANCER—HODGKIN'S DISEASE; CANCER—LEUKEMIA; CANCER—LYM-
PHOMAS (NON HODGKIN'S DISEASE); CYTOMEGALOVIRUS INFECTION; MONON-
UCLEOSIS, INFECTIOUS; PLAGUE; PNEUMONIA—VIRAL; TOXOPLASMOSIS
Fever with Severe Muscle Pains and Weakness
See: INFLENZA; POLIOMYELITIS
Fever with Rash
See: CHICKENPOX; MEASLES; RHEUMATIC FEVER; ROCKY MOUNTAIN SPOT-
TED FEVER; ROSEOLA; RUBELLA—GERMAN MEASLES, "THREE-DAY MEASLES";
SALMONELLOSIS—TYPHOID FEVER; SCARLET FEVER; TOXIC SHOCK SYNDROME
Fever with Rash and Sore Throat
See: MONONUCLEOSIS, INFECTIOUS; SCARLET FEVER
Fever with Skin Swelling, Redness and Tenderness
See: CELLULITIS
Fever with Sore Throat
See: ABSCESS, PERITONSILLAR; MONONUCLEOSIS, INFECTIOUS; PHARYNGI-
TIS—ACUTE; SCARLET FEVER; STREP THROAT; TONSILLITIS
Fever with Urinary Difficulties
See: PROSTATITIS—ACUTE; URINARY TRACT INFECTION—CYSTITIS; URI-
NARY TRACT INFECTION—ACUTE PYELONEPHRITIS

Fever with Vomiting and/or Diarrhea
See: COLITIS—ULCERATIVE; CROHN'S DISEASE; GASTROENTERITIS—ACUTE;
SALMONELLOSIS—SALMONELLA GASTROENTERITIS; URINARY TRACT INFEC-
TION—ACUTE PYELONEPHRITIS

TABLE 18 • HEARING LOSS

Loss of hearing can be sudden or gradual, and can range from mild and
almost unnoticed to very severe. There are two types: nerve deafness and
conductive deafness. With nerve deafness the acoustic nerve is unable to
receive the signals of sound and transmit them to the brain. Most often this
kind of deafness affects only certain pitches, and a person is able to hear in
some of the ranges of noise or sound. This type of deafness can be either
sudden or gradual in onset and congenital or acquired.

Conductive deafness or hearing loss, on the other hand, is caused by
something that interferes with the transmission of sound from the outside,
across the eardrum and the small bones of the middle ear to the nerve. This
can be a deformity, a collection of fluid or pus, or a problem with the bones
of the middle ear. This type of deafness can usually be helped by hearing
aids, while nerve deafness cannot. This type of deafness is also preventable
a good share of the time.

Hearing Loss, Mild to Severe
See: DEAFNESS; MEASLES; MENINGITIS; MUMPS; OTITIS MEDIA, (ACUTE IN-
FECTION)—WITH PERFORATION; OTITIS MEDIA—CHRONIC SECRETORY; OTO-
SCLEROSIS

Hearing Loss with Dizziness
See: ACOUSTIC NEURINOMA; ARTERIOSCLEROSIS; MENIERE'S DISEASE OR
SYNDROME; STROKE

Hearing Loss with Ringing in the Ears (Tinnitus)
See: ACOUSTIC NEURINOMA; MENIERE'S DISEASE OR SYNDROME; TINNITUS

TABLE 19 • HEART RATE CHANGES

The sensation of changing or irregular heartbeat is very bothersome for
people, especially if they have or think they have heart disease. Palpitations
are the sensations of the heart skipping a beat, beating irregularly or pounding
in the chest.

Most people have changes in the heart rate and rhythm as part of a normal
day, and palpitations may signal no disease at all. Others have this as a sign
of heart disease. When palpitations are pronounced or frequent, or if they are
associated with symptoms of light-headedness or difficulty breathing, it is important that a person seek prompt medical care.

Heart Rate Changes
See: CARDIAC ARRHYTHMIA (ALL TYPES)

Irregular Heartbeat

See: CARDIAC ARRHYTHMIA—ATRIAL FIBRILLATION
Rapid Heartbeat
See: CARDIAC ARRHYTHMIA—TACHYCARDIA (PAROXYSMAL SUPRAVENTRI-
CULAR [ATRIAL]); CARDIAC ARRHYTHMIA—VENTRICULAR FIBRILLATION
Slow Heartbeat
See: HEART BLOCK

TABLE 20 • HOARSENESS

Hoarseness, roughness or harshness of the voice arises when there is interference with the vibrations of the vocal cords. This is most often caused by inflammation of the vocal cords and surrounding areas, due either to infection or to irritation. Inflammation causes swelling of the lining tissues, so the vibrations are distorted.

Hoarseness can be caused, too, by growths on the vocal cords, which also interfere with their usual vibrations because of distortion. More unusual causes of hoarseness are paralysis of a vocal cord (several possible causes, not discussed in this book) and a few congenital abnormalities of the vocal cords and trachea (also not discussed in this book).

Hoarseness as a symptom can occur with abuse of the voice (screaming, for example). With this and other sudden causes, the symptoms are usually temporary. If hoarseness or change in the voice persists over several weeks, be sure to obtain a medical evaluation.

Hoarseness
See: CANCER—LARYNX; GROUP HYPOTHYROIDISM; LARYNGITIS; POLYPS—
VOCAL CORD

TABLE 21 • INFECTION

When an area of the body or the entire body is invaded by a microorganism (a germ)—such as bacteria, virus, fungus or parasite—an infection may occur. The infection may be limited to one small area of the body (called localized infection), or it may involve several or all areas and organs of the body (called generalized or systemic infection).

Infections are always potentially serious, because they can quickly spread to other areas of the body, destroying one body system after another if not swiftly diagnosed and treated. Because of this, a physician should be seen promptly whenever an infection is suspected.

Symptoms of infection include low-grade fever; pain or discomfort; swelling, tenderness, redness and warmth of an area; initial tenderness and swelling of lymph nodes near the infected area; and swelling of many lymph nodes if infection becomes generalized. If the infection is severe, shock and collapse can occur. (For more detailed information on infection, see "Infections: Special Considerations" in Section 2, "Multi-Systems Problems.")

Breast Infection
See: BREAST—MASTITIS

Ear Infections
See: OTITIS, EXTERNAL; OTITIS MEDIA—ACUTE
Eye Infections
See: CONJUNCTIVITIS (ALL TYPES); DACRYOCYSTITIS
Genital Infection, Female
See: VAGINAL INFECTIONS (this section)
Genital Infection, Male
See: BALANITIS; EPIDIDYMITIS; PROSTATIS—ACUTE; URETHRITIS
Gum Infections
See: GINGIVITIS; VINCENT'S INFECTION
Intestinal Infections
See: DYSENTERY—AMEBIC; DYSENTERY—BACILLARY; GASTROENTERITIS—
ACUTE; SALMONELLOSIS—SALMONELLA GASTROENTERITIS
Lung Infection
See: BRONCHIOLITIS; BRONCHITIS—ACUTE AND CHRONIC; DEVIL'S GRIPPE;
PNEUMONIA (ALL TYPES)
Infection with Lymph Node Swelling (Possible with any infection)
See: CYTOMEGALOVIRUS INFECTION; MONONUCLEOSIS, INFECTIOUS; PLAGUE;
TOXOPLASMOSIS
Skin and Nail Infections
See: ABCESS—BOIL; FUNGUS INFECTION—ATHLETE'S FOOT; IMPETIGO; LEP-
ROSY; PARONYCHIA (INGROWN NAIL)
Throat Infections
See: ABCESS—PERITONSILLAR ABCESS; MONONUCLEOSIS, INFECTIOUS;
PHARYNGITIS; STREP THROAT; TONSILLITIS; UPPER RESPIRATORY INFECTION
Urinary Infection—Chronic
See: CYSTOCELE; URINARY TRACT INFECTION—CYSTITIS
Vaginal Infections
See: CANDIDIASIS; CHLAMYDIA INFECTION; VAGINITIS

TABLE 22 • INFLAMMATION

Inflammation is one of the body's defense mechanisms against injury to its tissues. While it is often a defense mounted in response to threatened or real infection, inflammation also occurs when there is other trauma to tissues—heat injury, cold injury, crushing or antibody reactions from within.

When an "invader" appears on the scene, the body's response is to send white blood cells to the area to fight it. The blood vessels open up, and blood is sent to the area—causing redness and increased warmth. Swelling happens in response to injury to normal cells. And if the invader is a bacterial infection, white blood cells gather to engulf the invader and destroy it—producing pus. More distant from the site of entry, the lymph nodes, which act as another level of guard against harm, trap any products of infection or inflammation that pass by the local reaction, and they sometimes swell in the process. If the damage is severe, whether from infection or not, toxins may be released into the blood and cause fever.

The signs of inflammation, then, are: redness, swelling and warmth of an area; tenderness because of the swelling; enlargement of lymph nodes in the area of the original inflammation and perhaps in a distant area as well; and fever. These signs and symptoms are seen with any inflammation, not just with infection.

You can recognize many illnesses or problems that involve inflammation by their names. The ending -*itis* is used to refer to inflammation, with the location of the inflammation (in Latin or Greek) being the first part of the word.

Inflammation
See also: INFECTION (this section)

Inflammation of the Tendons of the Elbow
See: BURSITIS

Inflammation of the Eye
See: CONJUNCTIVITIS (ALL TYPES); DACRYOCYSTITIS; STY; VITAMIN DEFI-CIENCIES—VITAMIN B COMPLEX DEFICIENCY; VITAMIN DEFICIENCIES—VITAMIN C DEFICIENCY

Inflammation of the Genitals
See: BALANITIS; CANDIDIASIS; CERVICITIS; CHLAMYDIA INFECTION; URETH-RITIS; VAGINITIS

Inflammation of the Gums, Mouth, Tongue
See: GINGIVITIS; STOMATITIS (ALL TYPES); VITAMIN DEFICIENCIES—VITA-MIN B COMPLEX DEFICIENCY

Inflammation of One or More Joints
See: ARTHRITIS (ALL TYPES)

TABLE 23 • ITCHING

Itching is an uncomfortable sensation of skin irritation that can usually be eliminated by rubbing or scratching the irritated area. Itching is actually a sensation that is related to pain and is carried by the same nerve fibers.

Itching can be either limited to a small area of the skin or present over the entire body, and can be a minor, temporary problem or a serious, constant, nagging thing. The sensation is usually caused by skin irritation—a rash or irritant—and scratching, while relieving the itch temporarily, may cause further skin injury and start the "itch-scratch cycle" over and over. And there is a certain emotional component to itching—the thought of certain things (like ants crawling on you!) can start the sensation and cause you to scratch.

Although most itching is caused by local skin irritation in the form of rashes, general itching of the body without apparent rash should be a signal of a possible deep problem. This kind of itching is a result of a poisonous or toxic substance being present in the body in too large a quantity, usually because of failure of either the liver or kidney to remove it, or of an allergic reaction. Therefore, persistent itching, especially if there is no apparent rash, should prompt a thorough medical evaluation.

Itching with Sudden Breathing Trouble
See: ANAPHYLACTIC SHOCK

Itching of the Ears
See: ALLERGIC REACTIONS AND DISORDERS (ATOPY)—ALLERGIC RHINITIS; OTITIS, EXTERNAL

Itching of the Eyes
See: CONJUNCTIVITIS (ALL TYPES)

Generalized Itching Without Rash
See: CANCER—LIVER; CANCER—LYMPHOMAS; CANCER—PANCREAS; CIRRHOSIS OF THE LIVER; DIABETES MELLITUS; HEPATITIS (ALL TYPES); UREMIA

Itching of Feet or Toes
See: ALLERGIC REACTIONS AND DISORDERS (ATOPY)—CONTACT DERMATITIS; FUNGUS INFECTION—ATHLETE'S FOOT

Itching of Nose with Congestion
See: ALLERGIC REACTIONS AND DISORDERS (ATOPY)—ALLERGIC RHINITIS

Itching with Skin Rash
See: ALLERGIC REACTIONS AND DISORDERS (ATOPY)—CONTACT DERMATITIS; DERMATITIS—NEURODERMATITIS; LICE (PEDICULOSIS)—ALL TYPES; PSORIASIS; SCABIES

Anal Itching with Reddening of the Skin
See: ANAL PRURITIS; FISSURE, ANAL; HEMORRHOIDS; PINWORMS

Vaginal Itching
See: CANDIDIASIS; CHLAMYDIA INFECTION

TABLE 24 • JAUNDICE

Jaundice is a yellow color of the skin caused by accumulation of a substance called bilirubin. Bilirubin is a pigment that is a product of the breakdown of the red blood cells. It is normally changed in the liver to a chemical that can be excreted from the body through either the intestine or the kidneys. When the body is not able to excrete the bilirubin, it accumulates in the skin, leaving the yellow color.

Jaundice is most commonly caused by diseases of the liver, where inflammation or damage prevent the liver from being able to handle the bilirubin. However, there are two other groups of problems that also cause jaundice: breakdown of excessive numbers of red blood cells, as in certain types of anemia, and blockage to the drainage of bile into the intestine, as is seen in gallbladder disease, gallstones and certain tumors.

The appearance of jaundice is always a worrisome thing and needs to be evaluated by a doctor. Unlike some other symptoms, however, jaundice is rarely seen without other symptoms that help to point to the origin of the problem: the blood, the liver or the bile drainage system.

Jaundice
See: ANEMIA (SICKLE-CELL); CANCER—LIVER; CANCER—PANCREAS; CHO-

LECYSTITIS—ACUTE; CIRRHOSIS OF THE LIVER; GALLSTONES; HEPATITIS (ALL TYPES)

Jaundice with Enlargement of the Abdomen
See: CANCER—PANCREAS; CIRRHOSIS OF THE LIVER

Jaundice with Abdominal Pain
See: ANEMIA (SICKLE-CELL); HEPATITIS (ALL TYPES)

Jaundice with Loss of Appetite and Weight Loss
See: ALCOHOLISM; CANCER—PANCREAS; CIRRHOSIS OF THE LIVER; HEPATITIS (ALL TYPES); PANCREATITIS—ACUTE

Jaundice with Fever, Abdominal Pain and Loss of Appetite
See: CHOLECYSTITIS—ACUTE; HEPATITIS (ALL TYPES)

TABLE 25 • LUMP, TUMOR, GROWTH, THICKNESS

An abnormal growth can be a significant problem or a minor concern. Any newly found lump, whether painful or not, that does not disappear within a week or so should prompt a visit to a doctor for investigation. Most lumps and growths are not cancerous but rather represent the effects of an infection or a reaction to inflammation.

Lump, Tumor, Growth, Thickness
See: ABSCESS (ALL TYPES); BIRTHMARK (ALL TYPES); CYST
See also: SWELLING (this section)

Abdomen
See: FIBROID TUMOR, UTERUS

Anal Region
See: HEMORRHOIDS

Breast
See: BREAST—FIBROCYSTIC DISEASE; CANCER—BREAST

Eye
See: PTERYGIUM; STY

Bottom of Foot
See: WART—PLANTAR

Multiple Lymph Nodes
See: CANCER—HODGKIN'S DISEASE; CANCER—LEUKEMIA; CANCER—LYMPHOMAS; CYTOMEGALOVIRUS INFECTION; MONONUCLEOSIS, INFECTIOUS; PLAGUE; TOXOPLASMOSIS

Neck Lymph Nodes
See: LYMPH NODES—ENLARGED; MONONUCLEOSIS, INFECTIOUS; TUBERCULOSIS

Mucous Membranes
See: LEUKOPLAKIA; SYPHILIS

Nose
See: POLYPS—NOSE

Skin
See: ABSCESS—BOIL; CANCER—MALIGNANT MELANOMA; CANCER—SKIN; CYST; LEPROSY; SYPHILIS; WART

Throat
See: CANCER—LARYNX; POLYPS—VOCAL CORD

TABLE 26 • MOVEMENTS, ABNORMAL

Certain diseases or conditions are marked by their effect on the nervous and muscular system and lead to either excessive abnormal movements or lack of control of normal movements. Abnormal movements can involve a small part of the body, as in a tic disorder, or the entire body, as with a generalized seizure. Lack of control of normal movements leads to some of the characteristic problems seen with Parkinson's disease, while the addition of abnormal movements leads to some others. Abnormal movements can be quick and jerking, or writhing, and either rare or frequent. They may interfere completely with normal function or be a mild to moderate inconvenience.

Abnormal Movement of Body
See: CEREBRAL PALSY; SEIZURE; SEIZURE, FEBRILE; TIC
Abnormal Movement—Tremor
See: PARKINSON'S DISEASE
Abnormal Movement While Walking
See: PARKINSON'S DISEASE; SYPHILIS

TABLE 27 • NAUSEA

Nausea is a sensation of impending vomiting, or stomach upset, with a variety of causes. It is common as a symptom with many diseases but very prominent with a few of them. It can be very bothersome and persistent, leading to lack of food intake. As a symptom alone, it is not terribly helpful in determining what an illness might be, but if it is used in combination with other symptoms, the cause can become clearer.

Nausea
See: CANCER—LIVER; HEPATITIS (ALL TYPES); INDIGESTION; PREGNANCY—MORNING SICKNESS; RENAL FAILURE—ACUTE; UREMIA
Nausea with Abdominal Pain
See: ANGINA PECTORIS; APPENDICITIS; CORONARY ARTERY DISEASE; FOOD POISONING; GASTRITIS; GASTROENTERITIS—ACUTE
Nausea with Fever and Severe Headache
See: ENCEPHALITIS; MENINGITIS
Nausea with Heartburn
See: ESOPHAGITIS, PEPTIC; GASTRITIS; INDIGESTION; PREGNANCY—MORNING SICKNESS; ULCER—PEPTIC; ULCER—STOMACH
Nausea and Vomiting
See: GASTROENTERITIS—ACUTE; HEPATITIS (ALL TYPES); INDIGESTION; MOTION SICKNESS; PREGNANCY—MORNING SICKNESS

TABLE 28 · NUMBNESS

Numbness is a loss of sensation in a part of the body, most often caused by pressure on or swelling of the nerve that supplies the area. Nerve damage that produces numbness can be temporary or permanent. Numbness can also be caused by cutting a nerve or by damage to the brain or spinal cord. Persistent or recurrent numbness should be investigated by a physician.

Numbness of the Arm or Hand, Dull Pain
See: CARPAL TUNNEL SYNDROME; RAYNAUD'S DISEASE
Numbness of the Skin, Generalized
See: VITAMIN DEFICIENCIES—VITAMIN B COMPLEX DEFICIENCY
Numbness of the Skin, with Sores or Ulcers
See: LEPROSY; PERIPHERAL VASCULAR DISEASE; RAYNAUD'S DISEASE
Numbness of the Skin and Hands, with Pallor and Cold
See: FROSTBITE; RAYNAUD'S DISEASE

TABLE 29 · PAIN

Pain is one of the most obvious symptoms of illness or abnormality and can be of many characters. It can be constant or intermittent, sharp or dull, stabbing or boring, cramping or steady. It can stay in one location or move. Pain can be worse when moving or unchanged with position. It can originate from the area where it is felt or be referred—felt in another area that is served by the same nerves where the abnormality is.

Description and location of pain is one of the key factors in determining its origin. Pain is mediated by sensory nerves that pass through the spinal cord on the way to the brain. Most pain originates because of irritation of or pressure or stretch on the tiny nerve fibers that end in the skin or underlying tissue. It can, however, arise from pressure or inflammation of the nerve itself, even at the spinal cord.

Only certain tissues of the body are capable of "feeling" pain—some tissues do not have nerve endings for pain in them. For example, the brain does not "feel" pain—but the structures that cover it do (the meninges, blood vessels). In the abdomen the intestines are sensitive to stretching and distention—but not to cutting. The covering of the intestines and the lining of the abdomen (the peritoneum) is very sensitive to irritation from infection—and is the source of the pain in appendicitis. And finally, some people with lumbar disc problems can readily tell you about referred pain—their back condition causes serious pains down the back of the leg.

There is truth to the often-heard comment that some people are more sensitive to pain than others. No one is sure whether this is due to differences in nervous system function or to the presence in the brain of recently discovered hormones (called endorphins). These hormones, it is known, are similar to morphine and narcotics, in that they work as the body's own pain relievers. It is known that certain things will stimulate the production of more endorphins—the basis for certain pain-control regimens used for serious, intractable pain. Another reason for a difference in pain perception may relate to one's past experience with pain and how one learned to handle it. Each year more is learned about control of pain, one of the most perplexing problems of medicine.

Since pain is such a universal symptom, it is vital that you think hard about any pain that is persistent or severe and try to answer several questions about it:

1. Where exactly is the pain located?
2. What does the pain feel like? Steady, sharp, dull, boring, stabbing, burning, etc.?
3. Does anything that you do make it better or worse?
4. Have you ever had anything like it before?
5. What other symptoms are associated with it (so you can have some ideas about the kinds of illness that might be present)?

When you have the answers to all or most of these questions, you will find the sections below useful. The same questions and their answers will help your doctor determine the most likely possibilities for the source of your problem.

Abdominal Discomfort
See: CONSTIPATION; FLATULENCE; GASTRITITIS; HICCUPS; INDIGESTION
Abdominal Pain, Severe
See: ANEURYSM; APPENDICITIS; CANCER—LIVER; CANCER—PANCREAS; CANCER—STOMACH; CANCER—UTERUS (AND ENDOMETRIUM); CHOLECYSTI-TIS—ACUTE; COLIC—BILIARY; DIVERTICULAR DISEASE—DIVERTICULITIS; FOOD POISONING; GALLSTONES; GASTRITIS; KIDNEY STONES; PANCREATITIS—ACUTE; PELVIC INFLAMMATORY DISEASE; PERITONITIS; PLACENTAL ABRUPTION; PREG-NANCY—ECTOPIC; ULCER DISEASE—PERFORATION; ULCER DISEASE—PYLORIC OBSTRUCTION
Abdominal Pain with Diarrhea
See: COLITIS—IRRITABLE COLON SYNDROME; COLITIS—ULCERATIVE; CROHN'S DISEASE; DIVERTICULAR DISEASE—DIVERTICULOSIS; DYSENTERY—AMEBIC; DYSENTERY—BACILLARY; FOOD POISONING; GASTROENTERITIS—ACUTE; GIARDIASIS
Abdominal Pain with Fever
See: APPENDICITIS; DIVERTICULAR DISEASE—DIVERTICULITIS; FOOD POI-SONING; GASTROENTERITIS—ACUTE; PANCREATITIS—ACUTE; PELVIC INFLAM-MATORY DISEASE; PERITONITIS
Abdominal Pain with Vaginal Bleeding
See: ABORTION—INDUCED, COMPLICATIONS OF; ABORTION—SPONTA-NEOUS; DYSMENORRHEA; ENDOMETRIOSIS; PLACENTAL ABRUPTION
Pain in the Arm

See: ANGINA PECTORIS (LEFT ARM, WITH OR WITHOUT CHEST PAIN); BUR-SITIS; SPRAIN; STRAIN

Backache
See: ARTHRITIS—DEGENERATIVE JOINT DISEASE; ARTHRITIS—RHEUMA-TOID; BACKACHE; CURVATURE OF THE SPINE—KYPHOSIS; CURVATURE OF THE SPINE—SCOLIOSIS; DISC, RUPTURED; KIDNEY STONES; OSTEOPOROSIS; SPON-DYLOSIS; URINARY TRACT INFECTION—ACUTE PYELONEPHRITIS

Bone or Joint Pain, Severe
See: ARTHRITIS—RHEUMATOID; ARTHRITIS—SEPTIC; CANCER—BONE; CAN-CER—MULTIPLE MYELOMA; OSTEOMYELITIS; STRAIN; SYPHILIS; VITAMIN DEFI-CIENCIES—VITAMIN D DEFICIENCY

Chest Pain
See: ANEURYSM; ANGINA PECTORIS; CORONARY ARTERY DISEASE; DEVIL'S GRIPPE; DIVERTICULAR DISEASE—DIVERTICULOSIS OF THE ESOPHAGUS; PERI-CARDITIS; PLEURISY; PNEUMOTHORAX; SYPHILIS

Chest Pain with Shortness of Breath
See: ANGINA PECTORIS; PERICARDITIS; PNEUMONIA (ALL TYPES); PNEUMO-THORAX; SYPHILIS

Pain with Coldness in a Body Part, Paleness
See: FROSTBITE; HYPOTHERMIA; RAYNAUD'S DISEASE

Earache
See: MUMPS; OTITIS EXTERNAL; OTITIS MEDIA—ACUTE; OTITIS MEDIA, ACUTE—WITH PERFORATION; OTITIS MEDIA—CHRONIC SECRETORY "GLUE EAR"

Elbow Pain
See: BURSITIS

Eye Pain with Blurred Vision
See: CORNEAL ABRASION; FARSIGHTEDNESS; GLAUCOMA—ACUTE; RETINA, DETACHED

Facial Pain
See: ABSCESS—TOOTH; MUMPS; SINUSITIS—ACUTE AND CHRONIC

Foot and/or Leg Pain
See: BURSITIS; CRAMPS—LEG; FLAT FOOT; WART—PLANTAR

Genital Pain, Female
See: "VAGINAL PAIN" (below)

Genital Pain, Male
See: BALANITIS; CANDIDIASIS; CHLAMYDIA INFECTION; EPIDIDYMITIS; KID-NEY STONES; MUMPS—ORCHITIS; PROSTATITIS—ACUTE; URETHRITIS

Hand Pain with Numbness
See: CARPAL TUNNEL SYNDROME; RAYNAUD'S DISEASE

Head Pain
See: ANEURYSM; HEADACHE; HYPERTENSION; SINUSITIS—ACUTE AND CHRONIC; WHIPLASH

Headache with Fever and Stiff Neck
See: ENCEPHALITIS; MENINGITIS (ALL TYPES)

Headache with Fever and Vomiting

See: ENCEPHALITIS; GASTROENTERITIS, ACUTE; MENINGITIS; STREP THROAT
Headache with Visual Disturbance
See: ASTIGMATISM; CANCER—BRAIN; FARSIGHTEDNESS; HEADACHE; NEAR-
SIGHTEDNESS
Painful Intercourse
See: CANCER—CERVICAL; CANDIDIASIS; CERVICITIS; CHLAMYDIA INFEC-
TION; DYSPAREUNIA; ENDOMETRIOSIS; PROLAPSED UTERUS; TRICHOMONIASIS;
VAGINITIS
Pain in One or More Joints
See: ARTHRITIS (ALL TYPES); SPONDYLOSIS; SPRAIN
Pain in Joint(s) with Fever
See: ARTHRITIS—JUVENILE RHEUMETOID; ARTHRITIS—RHEUMATOID; AR-
THRITIS—SEPTIC; RHEUMATIC FEVER
Knee Pain
See: BURSITIS
Pain in Leg(s) with Swelling
See: SPRAIN; STRAIN; THROMBOPHLEBITIS; VARICOSE VEINS
Mouth Pain
See: ABSCESS—TOOTH; GINGIVITIS; HERPES SIMPLEX TYPE 1; STOMATITIS—
APHTHOUS; VINCENT'S INFECTION
Muscle Pain, Cramps
See: CRAMPS—LEG; PERIPHERAL VASCULAR DISEASE; PREGNANCY—MINOR
DISORDERS; UREMIA; VITAMIN DEFICIENCIES—VITAMIN B COMPLEX DEFICIENCY
Nail Pain (Finger or Toe)
See: PARONYCHIA
Neck Pain
See: SPONDYLOSIS; TETANUS; WHIPLASH
Pelvic Pain
See: ARTHRITIS—RHEUMATOID; DYSPAREUNIA; ENDOMETRIOSIS; PELVIC IN-
FLAMMATORY DISEASE; PREMENSTRUAL SYNDROME
Rectal Pain
See: FISSURE—ANAL; HEMORRHOIDS
Shoulder Pain
See: BURSITIS
Pain and Swelling Under or on the Skin
See: ABSCESS—BOIL; BREAST—MASTITIS; FROSTBITE; THROMBOPHLEBITIS;
VARICOSE VEINS
Sore Throat and Fever
See: DIPHTHERIA; LARYNGITIS; MONONUCLEOSIS, INFECTIOUS; PHARYNGI-
TIS—ACUTE; STREP THROAT; TONSILLITIS
Sore Throat with Hoarseness
See: CANCER—LARYNX; CANCER—THROAT; LARYNGITIS
Throat Pain with Swallowing Difficulty
See: CANCER—ESOPHAGUS; DIVERTICULAR DISEASE—DIVERTICULOSIS OF
THE ESOPHAGUS; FOREIGN BODY—ESOPHAGUS

Tooth or Jaw Pain
   See: ABSCESS—TOOTH; GINGIVITIS; MALOCCLUSION; MUMPS; PULPITIS; SIN-
USITIS—ACUTE AND CHRONIC; TEMPOROMANDIBULAR JOINT DISEASE; TETANUS
   Vaginal Pain
   See: CANDIDIASIS; CERVICITIS; CHLAMYDIA INFECTION; CYSTOCELE; PRO-
LAPSED UTERUS

TABLE 30 • PARALYSIS
   Paralysis is the inability to move or control a part of the body because of
damage to nerves. Nerve damage can result from infection of the nervous
system; injury to the brain, the spinal cord or the peripheral nerves; congenital
damage from accidents in the womb; or damage at the time of birth. Paralysis
can be present from birth, or it can be acquired as an older person. It is always
a serious problem that needs to be evaluated, but most often the damage
cannot be repaired.
   Paralysis or Weakness of One or More Body Parts
   See: CEREBRAL PALSY; MULTIPLE SCLEROSIS; MUSCULAR DYSTROPHY;
POLIOMYELITIS; STROKE

TABLE 31 • PEELING OF SKIN
   Peeling of the skin is a normal process that goes on day after day, every
day of our lives. The skin replaces itself frequently and is the tissue of the
body that undergoes the most rapid cellular division and replacement. Most
often, skin peeling that occurs during or after an illness is an indication that
the healing process of the skin is being completed. The "old skin" peels off
to reveal the new, repaired skin. Skin peeling can also occur as a response
to constant irritation of the skin—as happens with a chronic rash or irritation.
When peeling occurs, it is important to try to figure out which of these
processes is most likely to have taken place.
   Peeling of Skin of the Feet
   See: ALLERGIC REACTION AND DISORDERS (ATOPY)—CONTACT DERMATITIS;
ALLERGIC REACTIONS AND DISORDERS (ATOPY)—ALLERGIC DERMATITIS; FUN-
GUS INFECTION—ATHLETE'S FOOT
   Peeling of Skin over a Joint
   See: ARTHRITIS—GOUT
   Peeling of Skin with or After a Rash
   See: SCARLET FEVER; TOXIC SHOCK SYNDROME

TABLE 32 • RASH
   People most often think that a rash—a skin eruption—signifies measles
or another contagious disease. A rash, in fact, is often one of the more difficult
problems to diagnose and treat. A rash can result from infection (bacterial,

viral or fungal), or from contact with or sensitivity to irritating substances, or it can be inherited and be a unique part of someone's makeup. It can also signify that a serious, underlying problem has occurred. A rash can be the result of something as minor as dry skin or as serious as gangrene. It is the combination of symptoms that accompany a rash that determines its significance or points more specifically to certain problems and rule out others.

It is therefore important when a rash occurs to try to determine if any other symptoms are present as well. Other things to consider so you can better answer the doctor's questions are:

- Was there any contact with someone with a rash or contagious disease?
- Has there been a change in diet, contact with different substances (which may result in an allergic response) or a change in environment?
- Is the rash spreading or contained in one area?
- What does it look like exactly, and how long has it been there?
- Does the rash itch, hurt or burn?

Most often a physician must see a rash in order to determine its cause. Therefore, it is wise to seek the advice of a doctor if a rash: (1) persists for three or four days without improvement; (2) is spreading rapidly; (3) is terribly uncomfortable; (4) is associated with other symptoms that might indicate the need for evaluation (fever, headache, stiff neck, sore throat, listlessness, fatigue); (5) shows any signs of infection; or (6) its presence concerns you.

Dry, Scaly Rash
See: ALLERGIC REACTIONS AND DISORDERS (ATOPY)—ALLERGIC DERMATITIS; DERMATITIS—NEURODERMATITIS; FUNGUS INFECTION—RINGWORM; PSORIASIS; VITAMIN DEFICIENCIES—VITAMIN B COMPLEX DEFICIENCY

Oily or Greasy Rash
See: ACNE; SEBORRHEA

Wet, Weepy Rash
See: ALLERGIC REACTIONS AND DISORDERS (ATOPY)—CONTACT DERMATITIS; FUNGUS INFECTION—RINGWORM; HERPES ZOSTER

Rash with Dandruff
See: PSORIASIS; SEBORRHEA

Rash with Fever
See: CHICKENPOX; HERPES ZOSTER; MEASLES (RUBEOLA, "RED MEASLES"); ROCKY MOUNTAIN SPOTTED FEVER; ROSEOLA; RUBELLA—GERMAN MEASLES, "THREE-DAY MEASLES"; SALMONELLOSIS—TYPHOID FEVER; SCARLET FEVER; SYPHILIS

Hives (Urticaria)
See: ALLERGIC REACTIONS AND DISORDERS (ATOPY)—URTICARIA (HIVES)

Rash or Hives with Wheezing
See: ALLERGIC REACTIONS AND DISORDERS (ATOPY)—URTICARIA (HIVES); ANAPHYLACTIC SHOCK

Rash with Pain and/or Itching

See: ALLERGIC REACTIONS AND DISORDERS (ATOPY)—CONTACT DERMATI-
TIS; HERPES ZOSTER; LICE (PEDICULOSIS)—ALL TYPES; SCABIES (MITES)
Rash on Genitals
See: CANDIDIASIS; LICE (PEDICULOSIS)—CRAB LICE
Rash with Nail Abnormalities
See: FUNGUS INFECTION—RINGWORM; PSORIASIS
Rash on Nipple, with Itching and Burning.
See: ALLERGIC REACTIONS AND DISORDERS (ATOPY)—CONTACT DERMATI-
TIS; CANCER—BREAST

TABLE 33 · SEIZURE

A convulsive seizure is an abnormal set of movements that are caused by
an abnormal electrical discharge in the brain. The seizure can be generalized,
with jerking or twitching of the entire body, along with stiffening, or it can
be limited to one body part. It can be associated with complete unconsciousness, or the person can appear to be awake during part of the seizure. Certain
seizures involve only momentary lapses in awareness. Epilepsy is a chronic
problem that is characterized by the tendency to have seizures.

Seizures have a variety of causes. When a seizure occurs for the first time,
it is critically important that a cause be searched for. Of greatest concern are
the causes that can be corrected easily. Of additional concern is the stopping
of one seizure and the prevention of any future attacks.

If the doctor is to determine what kind of seizure occurred and what is the
likely cause, he or she needs an accurate description of what happened. If
you witness a seizure, try to pay attention to the following:

1. How did the seizure start, and what did it look like?
2. How long did it last?
3. What parts of the body jerked? Did the person lose consciousness?
4. How did the person act afterward?

When a seizure is brief (less than 10 or 15 minutes long), it usually does
not result in harm to the person, unless there was severe lack of oxygen. If
you are left to care for a person who has a seizure, first make sure the person
doesn't hurt himself or herself during the attack. Lay the person down on the
floor, but do not try to put anything between the teeth. Turn the person on
the side or on the abdomen, so secretions will drain out of the mouth. If a
seizure lasts longer than 15 minutes, summon help or go to an emergency
facility.

Most seizure disorders can be adequately controlled with medications,
which often must be taken for a lifetime. However, if the value of a medicine
that is taken for a lifetime were ever to be compared to a life with seizures,
most epileptics would tell you the medication is worth it.
Seizure

See: DYSENTERY—BACILLARY; SEIZURE; SEIZURE, FEBRILE; STROKE
Seizure in Pregnancy
See: TOXEMIA OF PREGNANCY—ECLAMPSIA

TABLE 34 • SEXUAL FUNCTION, PROBLEMS OF

Sexual problems are more common than many people realize. They are often not addressed as medical difficulties because of embarrassment or other reasons. While many sexual function problems are rooted in the emotions of the two partners, there are certain health problems that do interfere with the sex life. (Most notable on the list are prostatism, diabetes mellitus and alcoholism.) It is important that anyone with a significant sexual problem be evaluated physically instead of hiding the condition.

Sexual Function, Problems of
See: DYSPAREUNIA; EJACULATION, PREMATURE; IMPOTENCE; INFERTILITY, MALE AND FEMALE

TABLE 35 • SHOCK

Shock signifies an emergency where swift and immediate medical intervention is necessary. Essentially, shock results when the blood supply to vital organs is decreased. The blood flow to the skin and muscles ceases first, resulting in a pale look, with moist, clammy and cold skin. Then blood flow to the internal organs—intestines, kidneys, heart and brain—slows, leading to eventual collapse. Symptoms of shock are general weakness, nausea and vomiting, anxiety or panic, and thirstiness. Later light-headedness, difficulty breathing and eventually loss of consciousness follow. At this stage there is a risk of choking if vomiting occurs. Severe shock leads to death when the heart stops.

Shock is the body's response to injury, serious illness, overwhelming infection, blood loss or dehydration. Often if the cause receives immediate treatment, shock will be diminished, controlled or reversed.

When shock occurs, it is vital to remember that the situation (no matter what its cause) is potentially life-threatening. The paramedics or ambulance should be called, and the person should be kept calm. If vomiting occurs (and there are no head, neck or back injuries) the person should be rolled on his or her side so aspiration (inhaling vomitus into the lungs) does not occur. If the person stops breathing and the heart stops, CPR (cardiopulmonary resuscitation) should be started immediately. CPR can and should be learned by everyone. Classes are available through the American Heart Association, the Red Cross and other organizations.

Shock with Severe, Sudden Abdominal Pain
See: ANEURYSM; FOOD POISONING; GALLSTONES; PANCREATITIS—ACUTE; PLACENTAL ABRUPTION; PREGNANCY—ECTOPIC; ULCER DISEASE—PERFORATION; VARICES OF THE ESOPHAGUS

Shock with Severe Abdominal Pain and Vaginal Bleeding

See: PLACENTAL ABRUPTION
Shock with Diarrhea and Vomiting
See: CHOLERA; TOXIC SHOCK SYNDROME
Shock with Fever and Chills
See: SEPTICEMIA; TOXIC SHOCK SYNDROME
Shock with Severe, Sudden Chest Pain
See: ANEURYSM; CARDIAC ARRHYTHMIA—VENTRICULAR FIBRILLATION;
CORONARY ARTERY DISEASE; VARICES OF THE ESOPHAGUS
Shock with Severe, Sudden Head Pain
See: ANEURYSM; STROKE

TABLE 36 • SLEEP DISTURBANCE

There are numerous types of sleep disturbances, many of which are of a bothersome but not serious nature. However, sleep disorders cause serious problems for certain people, with many people truly suffering because of insomnia and other problems. In the past the solutions that had been suggested included medications and learning to live with the problem. As more studies are performed, not only are more sleep disturbances being better understood, but different solutions are being developed.

Nearly all illnesses can cause disturbed sleep. Most often, acute infections and chronic illnesses lead to a need for more sleep. Without these kinds of underlying problems, the true sleep disorders are uncommon. Among the most serious of the disorders is sleep apnea, which usually is recognized because of a serious snoring problem. Sleep disturbances of a chronic nature should be investigated medically, and in most cases "sleeping pills" should be avoided.

Disturbed Sleep
See: SLEEP DISORDERS—NIGHTMARES; SLEEP DISORDERS—SLEEP APNEA (ADULT); SLEEP DISORDERS—SNORING; VITAMIN DEFICIENCIES—VITAMIN B COMPLEX DEFICIENCY
Too Little Sleep (Insomnia)
See: SLEEP DISORDERS—INSOMNIA
Too Much Sleep
See: SLEEP DISORDERS—NARCOLEPSY

TABLE 37 • STIFFNESS

Stiffness of the joints is a common symptom, especially as people grow older. Although it is usually a symptom of joint degeneration or inflammation, it can occur as a result of acute inflammation of muscles and joints, with muscle spasm and tightness. Only a few of the causes of stiffness are serious, life-threatening problems: poliomyelitis and tetanus, for example.

Stiffness in the Back
See: BACKACHE; DISC, RUPTURED; SPONDYLOSIS
Stiffness in Hands

See: ARTHRITIS (ALL TYPES)
Stiffness in One or More Joints
See: ARTHRITIS—DEGENERATIVE JOINT DISEASE; SPONDYLOSIS
Stiffness in Muscles
See: HYPOTHERMIA; INFLUENZA
Stiffness in Muscles with Weakness
See: INFLUENZA; POLIOMYELITIS; TETANUS
Stiffness in Neck
See: SPONDYLOSIS; TETANUS; TORTICOLLIS (WRY NECK); WHIPLASH

TABLE 38 • SWALLOWING DIFFICULTY
Difficulty with swallowing can result from an actual blockage in the esophagus, pain or abnormalities of the muscles that are involved in the very complicated swallowing act. It can result from scar tissue that forms, limiting the amount of movement the esophagus can undergo.

In evaluating a problem of difficulty in swallowing, it is important to consider:

1. Is there pain associated? If so, where?
2. Is there a feeling of a lump in the chest or throat?
3. Do things get caught in the throat or cause gagging?

Difficulty Swallowing
See: ACHALASIA; CANCER—ESOPHAGUS; DIVERTICULAR DISEASE—DIVERTICULOSIS OF THE ESOPHAGUS; ESOPHAGITIS (PEPTIC OR REFLUX); FOREIGN BODY—ESOPHAGUS; HERNIA—HIATUS; MULTIPLE SCLEROSIS

TABLE 39 • SWELLING
Swelling is a symptom that can have many causes. It can be localized to a small area of the body as a response to inflammation, with redness and swelling as a part of the body's defense mechanism against infection. Swelling that occurs with inflammation is usually firm and tender to the touch.

Another form of localized swelling is that which occurs in response to injury of a body part. When there is injury or trauma to an area, swelling occurs, usually as a result of bleeding into the area. This type of swelling can appear bluish, or if deep enough, will not appear to be discolored. Swelling as a result of this kind of bruise can take some time to disappear.

More generalized swelling can result from edema, which is accumulation of water in the tissues without inflammation. This happens when there is a water or electrolyte (salt) imbalance in the body, when the kidneys do not function as well as they should, or when the heart is not strong enough to pump sufficient blood. It can also result from a blockage to the blood drainage from a part of the body. Edema swelling is usually soft, but when the tissues are pressed firmly, a dent can be left for a few seconds.

Protrusion of one part of the body is another cause of swelling. This kind of swelling is usually soft, and the protrusion can be pushed back into place until the swelling has disappeared. This is the type of swelling seen with hernias or ruptures.

If you have a problem with swelling, try to determine which type of swelling you probably have, then look at the section below and find the area of the body and the associated symptoms. As you read the areas to which you are referred, keep the distinction between the various types of swelling in mind.

Swelling
See also: DEFORMITY (this section); LUMP, TUMOR, GROWTH, THICKNESS (this section)

Generalized Swelling
See: EDEMA; NEPHRITIS—ACUTE AND CHRONIC; NEPHROTIC SYNDROME; PREGNANCY—MINOR DISORDERS; RENAL FAILURE—ACUTE; TOXEMIA OF PREGNANCY (ALL TYPES)

Swelling in or of the Abdomen
See: ASCITES; CIRRHOSIS OF THE LIVER; HEART FAILURE; NEPHROTIC SYNDROME

Swelling over Bone
See: CANCER—BONE; CANCER—MULTIPLE MYELOMA; OSTEOMYELITIS; VITAMIN DEFICIENCIES—VITAMIN D DEFICIENCY

Swelling of Breasts
See: BREAST—MASTITIS; PREGNANCY—MINOR DISORDERS; PREMENSTRUAL SYNDROME

Swelling of Face
See: MUMPS; NEPHRITIS—ACUTE; NEPHROTIC SYNDROME; POLYPS—NASAL; SINUSITIS—ACUTE AND CHRONIC

Swelling of Feet and Legs
See: EDEMA; PREGNANCY—MINOR DISORDERS; THROMBOPHLEBITIS; VARICOSE VEINS

Swelling in the Genital Region, Female
See: PROLAPSED UTERUS

Swelling in the Genital Region, Male
See: EPIDIDYMITIS; HERNIA—INGUINAL; HYDROCELE; MUMPS—ORCHITIS; SPERMATOCELE

Swelling of the Gums
See: GINGIVITIS; VINCENT'S INFECTION; VITAMIN DEFICIENCIES—VITAMIN C DEFICIENCY

Swelling in One or More Joints
See: ARTHRITIS (ALL TYPES); BURSITIS; SPRAIN; STRAIN

Swelling of One or More Lymph Nodes
See: CANCER (ALLTYPES); LYMPH NODES—ENLARGED; TUBERCULOSIS

Swelling of Lymph Nodes with Fever and Aches and Pains

See: CYTOMEGALOVIRUS INFECTION; MONONUCLEOSIS, INFECTIOUS; PLAGUE; RUBELLA—GERMAN MEASLES, "THREE-DAY MEASLES"; SYPHILIS; TOXOPLAS-MOSIS

Swelling of the Nail Area (Tissue Surrounding the Nail)
See: PARONYCHIA
Swelling in Neck
See: LYMPH NODES—ENLARGED
Swelling of Skin, with Fever
See: ABSCESS—BOIL; CELLULITIS
Swelling of Skin, with Itching and Rash
See: ALLERGIC REACTIONS AND DISORDERS (ATOPY)—CONTACT DERMATI-TIS; OTITIS, EXTERNAL
Swelling of Tongue, Mouth, Throat, with Difficulty Breathing
See: ABSCESS, PERITONSILLAR; ANAPHYLACTIC SHOCK

TABLE 40 • URINARY DISTURBANCES

Abnormalities of the urinary tract are brought to light with several quite distinctive symptoms, although these are very general—that is, they do not point directly to the heart of the problem. *Pain and burning* on urination are common and usually result from irritation of the lining of the urethra and bladder because of infection or an irritating urine (too concentrated, for example).

Urinary frequency—feeling the need to empty the bladder very often for very small amounts of urine—is another sign of irritation in the bladder and urethra.

Urgency is the feeling of needing to empty the bladder immediately— even if you had just done so.

Incontinence—loss of control of urine—is another symptom of irritation. So most of the symptoms we usually think of as relating to the urinary tract actually indicate irritation—from whatever cause.

Blood in the urine, like blood anywhere, is worrisome but can mean something as simple as a bladder infection or something as scary as bladder cancer. Two symptoms are usually indicative of prostate gland trouble in men—*urinary retention* (inability to urinate, even with a full bladder) and *hesitancy* (difficulty in starting the stream of urine). Urinary retention can occur in other situations as well, such as nervous system disorders and after anesthesia or certain medications.

As with other symptoms, it is the combination of the symptoms, along with the findings of a doctor's examination, that makes the diagnosis—but a review of each symptom will help you see how these symptoms can interact.
Blood in Urine
See: CANCER—BLADDER; CANCER—KIDNEY; KIDNEY STONE; URINARY TRACT INFECTION—CYSTITIS
Decreased Urination

See: NEPHRITIS—ACUTE AND CHRONIC; NEPHROTIC SYNDROME; PROSTAT-
ISM; RENAL FAILURE—ACUTE
Frequency (Frequent Urination)
See: CANCER—PROSTATE; CYSTOCELE; DIABETES MELLITUS; PROLAPSED
UTERUS; PROSTATISM; PROSTATITIS—ACUTE; URINARY TRACT INFECTION—
CHRONIC PYELONEPHRITIS; URINARY TRACT INFECTION—CYSTITIS
Frequency with Burning and Pain, Fever
See: PROSTATITIS—ACUTE; URINARY TRACT INFECTION—ACUTE PYELONE-
PHRITIS; URINARY TRACT INFECTION—CYSTITIS
Incontinence (Loss of Urine Control)
See: STRESS INCONTINENCE
Painful/Burning Urination
See: BALANITIS; CANDIDIASIS; CHLAMYDIA INFECTION; GONORRHEA; PROS-
TATITIS—ACUTE; TRICHOMONIASIS; URETHRITIS; URINARY TRACT INFECTION—
CHRONIC PYELONEPHRITIS; URINARY TRACT INFECTION—CYSTITIS
Difficulty Starting and Stopping Urination
See: PROSTATISM; PROSTATITIS; ACUTE—URINARY TRACT INFECTION—CYS-
TITIS

TABLE 41 • VISUAL DISTURBANCES

Disturbances of vision can be of great concern when they appear, either
alone or with other symptoms. The concern is to determine whether the
disturbances are related to an abnormality of the eye or whether they result
from chemical or physical changes elsewhere in the body.

Preservation of eyesight and eye function should be a top priority item for
everyone. Regular eye examinations, especially after the age of 40, may
detect certain eye diseases mentioned in this book *before* the disturbing symptoms of sudden loss of vision or blurring occur. They also serve to detect the
early stages of unpreventable, but treatable, eye problems, allowing a person
to plan for any future reduction in vision.

Blurred Vision or Dimness of Vision
See: CATARACT; MACULAR DEGENERATION; RETINOPATHY; VITAMIN DEFI-
CIENCIES—VITAMIN A DEFICIENCY
Blurred Vision when Looking at Close Objects
See: FARSIGHTEDNESS; PRESBYOPIA
Blurred Vision with Nausea, Headache and Dizziness
See: BOTULISM; HEADACHE; HEAT EXHAUSTION; HEATSTROKE
Blurred Vision with Redness, Pain, Burning, Itching of Eyes
See: CONJUNCTIVITIS; CORNEAL ABRASION; FARSIGHTEDNESS; GLAU-
COMA—ACUTE AND CHRONIC; PRESBYOPIA; VITAMIN DEFICIENCIES—VITAMIN
A DEFICIENCY
Double Vision
See: CANCER—BRAIN; CONCUSSION
Sudden Loss of Vision (In One or Both Eyes)

See: GLAUCOMA—ACUTE; RETINA, DETACHED; RETINOPATHY
Night Blindness
See: CATARACT; MACULAR DEGENERATION; NEARSIGHTEDNESS; VITAMIN DEFICIENCIES—VITAMIN A DEFICIENCY
Poor Vision
See: ASTIGMATISM; CANCER—BRAIN; CATARACT; COLOR BLINDNESS; FARSIGHTEDNESS; MACULAR DEGENERATION; NEARSIGHTEDNESS
Reduction in Side and Top Vision (Tunnel Vision)
See: GLAUCOMA—ACUTE AND CHRONIC; MACULAR DEGENERATION; RETINA, DETACHED; RETINOPATHY
Spots in Front of Eyes
See: CATARACT; FLOATERS; RETINA, DETACHED
Watery Eyes
See: CONJUNCTIVITIS (ALL TYPES)

TABLE 42 · VOMITING

Vomiting is one of those most unpleasant experiences brought about by any of a multitude of things. Seeing, smelling or tasting something unpleasant can result in vomiting, and it can even be a response to pain or anxiety. In other situations it occurs because of illness, poisoning, infection and a long list of different problems.

Vomiting, like many other major symptoms, may not be significant in itself (unless chronic or stained with blood). Most often it is one in a set of symptoms. Care should therefore be taken in trying to determine what other symptoms, if any, are present.

Vomiting of blood (bright red) usually indicates active bleeding and should signal the need for immediate medical intervention. Vomiting of blood that looks like "coffee grounds" usually indicates rather slow or presently inactive bleeding. (It looks like coffee grounds because it has been in the stomach's acids for a time.) This situation also requires prompt medical attention.

Anytime vomiting becomes severe (with one bout right after another), a doctor should be consulted. Because of the ever-present potential of aspiration (inhaling the vomitus into the lungs), which can be life-threatening, no one who is vomiting should be left unattended—even if he or she simply has the flu. Parents of very small children should take particular note of this, as should anyone caring for an elderly person.

The significance of vomiting, remember, will be dependent on any other symptoms present, so it is important to identify these in the event a physician's consultation becomes necessary.

Vomiting
See: CANCER—BRAIN; CANCER—LIVER; CANCER—PANCREAS; GASTROENTERITIS—ACUTE; MOTION SICKNESS; PREGNANCY—MORNING SICKNESS; UREMIA
Vomiting with Abdominal Pain
See: APPENDICITIS; FOOD POISONING; GASTROENTERITIS—ACUTE; HEPATI-

TIS (ALL TYPES); ULCER DISEASE—PYLORIC OBSTRUCTION; ULCER—PEPTIC
Vomiting of Blood
See: CANCER—STOMACH; NOSEBLEED; ULCER—PEPTIC; ULCER DISEASE—
MASSIVE HEMORRHAGE; VARICES OF THE ESOPHAGUS
Vomiting with Diarrhea
See: FOOD POISONING; GASTROENTERITIS—ACUTE; MOTION SICKNESS; SAL-
MONELLOSIS—SALMONELLA GASTROENTERITIS; TRAVELER'S DIARRHEA
Vomiting with Severe Fever and Headache
See: ENCEPHALITIS; MENINGITIS
Vomiting and Weight Loss
See: CANCER—BRAIN; CANCER—LIVER; CANCER—PANCREAS; CANCER—
STOMACH; CIRRHOSIS OF THE LIVER; HEPATITIS (ALL TYPES)

TABLE 43 • WEAKNESS
Weakness or a feeling of lack of strength is common to many problems but is especially prominent in certain of the more serious illnesses. While certain diseases are characterized by weakness of only some of the muscles, others are accompanied by generalized weakness as well as by a feeling of fatigue or tiredness. The problems listed in this group are those that involve true muscle weakness—not just fatigue.

Weakness might be caused by an abnormality of the muscle, with the inability of the muscle to contract. There may be a problem in the nerve that stimulates the muscle or a biochemical problem due to chronic illness. The damage may be paralysis of a muscle, inflammation of a muscle or nerve, or pressure on a nerve. In still other conditions the cause is not known.

When you are considering weakness as a problem, then, think about whether the muscles are truly weak—cannot perform—or are simply easily fatigued. Is the weakness limited to any particular part of the body? And as usual, what other symptoms are associated?
Muscle Weakness
See: CANCER (ALL TYPES); HYPERTHYROIDISM; HYPOTHYROIDISM; MULTI-
PLE SCLEROSIS; MUSCULAR DYSTROPHY;
Weakness with Chronic Cough and Shortness of Breath
See: BRONCHIECTASIS; HEART FAILURE; PNEUMOCONIOSIS; TUBERCULOSIS
Weakness with Diarrhea
See: BOTULISM; TRAVELER'S DIARRHEA
Weakness with Fever and Muscle Pains
See: INFLUENZA; POLIOMYELITIS
Weakness with Headache and Blurred or Double Vision
See: BOTULISM; CANCER—BRAIN; MULTIPLE SCLEROSIS
Muscle Weakness—Facial
See: BOTULISM; MULTIPLE SCLEROSIS; PARKINSON'S DISEASE; POLIOMYE-
LITIS; SYPHILIS
Weakness with Nervousness and Irritability
See: HYPERTHYROIDISM; STRESS

Weakness with Pallor
See: ANEMIA (ALL TYPES)
Weakness with Excessive Sweating
See: HEAT EXHAUSTION; HYPERTHYROIDISM

TABLE 44 • WEIGHT GAIN

While many people would like to blame weight gain on something other than overeating, it is not usually possible to do so. Simply, weight usually represents the addition of fat to the body, and fat is made when the number of calories eaten exceeds those burned through activity and metabolism. However, there are a few conditions that are associated with excess weight gain, often with the accumulation of body fluid (edema) rather than fat. It is important that a person take a careful look at the dietary intake when weight gain is a problem—and if the intake is honestly not excessive, seek medical evaluation.

Weight Gain with General Swelling
See: ASCITES; EDEMA; HEART FAILURE; NEPHRITIS—ACUTE AND CHRONIC; NEPHROTIC SYNDROME; RENAL FAILURE—ACUTE; TOXEMIA OF PREGNANCY; TOXEMIA OF PREGNANCY—PRE-ECLAMPSIA; UREMIA

Weight Gain with Swelling of the Abdomen
See: ASCITES; CIRRHOSIS OF THE LIVER

Weight Gain with Swelling of Legs and Feet
See: EDEMA; HEART FAILURE; HYPOTHYROIDISM; NEPHRITIS—ACUTE AND CHRONIC; NEPHROTIC SYNDROME; PREMENSTRUAL SYNDROME

TABLE 45 • WEIGHT LOSS

An absolutely complete list of the problems that cause weight loss would include almost every disease known to affect the human race. Conditions and diseases listed here are those in which weight loss is an especially prominent symptom. It seems to be an integral part of the human condition to reduce food intake when an illness occurs. Poor appetite due to upset stomach, nausea or vomiting is to blame in most minor, temporary illnesses. Often too, when people "just don't feel well," they tend not to eat. With a chronic or serious illness or condition, loss of appetite, nausea, vomiting and/or a nervous stomach can result in severe weight loss. On the other hand, there are some illnesses that increase the body's need for food, because they cause an increase in the burning of food for energy.

Severe weight loss in itself can be a real danger to one's well-being and is potentially life-threatening. It essentially represents "starvation" of the body because malnutrition has occurred. This can result in the destruction of one body system after another if the process is not stopped. Those with chronic illness must take special care to find ways to meet dietary needs, if at all possible. When not possible, nutrients and fluids can be given intravenously (by means of a special tube inserted into a vein).

Also weight loss without conscious dietary restriction may be a symptom of many diseases and conditions and should therefore signal the need for a physician's evaluation.

Weight Loss with Cough and Breathing Difficulty
See: BRONCHIECTASIS; CANCER—LUNG; PNEUMOCONIOSIS; TUBERCULOSIS
Weight Loss with Cough and Fever
See: BRONCHIECTASIS; TOXOPLASMOSIS; TUBERCULOSIS
Weight Loss with Diarrhea
See: COLITIS—ULCERATIVE; CROHN'S DISEASE
Weight Loss (Poor Weight Gain) in Infants
See: TOXOPLASMOSIS
Unexpected Weight Loss
See: ANOREXIA NERVOSA; CANCER (ALL TYPES)
Weight Loss with Vomiting
See: (ALL TYPES); HEPATITIS

TABLE 46 · MISCELLANEOUS

Certain disorders and diseases discussed in this book, while important and relatively common, do not lend themselves to extensive lists and lengthy discussion. They are included below to enable you to locate them.

Depression with Weakness
See: MULTIPLE SCLEROSIS; PARKINSON'S DISEASE; STRESS
Disorders of Aging
See: ARTERIOSCLEROSIS; ARTHRITIS—DEGENERATIVE JOINT DISEASE; ATHEROSCLEROSIS; CATARACT; HYPERCHOLESTEROLEMIA; HYPERLIPIDEMIA; MACULAR DEGENERATION; MENOPAUSE; OSTEOPOROSIS; PRESBYOPIA; PROSTATITIS
Disorders of Infant and Child Development
See: CELEBRAL PALSY; COLIC—INFANTILE
Disorders of the Skin, Hair and Nails
Hair Loss See: ALOPECIA—MALE PATTERN BALDNESSS; VITAMIN DEFIEICNCIES—VITAMIN A DEFICIENY; VITAMIN DEFICIENCIES—VITAMIN B COMPLES DEFICIENCY
Disorders of the Teeth
See: ABSCESS—TOOTH; CARIES (ALL TYPES); TEMPOROMANDIBULAR JOINT DISEASE
Intolerance of Cold
See: FROSTBITE; HYPOTHERMIA; HYPOTHYROIDISM; RAYNAUD'S DISEASE
Intolerance of Heat
See: HEAT EXHAUSTION; HEATSTROKE; HYPERTHYROIDISM; MENOPAUSE
Odors, Usual
See: BAD BREATH (HALITOSIS); BODY ODOR (BROMHIDROSIS)
Skin Changes—Stretch Marks
See: PREGNANCY—MINOR DISORDERS
Generalized Sweating
See: HEAT EXHAUSTION; HYPERTHYROIDISM; MENOPAUSE

Night Sweating (with Weight Loss and Cough)
See: TUBERCULOSIS
Prevention of Infection
See: IMMUNIZATION (VACCINATION)

SECTION FOUR

BIBLIOGRAPHY

Beeson, Paul B., M.D., and McDermott, Walsh, M.D., eds. *The Textbook of Medicine*. Philadelphia: W.B. Saunders Company, 1979.

Berkow, Robert, M.D., ed. *The Merck Manual*. 14th ed. New Jersey: Merck Sharp & Dohme Research Laboratories, 1982.

Boston Children's Medical Center, The, and Feinblum, Richard I., M.D. *Child Health Encyclopedia*. New York: Delacorte Press/Seymour Lawrence, 1975.

Dominguez, Richard H., M.D. *The Complete Book of Sports Medicine*. New York: Charles Scribner's Sons, 1979.

Freeman, Roger K., M.D., and Pescar, Susan C. *Safe Delivery: Protecting Your Baby During High-Risk Pregnancy*. New York: Facts On File, Inc., 1982.

Guyton, Arthur C., M.D. *Basic Human Physiology: Normal Function and Mechanisms of Disease*. 2nd ed. Philadelphia: W.B. Saunders Company, 1977.

Jackson, Douglas W., M.D., and Pescar, Susan C. *The Young Athlete's Health Handbook*. New York: Everest House, 1981.

Johnson, G. Timothy, M.D., and Goldfinger, Stephen E., M.D., eds. *The Harvard Medical School Health Letter Book*. New York: Warner Books, 1981.

Kempe, C. Henry, M.D., Silver, Henry K., M.D., and O'Brien, Donough, M.D., F.R.C.P., eds. *Current Pediatric Diagnosis & Treatment*. 7th ed. Los Altos, Calif.: Lange Medical Publications, 1982.

Krupp, Marcus A., M.D., and Chatton, Milton J., M.D., eds. *Current Medical Diagnosis & Treatment 1982*. Los Altos, Calif.: Lange Medical Publications, 1982.

Levitt, Paul M., et al. *The Cancer Reference Book*. New York: Facts On File, Inc., 1982.

Miller, Sigmund S. *Symptoms: The Complete Home Medical Encyclopedia*. New York: Avon Books, 1978.

Wakeley, Sir Cecil, Bt., and Bate, John, M.B., Ch.B. (Edin.), F.R.C.Path. *The Faber Medical Dictionary*. Philadelphia: J.B. Lippincott Company, 1975.

SECTION FIVE

INDEX OF
CROSS REFERENCES

Adenoiditis *see* TONSILLITIS.

Amebiasis *see* DYSENTERY—AMEBIC.

Anal Fissure *see* FISSURE—ANAL.

"Angel Kiss" *see* BIRTHMARK— "STORKBITE," "ANGEL KISS."

Anthracosis *see* PNEUMOCONIOSIS.

Aphthous Stomatitis *see* STOMATITIS—APHTHOUS.

Apnea *see* SLEEP DISORDERS—SLEEP APNEA.

Asbestosis *see* PNEUMOCONIOSIS.

Asthma *see* ALLERGIC REACTIONS AND DISORDERS (ATOPY)—ASTHMA.

Athlete's Foot *see* FUNGUS INFECTION—ATHLETE'S FOOT.

Atopy *see* ALLERGIC REACTIONS AND DISORDERS (ATOPY).

Atrial Fibrillation (auricular fibrillation) *see* CARDIAC ARRHYTHMIA—ATRIAL FIBRILLATION.

Bacillary Dysentery *see* DYSENTERY—BACILLARY.

Baldness *see* ALOPECIA—MALE PATTERN BALDNESS.

Bacteremia *see* SEPTICEMIA.

Biliary Colic *see* COLIC—BILIARY.

Bilious Attack *see* CHOLECYSTITIS—ACUTE; CHOLECYSTITIS—CHRONIC; COLIC—BILIARY; GALLSTONES; INDIGESTION.

Blackheads *see* ACNE.

Black Lung *see* PNEUMOCONIOSIS.

Blood Poisoning *see* SEPTICEMIA.

Infantile Colic *see* COLIC—INFANTILE.

Ingrown Nail *see* PARONYCHIA.

Inguinal Hernia *see* HERNIA—INGUINAL.

Insomnia *see* SLEEP DISORDERS—INSOMNIA.

Irregular Heartbeat *see* CARDIAC ARRHYTHMIA.

Irritable Bowel Syndrome (Irritable Colon Syndrome) *see* COLITIS.

Kidney Disease *see* NEPHRITIS—ACUTE; NEPHRITIS—CHRONIC.

Kidney Failure *see* RENAL FAILURE—ACUTE; UREMIA.

Kidney Infection *see* URINARY TRACT INFECTION.

Kyphosis *see* CURVATURE OF THE SPINE—KYPHOSIS.

La Turista *see* TRAVELER'S DIARRHEA.

Leaking Urine *see* STRESS INCONTINENCE.

Leukemia *see* CANCER—LEUKEMIA.

Lymphangioma *see* BIRTHMARK—LYMPHANGIOMA.

Lumbago *see* BACKACHE.

Mastitis *see* BREAST—MASTITIS.

Meat Packer's Lung *see* PNEUMOCONIOSIS.

Melena *see* BLACK STOOLS.

Menstruation, Difficult or Painful *see* DYSMENORRHEA.

Middle Ear Infection *see* OTITIS MEDIA (SPECIFIC TYPES).

Migraine *see* HEADACHE.

Miscarriage *see* ABORTION—SPONTANEOUS.

Mongolian Spot *see* BIRTHMARK—MONGOLIAN SPOT.

Montezuma's Revenge *see* TRAVELER'S DIARRHEA.

Morning Sickness *see* PREGNANCY—MORNING SICKNESS.

Mucous Colitis *see* COLITIS—IRRITABLE COLON SYNDROME.

Myocardial Infarction *see* CORONARY ARTERY DISEASE.

Myoma of the Uterus *see* FIBROID TUMOR—UTERUS.

Myopia *see* NEARSIGHTEDNESS.

Narcolepsy *see* SLEEP DISORDERS—NARCOLEPSY.

Nasal Polyps *see* POLYPS—NASAL.

Nephrosis *see* NEPHROTIC SYNDROME.

Neurodermatitis *see* ALLERGIC REACTIONS AND DISORDERS (ATOPY)—AL-
LERGIC DERMATITIS.

Nightmares *see* SLEEP DISORDERS—NIGHTMARES.

Nursing Bottle Mouth *see* CARIES.

Occupational Lung Disease *see* PNEUMOCONIOSIS.

Orchitis *see* MUMPS—ORCHITIS.

Osteoarthritis *see* ARTHRITIS—DEGENERATIVE JOINT DISEASE.

Palpitations *see* CARDIAC ARRHYTHMIA.

Paroxysmal   Supraventricular   (Atrial)   Tachycardia   (PAT) *see*

CARDIAC ARRHYTHMIA—PAROXYSMAL SUPERVENTRICULAR (ATRIAL) TACHYCARDIA.

Pediculosis *see* LICE (SPECIFIC TYPES).

Pellagra *see* VITAMIN DEFICIENCIES—VITAMIN B COMPLEX DEFICIENCY.

Peptic Esophagitis *see* ESOPHAGITIS (PEPTIC OR REFLUX).

Perforation—of Ulcer *see* ULCER DISEASE—PERFORATION.

Peritonsillar Abscess *see* ABSCESS—PERITONSILLAR.

Pertussis *see* WHOOPING COUGH.

Piles *see* HEMORRHOIDS.

Pink Eye *see* CONJUNCTIVITIS—ALLERGIC; CONJUNCTIVITIS—INFECTIOUS.

Pleurodynia *see* DEVIL'S GRIPPE.

Poison Ivy *see* ALLERGIC REACTION AND DISORDERS (ATOPY)—CONTACT DERMATITIS.

Poison Oak *see* ALLERGIC REACTIONS AND DISORDERS (ATOPY—CONTACT DERMATITIS.

Poison Sumac *see* ALLERGIC REACTIONS AND DISORDERS (ATOPY)—CONTACT DERMATITIS.

Port Wine Stain *see* BIRTHMARK—PORT WINE STAIN.

Pre-Eclampsia of Pregnancy *see* TOXEMIA OF PREGNANCY—PRE-ECLAMPSIA.

Pregnancy, Tubal *see* PREGNANCY—ECTOPIC.

Premature Ejaculation *see* EJACULATION, PREMATURE.

Premenstrual Tension *see* PREMENSTRUAL SYNDROME.

Pulmonary Embolism *see* EMBOLISM.

Pyloric Obstruction *see* ULCER DISEASE—PYLORIC OBSTRUCTION.

Quinsy *see* ABSCESS—PERITONSILLAR.

Red Eye *see* CONJUNCTIVITIS (ALL TYPES); CORNEAL ABRASION; GLAUCOMA—ACUTE; HERPES SIMPLEX TYPE 1, HERPETIC KERATITIS.

Red Measles *see* MEASLES (RUBEOLA, "RED MEASLES").

Reflux Esophagitis *see* ESOPHAGITIS (PEPTIC OR REFLUX).

Rheumatism *see* ARTHRITIS—DEGENERATIVE JOINT DISEASE; ARTHRITIS—RHEUMATOID.

Rheumatoid Arthritis *see* ARTHRITIS—RHEUMATOID.

Rickets *see* VITAMIN DEFICIENCIES—VITAMIN D DEFICIENCY.

Ringing in the Ears *see* TINNITUS.

Ringworm *see* FUNGUS INFECTION—RINGWORM.

Rubeola *see* MEASLES (RUBEOLA, "RED MEASLES").

Rupture *see* HERNIA—INGUINAL.

Ruptured Disc *see* DISC, RUPTURED.

Salpingitis *see* PELVIC INFLAMMATORY DISEASE.

Scoliosis *see* CURVATURE OF THE SPINE—SCOLIOSIS.

Scrotal Swelling *see* HERNIA—INGUINAL; HYDROCELE.